Medicinal Lichens

"Robert Rogers's *Medicinal Lichens* is a necessary addition not only to the libraries of herbalists but mycophiles as well!"

EUGENIA BONE, AUTHOR OF
MYCOPHILIA AND *HAVE A GOOD TRIP*

"When launching my documentary films like *Wild Harvest,* I prioritize consulting the world's leading experts, which is why I work with Robert. There is no one on this planet more qualified than Robert Rogers to continue to enlighten us all with his exhaustive yet engaging research into lichens and ethnolichenology. This book is a gift!"

SURVIVORMAN LES STROUD, SURVIVAL EXPERT,
FILMMAKER, AND AUTHOR OF *BEYOND SURVIVORMAN*

"The history of terrestrial life on Earth originates in symbioses, and one of the most astonishing basal relationships is that of what makes a lichen. In this extraordinary book, we find a portal into the taxonomy, ethnolichenology, pharmacopoeia, poetry, and chemistry of these essential organisms that have shaped life as we know it. A must-read!"

GIULIANA FURCI, FOUNDRESS AND
CEO OF THE FUNGI FOUNDATION

"Whether as food, medicine, or woodland curiosities, lichens demand our attention. Robert sheds necessary light on this mysterious group of composite organisms with detailed notes on edibility, therapeutic properties, Indigenous uses, and more for hundreds of North American species. Essential for the lichen enthusiast."

LANGDON COOK, AUTHOR OF *THE MUSHROOM HUNTERS*

"Lichens are my deep passion, and there are no books out there that can detail this type of medicine for me in the way that this one does. As an Indigenous person who grew up with my *kohkum* (grandmother) who was so versed in plant medicine, I always appreciate any time I get to spend with Robert and his fascinating knowledge. With a deeper connection to the plant world, Robert understands the medicines in the way my grandmother did, and the teachings in this book are invaluable!"

BRENDA HOLDER, CREE KNOWLEDGE KEEPER

Medicinal Lichens

Indigenous Wisdom and Modern Pharmacology

A Sacred Planet Book

Robert Dale Rogers, RH(AHG)

Photographs by Jason Hollinger

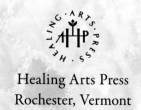

Healing Arts Press
Rochester, Vermont

Healing Arts Press
One Park Street
Rochester, Vermont 05767
www.HealingArtsPress.com

Healing Arts Press is a division of Inner Traditions International

Sacred Planet Books are curated by Richard Grossinger, Inner Traditions editorial board member and cofounder and former publisher of North Atlantic Books. The Sacred Planet collection, published under the umbrella of the Inner Traditions family of imprints, includes works on the themes of consciousness, cosmology, alternative medicine, dreams, climate, permaculture, alchemy, shamanic studies, oracles, astrology, crystals, hyperobjects, locutions, and subtle bodies.

Note to the reader: *This book is intended to be an informational guide. The remedies, approaches, and techniques described herein are meant to supplement, and not to be a substitute for, professional medical care or treatment. They should not be used to treat a serious ailment without prior consultation with a qualified health care professional.*

Cataloging-in-Publication Data for this title is available from the Library of Congress

ISBN 979-8-88850-024-8 (print)
ISBN 979-8-88850-025-5 (ebook)

Printed and bound in India by Nutech Print Services

10 9 8 7 6 5 4 3 2 1

Text design by Virginia Scott Bowman and layout by Debbie Glogover
This book was typeset in Garamond Premier Pro, Frutiger, and Stone Sans with P22 Mackinac Pro used as the display typeface

To send correspondence to the author of this book, mail a first-class letter to the author c/o Inner Traditions • Bear & Company, One Park Street, Rochester, VT 05767, and we will forward the communication.

Scan the QR code and save 25% at InnerTraditions.com.
Browse over 2,000 titles on spirituality, the occult, ancient mysteries, new science, holistic health, and natural medicine.

❧❧❧

I dedicate this book to Laurie Szott-Rogers, my true love.
Her support, gentle nudging, and encouragement
have made my life more complex, wondrous, and complete.
I also celebrate all the holobionts on the planet,
including humans whose bravery, tenacity,
diversity, and search for truth gives hope for
a more loving and sustainable world.

May the god of the tundra grant me lichen until I become lichen myself.

LAWRENCE MILLMAN

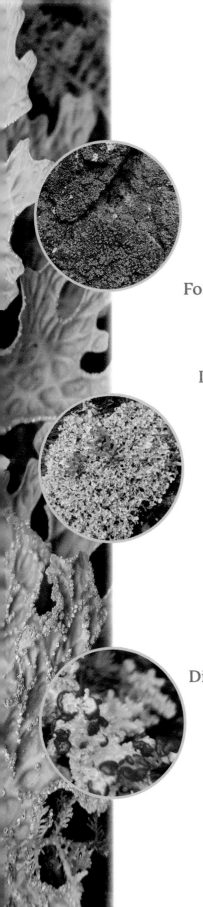

Contents

Foreword

by David Young, Ph.D.

I first met Robert Rogers in the early 1980s when I visited his clinic, the Strathcona Holistic Centre in Edmonton, Alberta, to seek help for asthma, which had caused me to be dependent upon an inhaler, which I carried with me all the time. After a lengthy interview, Robert concluded that I was suffering from food allergies. He put me on a strict diet, which involved avoiding all eggs, dairy, and wheat products. I soon began to feel better and discarded my inhaler forever.

Some years later, I invited Robert to accompany a field trip with some of my students at the University of Alberta. The purpose of the trip was to look for medicinal wild plants. Within the first fifty yards, Robert identified a couple of dozen medicinal plants by both their scientific and their common names, as well as what they were good for. This encyclopedic memory has served him well over the years.

In 1986, I organized a workshop for the conference "Knowing the North: Integrating Tradition, Technology and Science," sponsored by the Boreal Institute for Northern Studies at the University of Alberta. I invited Robert to give a talk at the workshop. His talk, "The Case for Alternative Medicine," was published in 1988 in *Health Care Issues in the Canadian North*, which I edited.

Some time later, I invited Robert to talk to my class on medical anthropology at the University of Alberta. After showing a film about Eduardo Calderon, the Peruvian healer, Robert talked about the time he spent with Eduardo in Peru. Robert formed a friendship with one of the students in the class, whom he eventually married. Robert and Laurie have been together for thirty-four years.

In 1984, I put together a team of researchers from the University of Alberta and the Provincial Museum of Alberta (now the Royal Museum of Alberta) to study the beliefs and healing practices of a Northern Cree healer, Russell Willier. This study, "The Psoriasis Research Project," resulted in the creation at the University of Alberta of the Centre for the Cross-Cultural Study of Health and Healing, to which Robert made various contributions over the years. Our research with Willier resulted in a University of Toronto Press publication by myself and two graduate students, Grant Ingram and Lise Swartz, *Cry of the Eagle: Encounters with a Cree Healer*. In 2011, I invited Robert to join me and Willier in researching and writing a sequel, *A Cree Healer and His Medicine Bundle*, published in 2015 by North Atlantic Books. Robert made a major contribution to the book by exploring the ingredients in the herbal medicines used by Willier that could account for the medicines' healing powers.

In 1994, I chaired the seminar "Culture, Health, and Healing: Establishing Intercultural Health Care in Canada," sponsored by the Intercultural Health Association of Alberta. I invited Robert to give a talk at the seminar, on herbal healing and homeopathy, in which he argued that the suppression of symptoms is one of the major causes of chronic illness.

In brief, Robert Rogers and I have had a fruitful relationship spanning many years. I especially appreciate the respectful manner in which he has gathered information from the Indigenous community and shared it in more than sixty books. Robert has had a major influence on the field of ethnomedicine. I am proud to have him as a friend and colleague.

Now to the book itself. In the introduction Robert makes the startling claim, which I have checked out and found to be accurate, that lichens have more in common with humans than with plants! Another interesting fact described by Robert is that lichens are composite organisms consisting of a symbiotic association of photosynthetic algae, cyanobacteria, fungi, and sometimes other things as well. There are 17,000 to 20,000 species of lichens on Earth, with around 5,600 of these located in North America. Lichens are among the earliest life forms on Earth, dating back 400 to 600 million years or longer. They can live for thousands of years.

The book consists of the introduction, medicinal lichen genera, lichen chemistry, and an extensive list of references. Medicinal Lichens discusses the many uses of lichens, with a focus upon North America and its Indigenous peoples. Lichen Chemistry consists of descriptions of the primary chemicals found in lichens and the action of these chemicals against medical problems.

Some of the uses are food for animals and humans, nesting materials for animals, dyes, cosmetics, perfume, alcohol, fiber, and others. Perhaps the most important use is for medicines. Lichens are also a potential source of antibiotics to treat pathogens resistant to antibiotics—a use that will become increasingly important in the future as antibiotic resistance becomes more prevalent.

Here is an example of the usefulness of lichens: black tree hair lichen (*Bryoria fremontii*) was dried, ground into a powder, and added to soup by the Indigenous people of Oregon. The Sahaptin of Oregon and Washington boiled it as a poultice for arthritis. The Shuswap mixed it with mud to chink log cabins. Various groups mixed it with other plant material to make vests, pouches, shoes, and leggings. Northern flying squirrels used it to make nests. Many other Indigenous groups used black tree hair lichens for various medicinal and other purposes. When describing the use of lichens for medicinal purposes, Robert frequently describes the chemical ingredients responsible for the desired effects.

The second chapter discusses lichen chemistry. To take one example, usnic acid is found in many lichen genera. Numerous studies suggest that usnic acid has antibacterial, antifungal, anti-biofilm, antioxidant, cytotoxic, photoprotective, antiviral, antiprotozoal, anti-inflammatory, analgesic, antiproliferative, antimitotic, and hepatoxic activity. It may be useful in the treatment of osteoporosis, lung cancer, influenza, and tuberculosis. A gargle of usnea tincture in water is extremely effective for strep throat, and usnic acid may be useful in treating free radical damage, myasthenia gravis, glaucoma, postural tachycardia syndrome, dementia, and various drug-resistant bacteria.

The book concludes with an index and list of references that represent a comprehensive summary of up-to-date research on lichens. In brief, this book is a valuable reference work for anyone interested in Indigenous knowledge, lichens, their chemistry, and their uses.

DAVID YOUNG, PH.D., Stanford University, was the director of the Centre for the Cross-Cultural Study of Health and Healing from 1984 to 1996 and is Professor Emeritus at the University of Alberta.

Acknowledgments

I wish to thank Jason Hollinger for his generosity of fantastic photographs, Stuart Crawford, Merlin Sheldrake, Andy MacKinnon, my wife Laurie Szott-Rogers, David Young, Langdon Cook, Nancy Turner, Lawrence Millman, Britt A. Bunyard, Tradd Cotter, Gina Mohammed, Eugenia Bone, Robin Marles, Trevor Goward, Giuliana Furci, Les Stroud, Dave and Brenda Holder, Duane Sept, Kevin Kossowan, and all my friends and colleagues in NAMA and the Alberta Mycological Society.

And of course all the people at Inner Traditions who made this manuscript into a work of art, including Richard Gossinger and my project editor Lisa P. Allen as well as Kayla Toher, Courtney B. Jenkins Mesquita, Erica Robinson, Virginia Bowman, and Debbie Glogover.

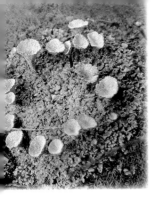

Medicinal Lichens
of North America

There is a low mist in the woods—
It is a good day to study lichens.

HENRY DAVID THOREAU

Well, any day is a good day to observe the lichens in your neighborhood. Rural or urban, desert or polar, on trees or rocks, on gravestones and monuments, they are everywhere! They favor gravestones, rock walls, cement sidewalks, telephone poles, traffic signs, rusty automobiles, windows, plastic, rubber, leather, and fence posts.

Lichens, along with mushrooms, molds, and yeasts, are members of the kingdom Fungi. Biologically, they are more closely related to humans than to plants. They are so unique they should be given their own kingdom or queendom—identifying them in terms of gender is also taxonomically challenging.

They are often neglected or ignored and have become to many humans an overlooked natural background in city and country. Lichens adapt to difficult ecologies, earning the term *extremophiles*.

Vincent Zonca (2023) offers his take on their role in our world:

Faceless, mineral and inert in appearance, lichen poses a moral and political problem: it inspires no spontaneous empathy. Like other "lower" beings, it has a hard time accommodating anthropomorphism . . . Must lichen be condemned to the scholarship of specialists or to our idealization of the marginal and compassion for antiheroes?

The neglect of lichens is symptomatic of human estrangement from nature. In the mid 1970s I read E. F. Schumacher's book (1973) *Small Is Beautiful*. It impacted me deeply on a personal level: how one's individual actions can make a difference. During the same time period I was living in a hippy commune, and began to understand the benefits of cooperation, and symbiotic, mutualistic interactions and energetics.

Our community created a private school, and my godson was an early student. Our walks together in the boreal forest must have rubbed off, as he later completed his Ph.D. in lichenology from Duke University.

But in the past fifty years, the unbridled pursuits of capitalism, optimizing gross domestic product growth, burning of fossil fuels, destruction of old growth forests, and destructive globalization have led to the extinction of numerous species. At present, Earthlings collectively consume the equivalent of 2.8 hectares of land per person, meaning we use the equivalent of 1.8 Earths to meet our present demand. Clearly, this practice is not sustainable.

Sandra Lawrence (2022) notes, "The canaries in this particular coal mine are quietly slipping into unconsciousness and not enough of us seem to be noticing."

Lichens are a metaphor for becoming more grounded, humble, and attuned to an awareness of the pressing need for a new ecology, and political change, by working on a local grounded level. This represents ancient wisdom, as well as a radical reactionary response. Lichens remind us of the need for positive environmental protection, and to learn lessons from history, not change them.

Lichens are both fragile and resistant. They have the capacity to adapt to changing environments yet are like the proverbial canary in the coal mine, foretelling impending danger. They grow slowly and are symbiotic, the exact opposite of Western society. "They invite us to leave the beaten paths, to cultivate slowness and patience to counter a consumerist ideal based on desires and the acceleration of time, to adopt a model of minimal growth to counter the hubris of exponential growth at any price" (Zonca 2023).

A collaboration between algae, cyanobacteria, bacteria, and fungi gives lichens the ability to survive and thrive in extreme conditions of temperature and lack of moisture.

Some lichens thrive around hot springs at temperatures above 200°C (392°F), while others thrive in cold extremes of minus 60°C (−76°F). The orange-colored elegant sunburst (*Xanthoria elegans*) lichen grows on rocks at

7,000 meters and survived eighteen months on the walls of the International Space Station. Lichens have been found as soon as four years after flowing lava has cooled.

They can go dormant during periods of drought and revive when moisture is available, swelling up and turning green as they absorb thirty times their weight in water! This process was named *reviviscence* by Claude Bernard in the mid-nineteenth century, and later *anabiosis*.

Today, the term *poikilohydric* is used, meaning the water regulation and content depend upon the lichen's environment. In hot, dry climates, lichens absorb small amounts of moisture from the atmosphere, as too high a content of water might simmer their tissue or interfere with carbon dioxide and nitrogen exchange.

The life span of lichens is difficult to determine. In the arctic and Antarctica, lichen growth may measure in the millimeters, while tropical lichens can grow several centimeters annually. It appears the slowest growers live longer, and some species, such as temperate-zone *Parmelia*, live only a decade or two. Semidormant lichens have been found in the arctic from 3,700 to 9,000 years old, while endoliths in Antarctic glacial ice may be up to 100,000 years old (Margesin et al., eds. 2008).

> *Some withered deciduous ones are left to rustle, and our cold immortal evergreens. Some lichenous thoughts still adhere to us.*
> HENRY DAVID THOREAU

The term *lichen* may derive from the ancient Greek word *leikhēn*, meaning "to lick." *Leprosy*, "what eats around itself," refers to this skin-related ailment's peeling appearance. The Latin *lichēn* may have derived from an ancient Greek word, and means "ringworm," a fungal skin infection.

This version of *lichen* was described more specifically by Hippocrates (460–371 BCE). Aulus Cornelius Celsus, a Roman physician, also used the term for "the papulae of an eroding, blistering eruption." Pliny the Elder described lichen as "synonymous with the impetigo of the Latins." Galen (129–217 BCE) described lichen as "a roughness of the skin, attended with much itching" (Zaghi and Griffin 2016).

Leikhēn is also the root of word *likanos*, meaning "the finger one licks," or the index finger. In turn, this name was given to a string on a lyre specifically played by the index finger.

The genus *Lepraria* and the term *leprosy* derive from the Greek *lepein*, "to peel." The autoimmune skin diseases lichen planus and lichen sclerosus stem from this root word. Even the Latin word *lepra* was denigrated by early Christian writers who used it to mean sin or heresy. No surprise there. On the other hand, it is related to the word "liken," which suggests comradeship, connectedness, contact, and affection.

But exactly how would one define the relationship between algae, cyanobacteria, and fungi?

Over time, various theories and metaphors have been proposed. Trevor Goward, a lichenologist at the University of British Columbia, suggests, tongue in cheek, that lichens are fungi that discovered agriculture. Other authors suggest lichen fungi are parasites that may become benevolent, or that lichen algae are solar panels for fungi—or the reverse, that fungi are greenhouses for algae growth.

One advantage of cyanobacteria is that it can fix atmospheric nitrogen into a useable form for plants and animals, leading to producing sugars. The fungi provide structure and protection.

Cyanobacteria, like humans, have a circadian rhythm. That is, they have a need for sleep, rest, and a restorative aspect. In humans, the recent discovery of the glymphatic tissue in the brain, with its ability to remove toxins from the brain during sleep, explains in part the ever-increasing levels of reduced mental health and increased levels of chronic neurological diseases. In terms of such rhythms, polar lichens possess internal clocks that help shift their adjustment to seasonal levels of sunlight.

Early authors depicted the fungus in the lichen as a sort of slave driver, or parasitic, describing the condition as helotism. Cooke (1893) wrote about the fungus, "It surrounds them as a spider its prey, with a fibrous net of narrow meshes, which is gradually converted into an impenetrable covering; but whilst the spider sucks its prey and leaves it dead, the fungus incites the algae found in its net to more rapid activity, nay, to more vigorous increase."

Lichens have a unique capacity to live where no other organisms can survive. The algae provide carbohydrates through photosynthesis, and the fungi in turn provide water, minerals and a complex thallus (a plant part that does not differentiate stems and leaves, lacks true roots, and lacks a vascular system) that prevents algae from drying out. Lichens with algae cannot absorb nitrogen and depend upon their rock or tree to make amino acids. How the algal, bacterial, and fungal elements communicate remains a mystery.

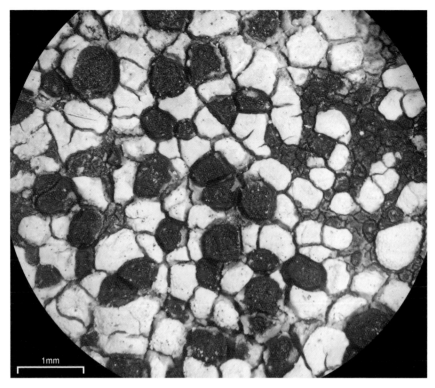

Rhizocarpon geographicum (Yellow Map Lichen)

Lichens are fascinating in that they create soil, by the breakdown of rocks, and provide plants with a means of growth. Lichens produce acid that breaks down stone, creating depressions to anchor themselves. When these fine crystals combine with decayed lichens, the first nitrogen-rich soil is formed.

Lichens are long-lived. The round-patched, light-green map lichens are up to five thousand years old. Yellow map lichen (*Rhizocarpon geographicum*) is estimated to live up to 8,600 years.

Fossils related to modern lichens are known from the Cretaceous period (145 to 66 million years ago) along with dinosaurs. Older lichen fossils from the Paleogene period (66 to 33 million years ago) have been found preserved in Baltic amber resin.

A letter to *Nature* magazine (Taylor et al. 1995) describes a lichen fossil (*Winfrenatia reticulata*) from thin sections dating to the Early Devonian epoch (400 million years old), from Rhynie Chert near Aberdeen, Scotland.

Evidence may be even older: Work by Yuan and Xiao (2005) identified fossil traces of algae-like cells wrapped in fungal threads, found in marine rock in southern China that could be 600 million years old.

A small number of lichens involve both algae and cyanobacteria, and it is possible that fungi may have "teamed up" with cyanobacteria around 1.5 billion years ago. It was the production of oxygen by cyanobacteria and chloroplasts that begin to change the planet by increasing the levels of exhaled oxygen in its atmosphere.

Nostoc is the most common genus of cyanobacteria in lichens. Kaasalainen et al. (2012) investigated 803 lichen thalli, representing twenty-three different cyanolichen genera. Mycocystins, which are potent toxins, were found in forty-two lichens. They are suspected to act as tumor promoters and are usually produced by bloom-forming cyanobacteria in freshwater ecosystems.

Various cystobasidiomycete yeasts (CBYs) are hosted in some lichens. Lendemer et al. (2019) searched for CBYs in 339 lichen species in the southern Appalachian Mountains. Nine taxa were present, representing 2.7% of all species tested. Seven of nine (remember the Star Trek character by that name?) are foliose and fruticose lichens. They are found in as many as two-thirds of known lichens (Lücking and Spribille 2024, 58).

Foliose derives from Latin *foliosus*, meaning "leaf," and are large, leafy lichens that are distinctly different on both sides. Examples are species of *Cetraria, Parmelia, Peltigera,* and *Xanthoria*. They tend to grow from their margins.

Crustose (crust) lichens generally grow flat on rocks, gravestones, old automobiles, and so on. Examples are found in species of *Graphis, Lecanora,* and *Rhizocarpon*. They do not have a bottom, per se, and grow from their margins.

The third major type of lichen are fruticose, derived from the Latin meaning "upright branch." They tend to be bushy, hairy or coral-like. Examples are found in the genus *Cladonia, Usnea,* and *Letharia*. They grow from their tips, and some have a strong central core.

Some lichenologists use the term *leprose* for powdery, shapeless fuzzy lichens. One example would be the genus *Lepraria*, the dust lichens, which appear as a granular powder.

Lungwort (*Lobaria pulmonaria*) and the *Collema* species can be classified as jelly lichens, due to their gelatinous, slimy texture when wet.

As an herbalist and ethnobotanist, I was misled in my university studies as to which came first: Of course, it was cyanobacteria (algae) needing a host (fungi) to sustain them on volcanic rock.

Blair Hedges of Pennsylvania State University suggests that aquatic algae evolved into a terrestrial form about 1.3 billion years ago. Their bright pigments helped reduce the harmful damage of ultraviolet radiation. The algae partner produced oxygen that entered the atmosphere, turning the planet into a hospitable environment, and led to development of land plants.

I have always thought the movement from fresh water to land was the beginning of setting an ecological landmass table for plants.

Nelsen et al. (2020) suggest that coupled with the absence of unambiguous fossil data, our work finds no support for lichens having mediated global change during the Neoproterozoic–early Paleozoic eras prior to vascular plants. Further, they suggest that ferns were present 100 million years before lichens. I would add, "Maybe." After all, did there not have to be soil and carbon dioxide for ferns to thrive? The absence of fossils may simply mean an absence of fossils.

It is presently thought there are about 17,000 to 20,000 species of lichens encrusting about 8% of the planet's surface. To date, approximately 5,600 species and 766 genera have been identified in North America.

They exhibit a wide range of colors, including green, gray, black, red, orange, yellow, lilac, pink, white, and brown. Lichens growing in shade tend to have a darker color, helping absorb as much ultraviolet (UV) radiation as possible, while the bright yellow-orange of rock lichens helps protect them from harmful radiation and allows them to absorb the portion of the color spectrum they can use. The same species will exhibit different color in sun or shade.

Amateur lichenologists may wish to invest in a hand lens with a UV light option. Many lichens fluoresce white, orange, or blue under the latter. Bright white suggests the presence of squamatic, divaricatic, evernic, alectoronic, or perlatolic acid. Orange and yellow suggest the presence of rhizocarpic acid.

Chemical testing is also relatively easy. For a potassium (K) test you can use caustic lye (potassium hydroxide) dry sticks from a chemical supply company, or purchase some Liquid Plumber. For a chloride (Cl) test, you can use bleach. Both are caustic, so be careful.

RECOGNIZING SYMBIOSIS

We are all lichens now.

SCOTT GILBERT

Merlin Sheldrake's (2020) *Entangled Life* contains a fascinating chapter on lichens. I contacted him with extra interest, as my English ancestry goes back to the Sheldrakes about three hundred years ago. His chapter "The Intimacy of

Strangers" contains a lot of great insight into lichens, which I will leave for the reader to follow up. I highly recommend the book.

He shares a few words about the Swiss botanist Simon Schwendener, who published a paper in 1869 presenting the idea of the "dual hypothesis of lichens." Schwendener suggested a notion that was radical for the times, that the fungal partners in lichens were "parasites, although with the wisdom of statesmen." The German botanist Heinrich Anton De Bary first noted the dualist nature in 1866, based in part on earlier work by Karl Wallroth, who observed what he called "gonidia" in lichens in 1825. de Bary defined *symbiosis* as "the shared life of organisms with different names." Several years earlier, in 1874, the term *commensalism* was first used.

Two Russian botanists, Andrei Famintsyn and Josep W. Baranetzky, isolated algae from *Xanthoria parietina* and *Pseudevernia furfuracea* and then cultivated them in a lab in 1867.

Terms like *mutualism* and then *symbiosis* (via the German *symbiotismus*) were coined during the 1870s and associated with lichens. The latter is from the Greek *symbiō-*, meaning "living together." The Belgian Pierre-Joseph Van Beneden spoke about mutualism in 1875 in his treatise, *Les Commensaux et les parasites dans le règne animal*. The term *mutualism*, according to Zonca (2023), first appeared in 1828, related to a society of silk weavers in Lyon, France.

The term *symbiotismus* was first mentioned by Albert Bernhard Frank in 1877 in his book on crustose lichens. He later discovered fungi on the roots of plants, and named them mycorrhizae, in 1885.

Charles Darwin wrote about natural selection, and the survival of an organism, based on the ability to adapt. The term *symbiosis* is sometimes referred to as "Darwin's blind spot" (Ryan 2002).

Merlin Sheldrake suggests the term *holobiont*. "Holobionts are the lichens of the world, more than the sum of their parts." Are we humans not also holobionts? We are a combination of mammal and microbial and fungal biomes, without which none could have a functional physiology. The disruption of our microbiome, through artificial and modified food, anti-inflammatory drugs, and overuse of antibiotics, herbicides, pesticides, and fungicides, has led to an increase in chronic and autoimmune disease.

Lynn Margulis (1938–2011) proposed that symbiotic interactions helped initiate evolution through horizontal transfer of genetic material between bacteria and eucaryotic cells. In 1974, she collaborated with James Lovelock on the Gaia hypothesis, suggesting our planet functions symbiotically and is self-regulating. Margulis and two colleagues (Guerrero et al. 2013) wrote the article "Symbiogenesis: The Holobiont as a Unit of Evolution," which was published soon after her death. The photobiont *Trebouxia lynnae* is named in her honor.

Margulis's groundbreaking work was initially met with considerable opposition from parts of the scientific community. Today, her hypothesis is widely accepted. All living beings live in symbiosis, and in interdependency with others. Her work was influenced by the Russian researcher Constantin Sergeïevitch Merejkovski (1855–1921), whose work involved the symbiotic origin of chloroplasts in diatoms and lichens.

Toby Spribille (2016), a lichenologist and professor at the University of Alberta (my alma mater), with his colleagues published a paper that turned the dualistic hypothesis by Schwendener on its head. He ground up a lichen and sequenced the DNA, finding more than algae and fungi, which suggested the presence of symbiotic partners. What was previously believed to be a contaminant turned out to be a single-celled yeast, found in many lichens. It is believed that bacteria and yeast "partners" are integral to the development of form, shape, and chemistry of each individual lichen. The significance of Spribille's finding is explored later in this book, in the context of the medicinal application of several endolichenic fungi and bacteria found within lichens. Spribille (2018) later found a fourth fungal partner in wolf lichen (*Letharia vulpina*).

Hawksworth and Grube (2020) suggested a new definition of lichen: "an autonomous ecosystem formed by the interaction of an 'inclusive' fungus, an extracellular organization of one or many photosynthesizing partners, and an indeterminate number of other microscopic organisms."

Lichens are amazing in their ability to reproduce from a broken piece, starting a new colony. Some lichens produce spores, which in the best case, land where other algae are waiting, in order create a new lichen. Lichens propagate asexually as well, with little bundles of fungal and algal material carried by the wind. In some cases, it is unclear how photobionts (algae) and mycobionts (fungi) find each other, turn out to be compatible, and choose to stay together, or not.

That brings me to my favorite lichen joke: Freddie Fungus met Annie Algae and they got together. They fell in love, soon married, but now it's on the rocks.

USES OF LICHENS

Linnaeus was not keen on lichens, calling them *rustici pauperrimi*, or "the poor trash of vegetation." However, lichens provide shelter, nesting material, and food for animals and humans. At least 46 species of North American birds use lichens for nesting material. It is estimated that one billion people consume lichens as part of their diet (Burlingame 2000). And about 15 different species of edible lichens are used for food in China (Choi et al. 2017).

Spruce grouse, deer, mouse, caribou, elk, mountain goats, bighorn sheep, pronghorn antelope, chipmunks, squirrels, voles, pikas, mice, bats, slugs, grasshoppers, butterflies, moths, spiders, beetles, and snails dine on lichens. In fact, various snail species prefer to eat different lichens, probably due to the ability to maximize energy and nutrients. Snail dietary preferences would also reduce competition for resources (Baur et al. 1994). Depending upon diet, terrestrial snails will sequester parietin and atranorin, while expelling (+)-usnic acid or alpha-collatolic acid in their feces (Hesbacher et al. 1995).

For sweet food, the green lacewing eats aphids that ants collect in "leaf jails." The green lacewing larvae secrete a sticky silk on their back and attach tiny pieces of lichen to it. They then sneak right by guard ants to feast. This works out well for lichens, too, as any pieces that fall off can start to grow.

Canadian naturalist Aleta Karstad reports identifying 20 types of lichens on one climb up a white spruce, each occupying a different zone (Bennet and Tiner 1993). When looking for lichens in the landscape, it is worth bearing in mind that each change in elevation of one thousand feet (300 meters) shifts the weather pattern by two weeks.

Other human uses of lichens include components of dyes, cosmetics, perfume, medicine, and poisons. In the past, lichens have been processed to provide alcohol, fiber for clothing, tanning compounds, hallucinogens, and aids for hunting and fishing, navigation, Egyptian mummies, rituals, and magic art. In Japan, lichens are added to paint to inhibit growth of mildew.

Lichens have inspired artists, poets, writers, and lyricists. From southwestern Quebec to northeastern Saskatchewan, on remote Laurentian Shield rock walls, are found lichenoglyphs created by Indigenous people. In such locations, dark, ancient lichens have been removed to reveal various symbols representing humans, animals, mythical creatures, sacred symbols, and spirit beings, such as the Algonquin spirit, Thunderbird, carved out of lichens on a cliff in northern Saskatchewan.

These works of art are not widely publicized, to help preserve them. Recently, the Mohawk Group of Calhoun, Georgia, presented carpet tiles designed to resemble various blooming lichens in their bright colors.

Lichens also produce hydrogen, a future source of green energy. When

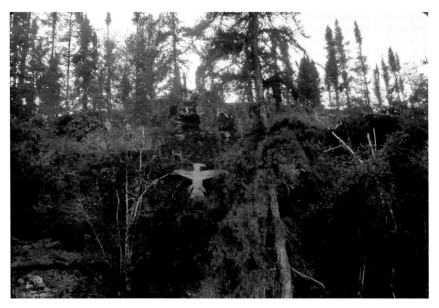

Thunderbird Lichenoglyph at Reindeer Lake, Saskatchewan
PHOTOGRAPH BY TIM JONES

there is light, lichens use a pathway that transfers electrons to hydrogenase, and under dark conditions they use the PFOR enzyme (pyruvate:ferredoxin oxidoreductase) and a fermentation process called the Arc system to supply electrons to hydrogenase. Both of these pathways then generate hydrogen. Combined with lichens' ability to survive extreme environments, this suggests they could be a unique and valuable natural factory producing hydrogen (Papazi et al. 2015).

In the far north, lichens have served as an emergency food. The rock tripe lichens, *tripes de roches*, lichens of *Umbilicaria* and *Lasallia*, could be boiled several times with water changes, or added to soup. Today the addition of baking soda somewhat improves their digestibility, which traditionally was done by adding wood ash to water or by predigesting the lichens in the rumen ("first stomach") taken from a caribou.

There are also beverages made with lichens: The Tarahumara (Rarámuri) of northern Mexico utilize *Usnea* species in the fermentation of corn beverages. (I vaguely remember one night overindulging in too much chicha beer in Cuzco, Peru. The altitude did not help.) A beverage called pozol is today produced with fermented corn and cacao beans.

Remember not to pick any lichen for medicine within 200 meters of a highway.

LICHEN DYES

Ye Lichens! touch'd by chemist's art,
Soft shades of various tint impart,
    That fashion's vesture dyes;
Torn from your sweet abode of shade,
To deck our fair—our commerce aid,
Your beauties soon in dust are laid,
    Ah! Never more to rise.

SARAH HOARE (1831)

Lichen dyes could take up an entire chapter. One great book to note is *Lichen Dyes* by Casselman (2011). *The International Fungi and Fibre Symposium*, which began in 1985 and is held annually around the globe, is another resource for those interested.

Consider the history of these uses: It is believed lichen dyes were first used in China about four millennia ago. The oldest recorded dye recipe was written in Greece, about 1800 years ago.

Later, in the British Isles, Harris, Shetland, Irish, and Donegal tweeds were formerly dyed with various lichens (*Parmelia* or *Roccella* sp.), "fixed" to more permanence using the addition of human urine. Factories would place "night water" barrels on the street corners of Edinburgh to receive donations of this ingredient. It really did matter on which side of town you resided. Highland tartan dyes, with blue and purple, were derived in this manner. As these sources were used up, lichens were imported from Norway and Sweden, then Cape Verde and the Canary Islands, and then parts of Africa and Peru, until the process ended in the early twentieth century.

PURPOSEFUL INGESTION OF LICHENS

At least one lichen possesses entheogenic (psychoactive) properties, including compounds identified as psilocybin and tryptamines. Wade Davis and Jim Yost (1983) were in the Ecuadorian Amazon in 1981 when elders mentioned the *Dictyonema huaorani* lichen, which they managed to collect. The Waorami (Huaorani) call it *neññendapñ*. It was added to a mixture of bryophytes when people wished to cast curses. As a drug, it is known as *kigiwai*, and ingestion creates headaches and confusion. It was also used to inflict sterility, by adding it to a young child's drink to induce barrenness.

The Akimel O'otham (Pima), meaning "river people," and Maricopa/ Pipaash of the Southwest pick a gray lichen with strong violet odor. Known as "earth flower," this lichen was mixed with tobacco either to act as a hallucinogen, or to attract women or bring good luck. Maybe all three!

A thick, yellow-green lichen on boulders of the Rocky Mountains is enjoyed as a narcotic by Indigenous people and by bighorn sheep. Young ewes, especially, enjoy a nibble, grinding their teeth or gums to scrape the lichen off the rocks. It may be a *Lecanora* species, as it's known that sheep in the deserts of Libya chew the lichen *L. esculenta* to the point of tooth loss. There is much speculation that this lichen is the wind-blown *manna* mentioned in the Bible.

A Menominee legend regards this lichen as scabs from the head of Mâ'nâpus, to keep his aunts and uncles from starving. Another version of the legend says that lichens were scabs from when Mâ'nâpus burned his buttocks, and they came off as he slid down a slanting rock (Smith 1923). Menominee/ Menomini (*manowinii*, meaning "wild rice people,") was a name given to the people by the Ojibwa.

Around 1300 CE the Spanish physician Arnaldus de Villa Nova discovered litmus, a word derived from the old Norse word *litmosi*, meaning literally "moss-dye." It became a way of testing the pH of materials. Orchil lichens (*Roccella* sp.) were overharvested in Europe for this purpose, and the resulting purple dye was valued for clothing.

Thousands of tons of oakmoss lichens have been harvested in Europe and Africa since at least the seventeenth century for perfumes, powdered wigs, and such. It is fortunate that only a few North American oakmoss lichens share these properties and are presently not harvested commercially. Let us hope that trend continues.

REPORTS OF THE MEDICINAL USE OF LICHENS

The first recorded use of lichens for medicine can be traced back to 1800 BCE, when *Evernia furfuracea* was found beneficial.

Numerous interesting laboratory and clinical trials have been conducted in the past decade (2012–2022), providing new information for readers and updating my previous work. Note that few human clinical trials have been conducted to date.

Lichens contain molecules such as polyketides that may help treat or decrease antibiotic-resistant infections. Estimates suggest about 50% of lichens exhibit promising antibiotic activities (Zambare and Christopher 2012). Various well-known pharmaceuticals, including erythromycin A, tylosin, monensin A, rifamycin, tetracyclines, and amphotericin B, were initially isolated from actinomycetes, which are bacteria. However, no new classes of antibiotics have been developed since 1987 (WHO 2020).

It is estimated that by 2050, the number of deaths from aggressive bacteria may exceed ten million per year. That works out to one person every three seconds worldwide, far exceeding projected deaths from cancer and diabetes combined. In 2019 there were an estimated 13.7 million infection-related deaths, with 7.7 million associated with 33 bacteria.

The acronym ESKAPE refers to the six most virulent bacteria species resistant to today's antibiotics. They are *Enterococcus faecium*, *Staphylococcus aureus*, *Klebsiella pneumoniae*, *Acinetobacter baumannii*, *Pseudomonas aeruginosa*, and *Enterobacter* species.

Antibiotic-resistant tuberculosis is another significant problem, discussed in more detail with usnic acid in the Lichen Chemistry chapter.

Staphylococcus aureus is the leading bacterial cause of death in 135 countries. It is estimated that 2% of the population carry methicillin-resistant *Staphylococcus aureus* (MRSA) in/on their body. In 2017, there were nearly 20,000 recorded infections in the United States, with a 30–40% mortality rate.

Another way to view this comes from the Global Burden of Disease (GBD) study: "Five leading pathogens—*Staphylococcus aureus*, *Escherichia coli*, *Streptococcus pneumoniae*, *Klebsiella pneumoniae* and *Pseudomonas aeruginosa*— were responsible for 54.9% of deaths among the investigated bacteria" (GBD 2023). The latter bacteria were responsible for 33,000 cases in 2017, resulting in 2700 deaths. They are particularly problematic for cystic fibrosis patients (Quave 2021).

There are other specific infections that raise enormous concern. For example, the microbe *Acinetobacter baumannii* causes severe infections, and in the hospital can survive for nearly two weeks on a dry surface. Carbapenem-resistant *Acinetobacter baumannii* (CRAB) hospitalized 8,500 American patients in 2017, killing 700. Multiple-drug-resistant and carbapenem-resistant *Klebsiella pneumoniae* is scary, with a mortality rate of 40–70% in infected patients; in those with alcohol addiction the mortality shoots up to 100%. Also, drug-resistant tuberculosis and gonorrhea (*Neisseria gonorrhoeae*) are on the rise. These infections rose to over 550,000 in the United States during 2018.

To address these concerns, consider that lichen compounds are revealing unique molecules that may lead to new antibiotics, or as adjunct medicines that are synergistic with older classes of antibiotics to which bacteria have become resistant.

Beyond such infections, various cancers worldwide account for approximately 13% of all deaths (Nguyen et al. 2014). Lung cancer and breast cancer accounted for 12% of new cases in 2018, with colon cancer third (Bray et al. 2018). Globally, 9.6 million people died of cancer in that year, and the number is predicted to reach 29.5 million by 2040.

At the present time, cancer treatments involve cytotoxic medicine, target-based agents, hormones and hormone antagonists, and immunomodulators (Liu et al. 2017). Seventy percent of these are derived from natural compounds or semisynthetic products (Katz et al. 2016).

Thus, it's good that lichens have much to offer in terms of compounds exhibiting antitumor, antioxidant, anti-invasive, antimigrative, antiproliferative, cytotoxic, and apoptosis (programmed self-death) potential.

Before you start writing to me about using lichens as medicine, I need to clearly state my position on the use of lichens for human and animal health. Although I have personally collected and produced alcohol extractions of usnea species of the boreal forest for my own use, the chemistry of lichens can be replicated synthetically, with few exceptions.

The delightful and insightful book *The Lichen Museum* (Palmer 2013) reminds us that lichens refuse to grow in laboratories, and that asking how they can be useful to humans is the wrong question. Palmer suggests their refusal should be considered a lesson for us. Their slow growth also makes them resistant to commercial and industrial harvest and exploitation. Instead, the unique secondary metabolites of lichens can be produced by engineering lichen gene clusters with cultivated bacterial or viral hosts (Calcott et al. 2018).

So let us take a deep dive into the world of lichens. Note that DNA and genetic research are redefining and renaming binomials, that is, the two-word taxomonic classification for lichens and other organisms. I provide my most up-to-date Latin genus and species here, but these will change with time.

As Zonca (2023) reminds us, "Someone who takes an interest in lichens, who takes the time and trouble to stop in front of a wall, to circle a tree trunk, to climb a roof and to approach it close up, is thus seen as eccentric, enlightened, unnerving." Sounds like me! And maybe you!

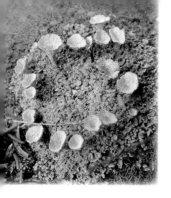

Medicinal Lichens

....

Acarospora to *Xylopsora*

Romance and poetry, ivy, lichens and wallflowers need rain to make them grow.

NATHANIEL HAWTHORNE

ACAROSPORA

Cobblestone Lichen   Soil Paint Lichen

Geographic Range: Canada, the U.S. Southwest, Mexico

Habitat: rocks, full sun, dry soil

Medicinal Applications: antimicrobial, antioxidant, cancer

Notable Chemicals: atranorin, chloroatranorin, epanorin; and gyrophoric, norstictic, rhizocarpic, stictic, and usnic acid

There are an estimated seventy-four species of *Acarospora* lichens found in North America. The genus name may derive from the Greek *akarpos*, meaning "sterile or bearing no fruit," and *spora*, "sowing or seed."

The Yuman people of northern Mexico know this genus as *Uja' tebiyauup*, with *uja'* meaning stone, and *tebiyauup* for flower. In Spanish it is known as *Flor de Piedra*. This was the term also used for *Caloplaca* and *Lecanora* species.

Brown cobblestone lichen (*Acarospora fuscata*) grows on granite rocks in full or partial sun from Alaska diagonally across northern Manitoba to New England, and south to Arizona and New Mexico. The name *fuscata* may derive from the Latin *fuscus*, meaning "dark gray" or "dusky."

It contains atranorin, chloroatranorin, stictic, norstictic, usnic and gyrophoric acid, which possess antioxidant and anti-microbial activity. This lichen's component gyrophoric acid, in vitro, shows activity against the gram-positive bacteria *Bacillus mycoides*, *B. subtilis*, and *Staphylococcus aureus*, gram-negative

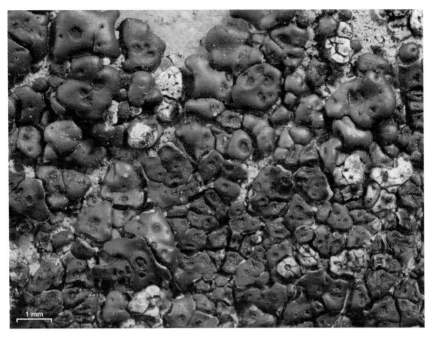

Acarospora americana (Dusty Cobblestone Lichen)

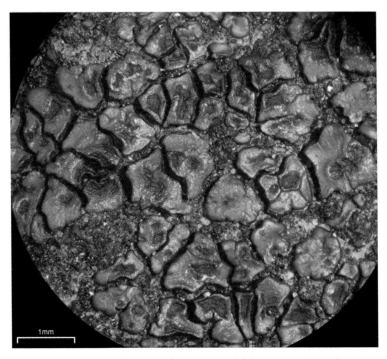

Acarospora fuscata (Brown Cobblestone Lichen)

bacteria including *Escherichia coli* and *Klebsiella pneumoniae*, and various fungi including *Penicillium purpurescens* and *P. verrucosum*.

Extracts in vitro express strong activity against A549 (lung), Fem-x (melanoma), LS174 (colon), and K562 (chronic myelogenous leukemia) cancer cell lines (Kosanic et al. 2014).

Bright cobblestone lichen (*Acarospora socialis*) is commonly found on desert rocks in Arizona and California. *Socialis* refers to growing in clumps. Work by Yeash et al. (2017) found ethanol extracts to exhibit significant DPPH antioxidant scavenging activity.

This lichen contains epanorin, a secondary metabolite that inhibits proliferation of MCF-7 (breast cancer cells) by inducing cell cycle arrest in G0/G1.

Work by Palacios-Moreno et al. (2019) found a lack of cytotoxicity in normal cell line HEK-293 and human fibroblasts, suggesting potential antineoplastic activity, without harm to normal cells.

Lichens are symbiotic, but they can become parasitic. The soil paint lichen (*Acarospora schleicheri*) is found on dry soil from Saskatchewan to Mexico. It contains rhizocarpic acid, which gives its yellow color. The related *Acarospora stapfiana*, also yellow, parasitizes the desert firedot lichen (*Caloplaca trachyphylla*).

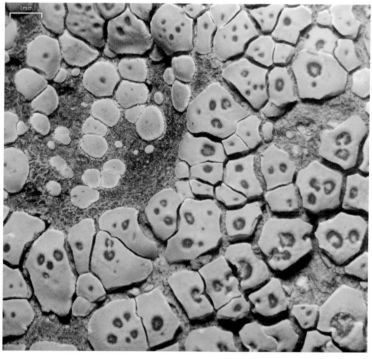

Acarospora socialis syn. *A. radicata* (Bright Cobblestone Lichen)

ACROSCYPHUS
Mountain Crab Eye Lichen

Warning: Do not pick!

Mountain crab eye lichen (*Acroscyphus sphaerophoroides*) is found at only eight sites in British Columbia, and is Red Listed (critically endangered) according to the International Union for Conservation of Nature. It is rarely found in Alaska and Washington in coastal mountains, associated with fallen or dead mountain hemlock trees in fens and bogs. Observe but do not pick.

Methanol extracts show low to moderate activity against 11 bacteria (*Bacillus subtilis, B. cereus, Enterobacter aerogenes, Escherichia coli, Klebsiella pneumoniae, Micrococcus luteus, Proteus mirabilis, Pseudomonas aeruginosa, Salmonella typhimurium, Staphylococcus aureus, Streptococcus pneumoniae*) and eight fungi (*Aspergillus flavus, A. nidulans, A. niger, A. sulphuricus, A. terreus, Candida albicans, Cryptococcus albidus, Trichophyton rubrum*) (Nayaka et al. 2010).

ALECTORIA
Caribou Moss   Crow Whiskers   Green Witch's Hair Lichen

Geographic Range: coastal, subarctic and arctic North America

Habitat: lower forest canopy

Practical Uses: clothing, fire starter (discouraged)

Medicinal Applications: arthritis, lung conditions, skin conditions, tumors

Notable Chemicals: alectosarmentin, arabitol, chloroatranorin, dibensofuranoidlactol, diffractaic acid, mannitol, and alpha-collatolic, physodic, squamatic, and usnic acid

Like rock or stone, it is o'ergrown
With lichens to the very top,
And hung with heavy tufts of moss,
A melancholy crop.

WILLIAM WORDSWORTH

There are eight species of *Alectoria* in North America, among them caribou moss (*Alectoria ochroleuca* and *Alectoria nitidula*), crow whiskers (*Alectoria sarmentosa*), and green witch's hair lichen (*Alectoria ochroleuca*). Alectoria originally meant a magical talisman stone found in the stomach or liver of a cock or capon. It could also allude to Alecto, one of the three furies in Greek mythology—the goddess of vengeance. This is less likely.

Alectoria and *Usnea* species with reflecting usnic acid pigments are usually found in the lower forest canopy. The dark *Bryoria* species (described later) dominate the upper canopy (Färber et al. 2014). *Sarmentosa* means "creeping" or "vine-like." *Ochroleuca* derives from *ochro*, meaning ochre (brown-yellow), as in the clay used to protect skin from sun and insects, and *leuca* (white).

Crow whiskers (*Alectoria sarmentosa*) lichens were used medicinally in an unspecified manner (Turner 2004). The Saanich call it *k'aalts'idaa llisga*, meaning "crow's mountain goat wool," in reference to the Tsimshian, who collected mountain goat wool attached to bushes.

Both *Alectoria* and *Bryoria* species lichens were utilized for clothing, by weaving them into other materials. This was usually done by combining them

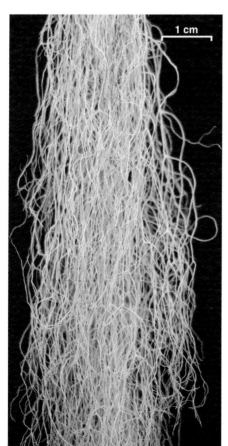

Alectoria sarmentosa ssp. *sarmentosa* (Crow Whiskers)

with cedar or silverberry/wolf willow bark to manufacture vests, leggings, and moccasins. Fireweed seed fluff was sometimes spun together with mountain goat wool to produce waterproof apparel.

The lichen was also used to strain impurities out of hot pitch from conifers, when making medicine.

The Nuxalk (Bella Coola) of British Columbia call this *suts' wakt*, or *ipts-aak*, meaning "limb moss." When found on red alder, it is warmed and applied to a broken boil or festering sore (Smith 1929; Turner 1973). The long hair was utilized for false whiskers and hair on dance masks.

The Ditidaht (meaning "people along the coast") of southwestern Vancouver Island know the lichen as *p'u7up*. They applied the lichen to wounds and used it for sanitary napkins and baby diapers (Turner et al. 1983).

The Haida name is *kwii7aawaa*, "cloud," referring to the cumulus clouds mentioned in legend. They used the lichen in a variety of ways.

In the Ts'msyen language, this lichen and *Usnea* species were known as *iimgmgen*, or "whiskers of the tree."

The Salish or Flathead (*Salish,* meaning "the people") of Montana call it *sqaliö*, and combine it with pineapple weed (*Matricaria discoidea*) in a tea to ensure the placenta is totally expelled after giving birth (Stubbs 1966).

In Washington and Oregon, both the Umatilla (*Imatalamiáma*) and the Cayuse used this lichen. The name Cayuse may derive from the French-Canadian fur traders, who called the tribe *Cailloux*, meaning "rock people," or from *Kyuuse*, a name given them by the famous Scottish botanist David Douglas. This lichen often hangs from the Douglas fir tree, named in this botanist's honor.

The Umatilla and Cayuse both boiled and applied the compress to open sores, arthritic pain, and *achash-pama* (an eye problem). It is known as *laxpt* or *mak'hl* (Hunn 2005).

The lichen contains dibensofuranoid lactol, usnic acid, physodic acid, 8'-O-ethyl-beta-alectoronic acid, alectosarmentin, alpha-collatolic acid, squamatic acid, mannitol, arabitol, and physodic acid. Mannitol and arabitol are antitumor polysaccharides.

Green witch's hair covered a sick person in steam baths to hold the heat, used this way by the Sugpiaq ("the real people") or Alutiiq people of Alaska. (The name Alutiiq may derive from Aleut, the name given to the Indigenous tribe by Russian fur traders and settlers.) Since it contains mannitol, compare this to the use of mannitol dry powder, which has been found to improve some measures of lung function in cystic fibrosis patients compared to a control (Nevitt et al. 2020). Relatedly, inhaled mannitol (Bronchitol) is licensed in Australia as a safe and efficacious support for patients with cystic fibrosis. The main catch is the prohibitive cost of $40,000 Australian per year. (Warren et al. 2019).

The Inuit call this lichen "green beard" or *tinqaujait*, meaning, "what looks like pubic hair." It may have been used to staunch bleeding from wounds (Wennekens 1985).

Artists and poets have long correlated lichens like this one with a bushy female mons veneris. It makes a handy, quick fire-starter in wilderness emergencies. Use for the latter purpose is discouraged, as the lichen is only abundant on trees at least a century old.

Both witch's hair lichen (*Alectoria sarmentosa*) and green witch's hair lichen (*A. ochroleuca*) show significant activity against motility of human non-small-cell lung cancer cell lines (Yang et al. 2016).

Green witch's hair lichen was used in Russia during the 1930s to produce a molasses-like syrup, yielding glucose at 82% of dry weight. It was also used by distillers to produce alcohol (Rogers 2011).

Green witch's hair lichen (*Alectoria ochroleuca*) contains (−)-usnic acid. Extracts from the lichen inhibit the growth and proliferation of breast (T-47D) and pancreatic (Capan-2) cancer cell lines (Einarsdóttir et al. 2010).

Witch's hair ethanol extract contains usnic acid, physodic acid, and alectosarmentin, an antimicrobial (Gollapudi et al. 1994). It also contains diffractaic, thamnolic, barbatic, alectoronic, and chloroatranorin acids.

Later work by Cobanoglu et al. (2010) found *Alectoria sarcomtosa* lichen extracts inhibit three species of bacteria.

Gray witch's hair lichen (*Alectoria nigricans*, now *Gowardia nigricans*) has a similar common name but is no longer considered part of this group. It grows on the ground and low branches throughout the arctic and British Columbia. It lacks yellow due to an absence of usnic acid but does contain alectorialic acid.

Green witch's hair lichen and *Alectoria nitidula* (*Bryoria nitidula*) were known as caribou moss by the Inuit and were offered to young fawns to try to get them to eat from people's hands (Moerman 2010). *Nitidula* is the diminutive of *nitidus*, meaning "somewhat elegant" or "trim."

Work by Ingólfsdóttir et al. (2000) found these lichen extracts active against leukemia cancer cell lines and to exhibit quinone reductase activity. Quinone reductase is an enzyme inside cells that makes certain molecules less toxic, aiding cellular detoxification.

AMANDINEA

Button Lichen

Button lichen (*Amandinea* sp. syn. *Buellia*) extracts show little cytotoxicity but inhibit lipopolysaccharide (LPS)-induced release of pro-inflammatory cytokines. The extracts reduced the cytosolic p-1$_k$B-a level and the level of nuclear factor p65 (Kim et al. 2020). The genus name may derive from the Latin *amanda*, meaning "to be loved."

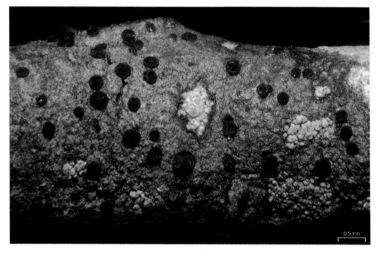

Amandinea polyspora (Button Lichen)

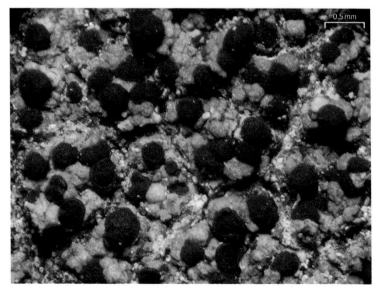

Amandinea punctata (Tiny Button Lichen)

AMYGDALARIA
Powdery Almond Lichen

Powdery almond lichen (*Amygdalaria panaeola* syn. *Biatora panaeola* syn. *Lecidea panaeola*) is confined to rocks on coastal areas of Alaska and Newfoundland south to the northeastern United States. *Panaeola* derives from the Greek meaning "variegated."

This lichen contains gryphoric acid, confluentic acid, and derivatives. Its black tumor-like growths called cephalodia are groups of blue-green algae. Confluentic acid shows selective inhibition of monoamine oxidase (MAO)-B with an IC50 value of 0.22 µM (Endo et al. 1994).

Powdery almond lichen produces a fluorescent yellow-green pigment called panaefluoroline B in the cultured mycobiont (Kinoshita et al. 2015).

ARTHONIA
Bloody Comma Lichen

The *Arthonia* genus is quite large, containing at least 110 species in North America. Bloody comma lichen (*Arthonia cinnabarina*) is a pink–purple species,

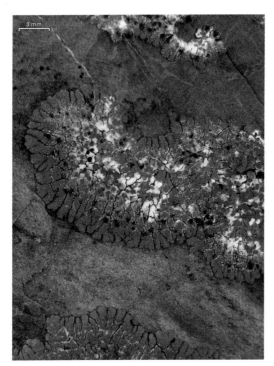

Arthonia molendoi

found on bark in isolated parts of Appalachia and throughout Florida and the Gulf Coast. The genus name may derive from the Greek *arthon*, meaning "joint." (Inflammation of a joint is known as arthritis.) *Cinnabar* is the ancient name for red mercury sulfide pigment. It is worth noting that mercury, sulfur, and salt are the three major elements engaged in alchemy.

Work by Yamamoto et al. (2002) identified arthoniafuranes A and B. Previous work identified bostrycoidin and 8-O-methylbostrycoidin in culture. Bostrycoidin shows activity against gram-positive and gram-negative bacteria, as well as against bovine and avian tuberculin mycobacteria.

The related *A. impolita* syn. *A. pruinata* syn. *Pachnolepia pruinata* contains arthoniaic acid.

ASAHINEA
Rag Lichen

Geographic Range: extreme northern arctic, from the interior of Alaska to Baffin Island
Habitat: rocks, decaying vegetation
Medicinal Applications: neurogenerative conditions
Notable Chemicals: asahinin, atranorin, cynodontin, islandicin, and haematommic and usnic acids

There are only two *Asahinea* lichen species in North America.

Arctic rag lichen (*Asahinea chrysantha* syn. *Cetraria chrysantha* syn. *Platysma septentrionale*) is found in the extreme northern arctic, from the interior of Alaska to Baffin Island. It contains usnic acid, atranorin, ß-collatolic acid, cynodontin, haematommic acid, islandicin, asahinin, and 1,5,6,8-tetrahydroxy-3-methylanthraquinone. Islandicin is structurally related to emodin, and is mutagenic for *Salmonella typhimurium* (Liberman et al. 1980).

The recent COVID-19 viral pandemic has led to research into antagonists of viral protein. Work by Mahrosh et al. (2021) found islandicin to be one of the ten best ligands for antiviral activity, out of 200 ligands examined.

The anthraquinone cynodontin is a potent antifungal inhibitor of *Sclerotina minor, Sclerotina sclerotiorum*, and *Botrytis cinerea* (Chrysayi-Tokousbalides and Kastanias 2003).

Yellow rag lichen (*Asahinea scholanderi*) grows on rocks and decaying vegetation above the Arctic Circle. The genus is named in honor of the

Japanese lichenologist Yasuhiko Asahina. The species name honors the Swedish lichenologist Per Frederik Thorkelsson Scholander (1905–1980). He spent time in Greenland and helped revise the many *Umbilicariaceae* genera.

    Work by Urena-Vacas et al. (2022) found extracts from this species to be the best inhibitors of acetylcholinesterase and butyrylcholinesterase, out of fourteen lichen samples. Inhibition of these enzymes is one approach to addressing neurodegenerative conditions, including Alzheimer's disease.

    Cetraria cucullata, mentioned again later, also showed inhibition of enzymes involved in neurodegenerative disorders. The major secondary metabolites identified were alectoronic and alpha-collatolic acid.

    In a conference paper, Varol et al. (2015) presented their findings on the anticancer and anti-angiogenic activities of alpha-collatolic acid. Angiogenesis is the process by which tumor cells develop blood vessels to feed themselves. Anti-angiogenic drugs, of which eleven have been approved by the Food and Drug Administration (FDA), were trialed. Only four led to FDA approval for marketing. The problem is complex, as the restriction of blood vessel development can affect normal vessels rather than tumor cells prone to mutation. Research is ongoing.

ASPICILIA

Rim Lichen

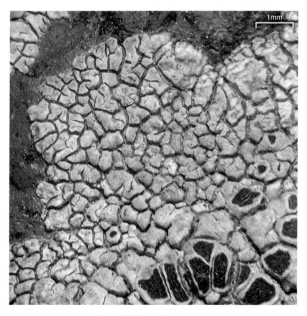

Aspicilia arizonica

There are sixty-one species of *Aspicilia* in North America, although many have been moved to the *Lecanora* genus or vice versa.

Rim lichen (*Aspicilia fruticulosa* syn. *Circinaria rogeri*) is somewhat rare, but is found in eastern Montana, southern Idaho, and eastern Oregon. *Aspicilia* derives from the Greek, meaning "shield concave," and *fruticulosa* for "an abundance of fruit."

This lichen has traveled to space and back. The Lithopanspermia space experiment, launched in 2007, included this lichen species, exposing it to space vacuum, as well as to cosmic and solar radiation. Upon return to Earth, the lichen was capable of self-repair of all the space-induced damage (Raggio et al. 2011).

BAEOMYCES
Brown Beret Lichen

There are only three species of *Baeomyces* lichens in North America.

Brown beret lichen (*Baeomyces rufus*) is the most common, found on mineral soil or shaded rocks. It contains stictic and norstictic acid. It contains the lichenized algae *Elliptochloris bilobata*, which accumulates sugars in response to cold acclimation (Miguez et al. 2017).

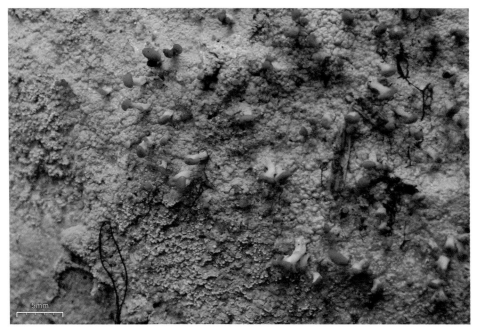

Baeomyces rufus (Brown Beret Lichen)

BIATORA
Dot Lichens

Geographic Range: from Alaska to Newfoundland and south to
    New England, with disparate growth in Appalachia and Colorado
Habitat: mossy regions on rocks
Medicinal Applications: leishmania
Notable Chemicals: atranorin, gyrophoric acid, and ß-orcinol
    depsides, especially argopsin

Dot lichen (*Biatora vernalis*) is common in the arctic, and is rarely found below the 40th parallel. It prefers mossy regions on rocks, rarely on tree bark. The species name is derived from the Latin *vernus*, meaning "of the spring." Work by Printzen and Lumbsch (2000) found molecular evidence that *Biatora* diversification began as early as the Late Cretaceous period.

The lichen contains gyrophoric acid, atranorin, and ß-orcinol depsides, especially argopsin (1'-chloropannarine). Argopsin exhibited antileishmania activity in vitro (Fournet et al. 1997).

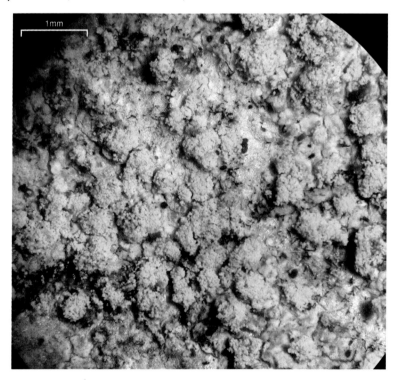

Biatora printzenii

Lichens are extremely sensitive to environmental changes, including pollution. In the 1970s, the first of many Athabasca Oil Sands projects began operations in northeastern Alberta, my home province. A lichen project was initiated to monitor the ecological impact of the new industry.

Mors Kochanski, my noted friend and a survival/bushcraft expert, co-edited and published *Wilderness Arts & Recreation* back in those days. He left us a few years ago, but the hundreds of people he educated in living with nature continue his legacy to this day. His favorite quote about walking and thriving in the boreal forest was "The more you know, the less you carry."

In volume one of *Wilderness Arts & Recreation*, in issue four, there is an article by Dar Tost in which the oil company Syncrude vows to take environmental responsibility and to monitor their levels of sulfur dioxide. Fifty-six lichen plots over 40 square kilometers were established for this monitoring.

About ten years ago, I asked the company for information about the project, and after a six-month runaround, I was told the study had been shut down, due to the death of all the lichens. No surprise there!

BRYORIA

Horsehair Lichens

Geographic Range: North America

Habitat: mainly on conifers and birch

Practical Uses: clothing, food, paint

Medicinal Applications: cancer, swelling

Notable Chemicals: atranorin, barbatolin, and alectorialic, barbatolic, fumarprotocetraric, gyrophoric, lobaric, protocetraric, stictic, usnic, and vulpinic acids

Twenty-four species of *Bryoria* are found in North America. The genus name derives from the Greek *bryon* meaning "moss or lichen."

In 2014 a study on lead, polycyclic aromatic hydrocarbons (PAHs), and sulfur and other elements was conducted on three boreal forest sites in the region. *Bryoria furcellata*, *Hypogymnia physodes*, and three other lichens were monitored along a 100-kilometer distance gradient (Graney et al. 2017). Although *Hypogymnia physodes* is the most tolerant of sulfur dioxide pollution, it was chosen by scientists as the best monitor. Again, no surprise at this lack of rational planning! When sulfur dioxide levels in the air are above 30 µg/m^3, lichen growth is adversely affected. Sulfur interferes with chlorophyll survival and inhibits photosynthesis of sugars.

Most lichens are very susceptible to climate change and environmental pollutants. Wilhelm Nylander (1866), a botanist from Finland, first noted the connection between pollution and lichen growth on trees in Paris, more than 160 years ago. "However, most lichens seem to flee the cities, and those that one does encounter there are often only partially developed, in a sorediferous state or completely sterile . . . Lichens constitute a kind of very sensitive hygiometer."

PAHs accumulate in the algal layer of lichens, and once absorbed remain in this layer and not in the fungal hyphae. The PAHs cannot be washed off (Augusto et al. 2015).

On the other hand, sunburst lichen (*Xanthoria parietina*) is a nitrophile, meaning it thrives on the excess nitrogen in our cities' atmosphere, becoming more abundant. Of course, all lichens take up nitrogen from the air, and when they degrade, they release this nitrogen, which in nitrogen-poor soils acts to benefit plant growth.

Zonca (2023: 111) summarizes, "It is estimated that twenty-five to forty percent of lichens will disappear from the earth's surface in the next sixty-five years, due to climate change and increasing development."

Gray horsehair lichen (*Bryoria capillaris*) is known to the WSÁNEĆ (Saanich) of Vancouver Island as *hlk'am.aal kaj*. The species name derives from the Latin *capillus*, meaning "hair." It contains alectorialic and barbatolic acid.

"Both Swanton (1905a) and Newcombe (1901) refer to a plant called *skiida wasliia* and *gudgina wasliaa* ('a lichen') respectively . . . Swanton says that it was steamed with deer bones (apparently as a food)" (Turner 2004). It was burned into an ash to produce black paint for wood.

Imazalil is a fungicide used in clinical and agricultural settings. It is seriously toxic to vertebrates, including humans. A study by Turkez et al. (2014) found that water extracts of gray horsehair (*B. capillaris*) protect human lymphocytes from genetic damage, caused by the fungicide. A prophylactic, proprietary product to help protect farmers and ranchers who use the product would be useful.

Work by Tas et al. (2017) found extracts of *Bryoria capillaris* active against both gram-positive and gram-negative bacteria, with weak antiproliferative activity.

Black tree hair lichen, or edible horsehair lichen (*Bryoria fremontii*), is common on pine, larch, and Douglas fir trees in western North America. The species name is probably in honor of John C. Frémont (1813–1890), an early pioneer, botanist, and author. It is considered British Columbia's unofficial provincial lichen. The black spruce forests of northern Saskatchewan produce over 500 kilograms of this lichen per hectare.

Traditional Uses

As the name suggests, horsehair lichen is edible, and it was an important fire-pit food. It is said to taste like acorns. Indigenous people of Oregon call it *wa kamwa*. They would dry the lichen, grind it into a powder, and add this to soups. Youngsters were often sent up into the trees to throw down the lichen, or long poles were used to detach it. In a good location, five or six trees yielded enough harvest for one family for the year.

The lichen was baked with root vegetables in layers of skunk cabbage and sheets of bark. The fire pits were about ten square feet and two feet deep. After covering the layers of lichens, onions, camas, and other vegetation with sand, a fire was built over the top and allowed to burn down for twenty-four to forty-eight hours. Work by Crawford (2007) suggests the complex carbohydrates are mainly indigestible, but the lichen absorbs fructose from camas bulbs. When dried, the loaves from this process keep indefinitely.

When cooked alone this lichen was considered a tonic for the sick. The Salish (Flathead) of Montana used several names for the lichen, including *caumtemkan, st'telu, skolapkan, skolke,in? sqatlo*, and *sawtemqen* (Turney-High 1937; Stubbs 1966; Hart 1974).

The Ichishkiin Sínwit (Sahaptin), along the Columbia River between Oregon and Washington, boiled $k^{lw}inc$ as a poultice for arthritis (Hunn 1990).

In Montana, the Nimi'ipuu (meaning "we, the people") or Nez Perce (meaning "pierced nose") know this lichen as *ho.pop* or *hóopop*. When decocted, the broth from it was given to treat upset stomach, indigestion, and diarrhea (Hart 1976; Marshall 1977). (As a side note, although Nez Perce was the name given to this group by French-Canadian fur traders, a pierced nose was never their practice.)

The Nlaka'pamux (also known as the Thompson or Thompson River Salish) know black tree hair lichen as /wi?e, or *wi-uh*. The lichen was heated on rocks around a fire and applied to fresh wounds, after warts were cut off (Teft and Boas 1900; Turner et al. 1990). The Nlaka'pamux prepared a pudding with the lichen and various *Allium* species and berries, forming a black, chewy mass. "Now called 'black tree-lichen,' it is still being prepared by the *Nlaka'pamux* of south-central British Columbia (in modern ovens, these days) and served as a kind of taffy candy called *we'ia*, or *wíla*, with the texture and appearance, if not the flavor, of licorice" (Brodo et al. 2001).

When steam-pit cooked, a twenty-centimeter-thick layer of this mixture reduces after steaming to a thickness of four centimeters. Dried cakes of this were carried on long journeys. Pregnant women would not eat the lichen bread for fear of turning their babies a dark color.

The Tsilhqot'in or Chilcotin, "people of the river," living near Williams Lake, British Columbia, know *Bryoria* species as *texa* or *taxa*. They burned this lichen, along with their own hair, into ash, which was then rubbed into the scalp to stop hair from turning gray (Kay 1995; Turner 2004a).

The neighboring Okanagan (Sylix) call this lichen *skwelip*, or sqʷel'íp. They mixed it with wild berry juice and simmered the mixture into a syrup that was given to recently weaned babies (Gabriel and White 1954). The Okanagan would also cook it with false Solomon's seal rhizomes, while others would sweeten it with a unique sugar called trehalose, found on Douglas fir needles.

Bryoria species have been applied as a poultice to reduce swellings, either decocted or in dry form, by the Atsugewi of California (Garth 1953).

Trehalose exhibits benefit in diabetes and possibly in Huntington's disease (Rogers 2019). The sugar crosses the blood–brain barrier. Trehalose ameliorated diabetic cardiomyopathy in an in vivo study in mice (Liu et al. 2021). Evidence suggests it works via the PK2/PKR pathway. The rare sugar also promotes functional recovery in mice with spinal cord injury, via the suppression of ferroptosis, an oxidizing cell death iron-dependent pattern. In work by Gong et al. (2022), trehalose reduced the degeneration and iron accumulation of neurons, by inhibiting the production of ferroptosis and the molecules called reactive oxygen species (ROS). Survival of neurons and improved recovery of motor function were noted.

In a different approach, this lichen was dried, powdered, mixed with animal fat, and then rubbed into the belly button of a newborn to prevent infection (Turner et al. 1980).

Another name for the lichen is black moss, and the Okanagan (Sylix) have a story about how Coyote created it for food. As told by Mourning Dove (1933):

> Coyote tries to catch some swans for himself and his son to eat. The swans fool him by playing dead, and he catches them easily. He then ties his son to the "dead" swans (so that he won't stray) and climbs up a pine tree to get

the pitchy top to use as a fire drill so that he can cook the swans. But the swans suddenly come back to life and fly away with Coyote's son still tied to them. Witnessing this from high up in the tree, Coyote tries to climb down in order to save his son, but his long hair braid becomes entangled in the tree branches. In frustration, Coyote cuts off his hair braid and drops to the ground. He then transforms his hair into sqʷel'íp, saying, "you shall not be wasted, my valuable hair. After this you shall be gathered by the people. The old women will make you into food."

A similar story from the Shuswap (Secwépemc) involves Coyote being misled by a spider, with the same resultant entanglement and use of the lichen as food (Bouchard and Kennedy 1979): Spider saw Coyote hanging from a tree, and asked him why he tries to copy others, and said that he had been sliding on his web for a long time. Spider helped untangle Coyote and put him back on solid ground, noting that his fur hanging from the branches will become black tree moss and will be gathered by people to cook and eat.

The Coeur D'Alêne (Schitsu'umsh, meaning "those who were found here") people prepare this lichen as food and call it *skola'pken*. The interior Salish/Flathead group call it *wila*. The northern Secwépemc (Shuswap) name is *wi-luh*. It was gathered and mixed with mud to chink log cabins. Several Indigenous tribes of the province wove the fiber with other plant material, such as wolf willow, to make vests, pouches, shoes, and leggings.

By the way, northern flying squirrels use this lichen to make cozy nests.

Stuart Crawford wrote a thesis for his Master of Science degree called "Ethnolichenology of *Bryoria fremontii*" for the University of Lethbridge in 2001. It contains a wealth of information on the widespread use of this specific lichen.

Pale-footed horsehair lichen (*Bryoria fuscescens*) is widespread, from the northern tip of Alaska across to Newfoundland, and south to Arizona. The species is derived from the Latin *fucus*, meaning "gray brown" or "dusky." It contains fumarprotocetraric acid and atranorin. Work by Cobanoglu et al. (2010) found that extracts from pale-footed horsehair lichen inhibited all three bacterial strains on which they were tested.

Nemania is an endolichenic fungus that lives inside the thallus of pale-footed horsehair lichen (*Bryoria fuscescens*). Compounds isolated from *Nemania*, including radianspenes C-D and dahliane D, inhibit proliferation of lung cancer (H1975) cell line (Varli et al. 2022). This cell line was derived from a nonsmoking female with non-small-cell lung cancer.

Shiny horsehair lichen (*Bryoria glabra*) is mainly a West Coast species. It was gathered and burned into a black powder that was mixed with fat as a wood paint.

Horsehair lichen (*Bryoria trichodes*) is found on the West Coast in Alaska and southward, as well as around the Great Lakes. The Sugpiaq/Alutiiq of Alaska call it *nakuraartum nuyii*, or *napamungagua'i*. It was used in a similar manner to *Alectoria ochrolechia* to staunch bleeding wounds, or was piled on sick people in steam baths, to hold in the heat (Wennekens 1985). The Colville (Sinixt:Enselxcin) of eastern Washington mixed the dry lichen with animal grease and rubbed it into the navel of a newborn to prevent infection.

Horsehair lichen is common in central Saskatchewan and British Columbia, but is mainly found in northeastern North America. Indigenous people of the northern boreal forest heat horsehair lichens into a powder, to sprinkle on burns. The Nimi'ipuu (Nez Perce) used the lichen to treat diarrhea and indigestion. *Bryoria trichodes* ssp. *americana* is found on the Pacific Coast.

Medical Uses

Bryoria species extracts inhibit mixed lymphocyte reaction via the suppression of IL-2 receptor alpha chain expression in D8$^+$ T cells. This suggests potential development of an immunosuppressive compound for organ transplants (Hwang et al. 2017).

Barbatolic acid, isolated from *Bryoria capillaris*, is a promising anti-angiogenic and anti-migratory compound showing activity against HCC1428 and T-47D breast cancer cell lines. HCC1428 is a cisplatin-resistant BRCA2 mutated breast cancer adenocarcinoma cell (Varol 2018).

Horsehair lichen contains atranorin, and alectorialic, usnic, fumarprotocetraric, confumarprotocetraric, stictic, lobaric, gyrophoric, vulpinic, and barbatolic acids. Various fractions from this lichen were tested by Karagoz et al. (2018), who found barbatolic and alectorialic acids were effective antimicrobials in liquid, but not in solid, media.

Horsehair lichen also exhibits an antiproliferative effect on PC-3 (human prostate) cancer cell lines (Goncu et al. 2020).

Cyclosporin A, a drug that counters rejection among differing cells (as in transplants), was discovered from work with the asexual anamorph of the fungus *Cordyceps subsessilis* (*Tolypocladium inflatum*) in the 1970s. The initial soil samples containing this fungus were found in Wisconsin and Norway. In nature this organism had to compete with other molds, but instead of killing them, it made their hyphae branch repeatedly. Thus, instead of growing longer, the hyphae tied up the mold colonies into knots that could not spread.

Cyclosporin A has changed organ transplant viability by interrupting T cells before they can attack foreign tissue. Over time, however, cyclosporin injures the kidneys. Rogers (2020) reported that "The use of *C. sinensis* [*Ophiocordyceps sinensis*] with low doses of cyclosporine, shows benefit in kidney transplant patients, and less complications than drug alone. Levels of IL-2 were similar but the anti-inflammatory cytokine IL-10 was significantly higher in cordyceps group (Ding et al. 2011)." The immune suppression, however, makes patients more vulnerable to a pathogenic bacterium, *Aspergillus fumigatus*.

Spiny gray, or Nadvornik's horsehair lichen (*Bryoria nadvornikiana*) is found in variable spots. The species name honors the Czech lichenologist Josef Nádvornik (1906–1977). Several genera and species of lichens are named in remembrance of his work.

Spiny gray lichen ranges across the boreal forest on birch and conifers, as well

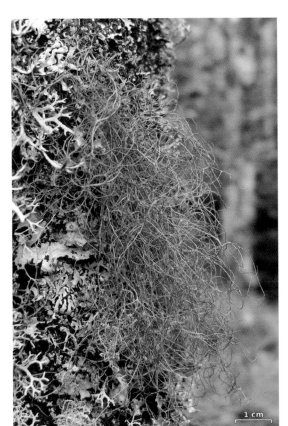

Bryoria nadvornikiana
(Spiny Gray, or Nadvornik's
Horsehair Lichen)

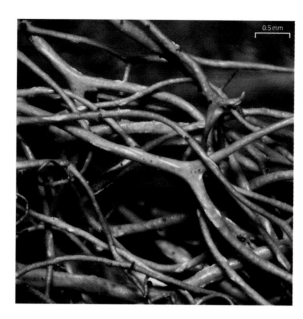

Bryoria tortuosa
(Yellow Twist
Horsehair Lichen)

as on rock cliffs, especially in humid areas with waterfalls and lakes. It contains atranorin, barbatolin, barbatolic, alectorialic and fumarprotocetraric acids, as well as 6-formyl-5,7-dihydroxyphthalide. It contains cystobasidiomycete yeasts, a relative rarity in lichens (Lendemer et al. 2019).

The inedible yellow twist horsehair lichen (*Bryoria tortuosa*) is found in British Columbia and south down the Pacific Coast, hanging from pine and oak trees. It contains vulpinic acid, a toxic substance also found in wolf lichen (*Letharia vulpina*). The difference in constituents may be due to a different symbiont, or algae. Tortuosa derives from *tortuoso*, meaning "twisting or winding." Indigenous peoples knew to avoid cosuming this *Bryoria* species.

BUELLIA
Button Lichens

There are approximately seventy-two button (*Buellia* sp.) lichens in North America. They contain various compounds, including norstictic acid, atranorin, and xanthones. They are found mostly on rock, but a few grow on wood, bark, or the ground, and they sometimes are parasitic on other lichens.

Seaside button lichen (*Buellia halonia*) is confined to coastal rocks in Southern California. It contains arthothelin and various xanthones.

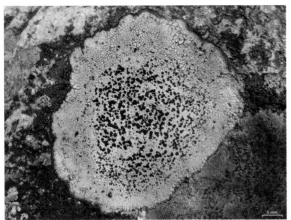

Buellia spuria

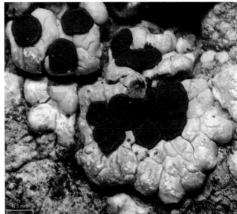

Buellia dispersa

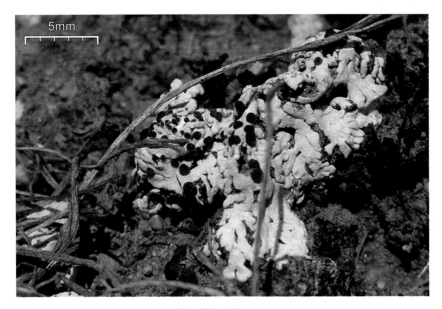

Buellia elegans

CALOPLACA

Firedot Lichens

Geographic Range: wide range from northern Alaska to Florida

Habitat: most grow on rocks or soil

Medicinal Applications: antifungal, antimicrobial, antioxidant, breast cancer, hyperglycemia, polio, prostate cancer

Notable Chemicals: chrysophanal and chrysophanol

Retiring lichen climbs the topmost stone, and 'mid the air ocean dwells alone.

ERASMUS DARWIN (1791)

Caloplaca species number around 133 in North America. The genus name derives from the Greek *kalos*, meaning "beautiful," and the Latin *placates*, "pleasing."

A new species was discovered in 2007 on Santa Rosa Island, California, and was named *Caloplaca obamae*, in honor of Barack Obama, a two-term U.S. president.

Jewel lichen (*Caloplaca biatorina*) is a bright orange species found on rocks, wood, even parasitizing other lichens. Work by Valadbeigi (2016) identified *Caloplaca biatorina*'s inhibitory activity for alpha-glucosidase. This enzyme hydrolyzes oligosaccharides and disaccharides into glucose, which is absorbed through the gut wall. Inhibition helps reduce blood plasma glucose and post-prandial hyperglycemia. Other work by Valadbeigi in the same paper examined this lichen's chemical composition, antimicrobial and antioxidant activity, and brine shrimp toxicity.

Gray-rimmed firedot lichen (*Caloplaca cerina*) is widespread throughout North America, except for the extreme South. Its bright yellow to orange dots

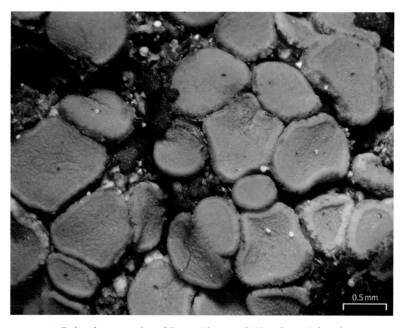

Caloplaca cerina (Gray-Rimmed Firedot Lichen)

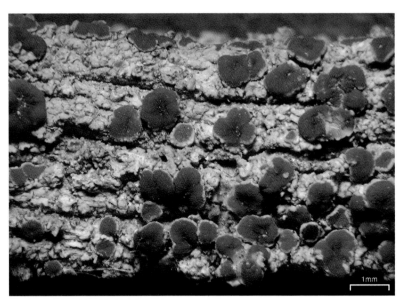

Caloplaca arizonica syn. *Gyalolechia epiphyta*

are common on the bark of poplar and elm trees. *Cerina* may derive from the Latin *serenus*, meaning calm, as in serene. This lichen contains parietin, possessing antifungal activity (Manojlovic et al. 2005).

An essence of *Caloplaca flavescens* syn. *Variospora flavescens* lichen helps to redefine the contact with the outside world, and promotes a healthy skin as described on an energy level as well. The essence is suggested for people who are too thin-skinned in their relationships, according to PHI Essences. *Flavescens* means "yellowish."

Firedot lichen (*Caloplaca pusilla* syn. *Calogaya pusilla*) is a granite rock lichen found in Europe and parts of the United States. *Pusillus* means "very small." This lichen, when grown on G-LBM medium, exhibits high potency in decreasing the viability of MCF-7 (human breast), PC-3 (prostate), and HeLa (cervical/epithelial) cancer cells. Increased concentrations induced apoptosis (Felczykowska et al. 2017).

Caloplaca rheinigera contains chrysophanal and chrysophanol (chyrosophanic acid). Chrysophanol is unique anthraquinone with anticancer, hepatoprotective, neuroprotective, anti-inflammatory, anti-ulcer, and antimicrobial properties (Prateeksha et al. 2019). It blocks the proliferation of SNU-C5 colon cancer cell lines, but not the proliferation of other more common lines, including SW480, HCT116, and HT29. When chrysophanol was combined with the MTOR inhibitor rapamycin, cell proliferation was greatly decreased (Lee et al. 2011).

Chrysophanic acid reduced testosterone-induced benign prostatic hyperplasia in a rodent study, by suppressing 5-alpha-reductase and extracellular signal-regulated kinase (Youn et al. 2017). The description of candleflame lichen, in the following, offers more on 5-alpha-reductase benefits. The compound inhibits the replication of poliovirus types 2 and 3 in vitro (Semple et al. 2001).

The related *Caloplaca obesimarginata* and *C. kamczatica* of the Pacific Northwest contain methyl parietinate.

Caloplaca saxicola has been identified by Edwards et al. (2003a) as a possible surface or subsurface potential form of life on Mars. They also identified *Acarospora chlorophana* (syn. *Pleopsidium chlorophanum*) and *Xanthoria elegans* as other possible biomarkers. The species name *Saxicola* may derive from the Latin *saxum* "rock" and *inola*, meaning "dwelling in."

CANDELARIA
Candleflame Lichen

Candleflame lichen (*Candelaria concolor* syn. *Teloschistes concolor* var. *effusa*) is widespread on nutrient-rich substrates throughout western Canada and most of the United States. The common name and genus derive from the Latin *candela*, referring to the color of wax used in earlier times. *Concolor* alludes to having the same color.

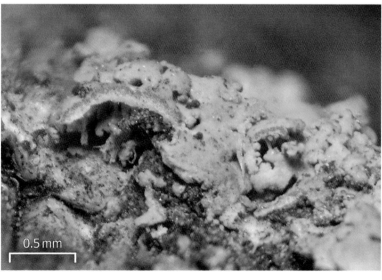

0.5 mm

Candelaria concolor (Candleflame Lichen)

This lichen produces colonies on rain tracks of tree bark or branches. It contains the yellow compound calycin, which has shown activity against the main protease of the SARS coronavirus (Joshi et al. 2021). Candleflame lichen also contains callopismic acid (ethylpulvic acid), stictaurin (dipulvic) acid, barbatic acid, dipulvic dilactone, tetronic acid derivatives, vulpinic acid, and 5-chloroatranorin. It also contains physcion (parietin), which provides a bright orange color.

In addition to its color, physcion is a novel inhibitor of 5-alpha-reductase that promotes hair growth in vitro and in vivo, improves hair follicle morphology, and increases follicle count (Lao et al. 2022).

CANDELARIELLA

Egg Yolk Lichen   Goldspeck Lichen

Geographic Range: wide range in North America from high arctic to Arizona

Habitat: hardwoods, bark

Practical Uses: yellow dye

Medicinal Applications: cancer, sunscreen, tumors

Notable Chemicals: calycin, methanol, and physodic acid

It is somewhat of a lichen day. The bright-yellow sulfur lichens . . . look novel, as if I had not seen them for a long time. Do they not require cold as much as moisture to enliven them?

HENRY DAVID THOREAU

The genus *Candelariella* has 22 species.

Powdery goldspeck lichen (*Candelariella efflorescens*) is a very common yellow lichen found on various hardwoods. It is tiny, but tenacious. Along with *Parmelia, Xanthoria*, and *Melanelia* species, it will often be found in corticolous communities on trees in eastern North America. It contains calycin.

Methanol extracts (80%) of common goldspeck or egg yolk lichen (*Candelariella vitellina*; vitelline is the membrane that separates the egg yolk from the albumen) exhibit increased invasion of tumor cells in vivo and increased apoptosis potential. No cytotoxicity to normal human peripheral lymphocytes was noted (El-Garawani et al. 2019).

An extract of *Candelariella vitellina* ameliorated mitomycin toxicity by reducing the apoptotic cells and normalizing cell cycle phases. It ameliorated the diminished mitotic index and DNA single-strand breaks caused by a chemotherapy drug. In vivo work with female Swiss albino mice showed the same pattern of anticancer activity but was dependent on p53 expression.

The lichen extract showed low cytotoxicity toward normal human lymphocytes but exhibited antioxidant and antihelminthic potential (El-Garawani et al. 2020).

Rotavirus is a major viral pathogen that causes diarrhea in young children and infants, worldwide. Each year, over 450,000 children, younger than five years old, die due to this virus. Work by Elkhateeb et al. (2020) found methanol extracts of this lichen showed in vitro inhibition of rotavirus. The same study found cytotoxicity against human colon (HCT116) cancer cells, the third most common cancer and fourth most common cause of mortality.

Calycin, the yellow pigment that *Candelariella vitellina* exudes for sun protection, was formerly used for dyes. The lichen also contains physodic and physodalic acids.

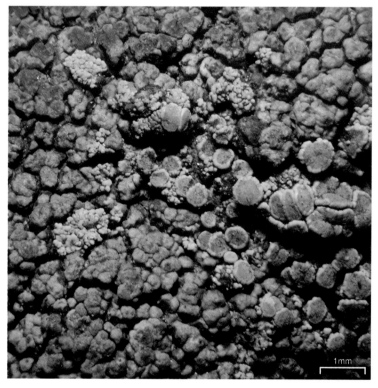

Candelariella vitellina
(Common Goldspeck or Egg Yolk Lichen)

CANOPARMELIA
Shield Lichens

Geographic Range: Southeastern United States

Habitat: tree bark of conifers and hardwoods

Medicinal Applications: antihelmintic, breast cancer

Notable Chemicals: divaricatic and perlatolic acids

Canoparmelia has only 7 species.

Carolina shield lichen (*Canoparmelia caroliniana* syn. *Pseudoparmelia caroliniana*) is confined to hardwood and coniferous bark in the southeastern United States. It contains perlatolic acid, which is highly cytotoxic to MCF-7 (breast) cancer cells, and is less aggressive but still active against HepG2 (hepatocarcinoma) cell lines (Garrido-Huéscar et al. 2022).

Both Carolina and Texas shield lichens are cyanobacteria deprived, but contain nitrogen-fixing bacteria that belong to the gamma-proteobacteria group.

Work by Liba et al. (2006) with shield lichen found the release of amino acids, phytohormones, 3-indoleacetic acid, and 64% solubilized phosphates and 30% ethylene.

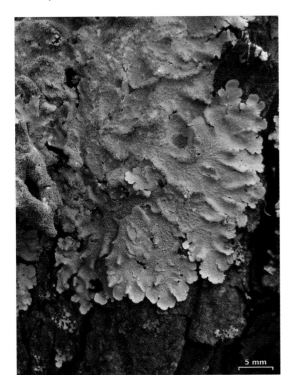

Canoparmelia caroliniana
(Carolina Shield Lichen)

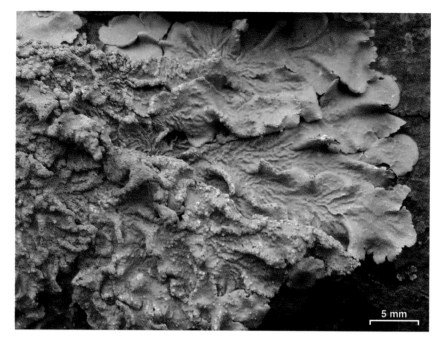

Canoparmelia texana (Texas Shield Lichen)

Texas shield lichen (*Canoparmelia texana* syn. *Pseudoparmelia texana*) is rare in Texas, but plentiful in parts of the southeastern United States. It grows on hardwood and conifer bark and is rich in divaricatic acid and 3ß-acetoxyhopane-1ß,22-diol.

Work by Silva et al. (2021) evaluated the in vitro effect of divaricatic acid, which is found in Texas shield lichen, on *Schistosoma mansoni* worms, and on snails, an intermediate host. Extensive damage to the organisms was observed, such as peeling, erosion, bubbles, edema, damage and loss of tubercles and spines, fissures, and tissue ruptures. No cytotoxicity of this acid was noted, however, in human peripheral blood mononuclear cells.

This blood fluke lives in mesenteric veins near the intestine and is the leading cause of schistosomiasis in tropical regions of Africa, the Middle East, the Caribbean, and northern South America. It is carried in fresh water, initially in snails (*Biomphalaria glabrata*), and is transmitted to humans. The World Health Organization (WHO) estimates some 236 million people were affected by the disease in 2021. The drug praziquantel is on the WHO List of Essential Medicines, with risk/benefit status described. This drug is the most effective at this point, but new approaches are needed to prevent drug-resistance.

CETRARIA

Curled Shield Lichen   Iceland Lichen

Curled Snow Lichen   Spiny Heath Lichen

Geographic Range: Northern United States, Canada

Habitat: among heath plants, in alpine meadows and higher elevations

Practical Use: food

Medicinal Applications: antibacterial, cancer, cough, gastrointestinal diseases, heart attacks, lung disease, mucus, nausea, neurodegenerative conditions, vaginal irritation, type 1 diabetes

Notable Chemicals: allomelanin; and cetraric, fumarprotocetraric, gyrophoric, lichenesterinic, lichenostearic, norstictic acid, protocetraric, protolichesterinic, allo-protolichesterinic, and usnic acids

Warnings: contraindicated for excess mucus, fever, ulcers

A woman's love, like lichens upon a rock, will still grow wherever charity can find no soil to nurture itself.

CHRISTIAN NESTEEL BOVEE

There are nine *Cetraria* species in North America.

Medical Uses

Work by Yarli et al. (2023) identified the endolichenic fungus *Jackrogersella* sp. EL001672 from a *Cetraria* lichen. This led to the isolation of 1'-O-methyl-averantin in culture. Both the extract and isolated compound showed cyto-toxic effects against colorectal (CRC) cancer cell lines, by regulating the Sonic Hedgehog and Notch signaling pathways. Note that colorectal cancer is the sec-ond most diagnosed disease in men and women, with a lifetime risk of over 4%.

Spiny heath lichen (*Cetraria aculeata* syn. *Coelocaulon aculeatum*) grows among heath genus plants in the high arctic and in elevated alpine meadows south to Colorado. It contains norstictic and protolichesterinic acids. Extracts of this lichen were found to strongly inhibit *Escherichia coli* WP2 strain, and Ames *Salmonella* strains TA1535 and TA1537. Antimutagenic and antioxidant activity is thought responsible for this inhibition (Ceker et al. 2018). An acetone extract showed significant antigenotoxic activity against *Salmonella typhimurium*, but no cytotoxicity against mammalian cancer cells (Zeytinoglu et al. 2008).

Early work by Türk et al. (2003) found this lichen and protolichesterinic acid to exhibit activity against *Escherichia coli, Staphylococcus aureus, Aeromonas hydrophila, Proteus vulgaris, Streptococcus faecalis, Bacillus cereus, B. subtilis, Pseudomonas aeruginosa*, and *Listeria monocytogenes* bacteria. Drug-resistant *Aeromonas hydrophila* is a gram-negative, opportunistic aquatic pathogen. It causes significant problems in fish farming, and is also found in meat, dairy, and vegetables (Stratev and Odeyemi 2016).

Curled snow lichen (*Flavocetraria cucullata* syn. *Cetraria cucullata*), formerly classified in the *Cetraria* genus, was one of fourteen species tested by Urena-Vacas et al. (2022) for possible health benefit. The lichen contains protolichesterinic acid and usnic acid. This lichen was found to be one of the best inhibitors of acetylcholinesterase and butyryl-cholinesterase, suggestive of benefit in neurodegenerative conditions. It also contains the unusual compound bisnovcristazarin.

The formation of beta-amyloid plaque in the brain and the prevention or dissolving of this fatty tissue that prevents neuron firing have occupied the attention of pharmaceutical companies for decades. More than 300 drugs have been developed and trialed against this plaque with little success. One Japanese study cut open the beta-amyloid plaques and in 70% of them found the herpes simplex virus! Leaky gut and leaky brain allow transport across the blood–brain barrier of this virus and numerous other pathogens (Rogers 2019). Therefore, the following effects have been noted with interest. The brain responds to this invasion by using fats to incapsulate the virus to prevent further damage.

Curled snow lichen exhibits antibacterial activity against *Bacillus subtilis, B. mycoides, Sarcina lutea, Streptococcus pneumoniae, S. pyogenes, S. viridans, Staphylococcus aureus*, and *S. albus* (hemolytic) (Burkholder and Evans 1945).

The snow-bed Iceland lichen (*Cetraria delisei* syn. *Cetrariella delisei*) contains hiascic acid and gyrophoric acid. This lichen exhibited 82% inhibition of aromatase at 40 µg/mL. Aromatase inhibition is known to help prevent or reduce the overgrowth of hormone-sensitive cancer cell lines.

Iceland lichen (*Cetraria ericetorum*) is found from Yukon to Newfoundland, and along the Rocky Mountains to Arizona at higher elevations. It does not contain fumarocetraric acid, but instead, lichenesterinic acid and allo-protolichesterinic acid.

The related *Cetraria halei* syn. *Tuckermannopsis americana* contains alectoronic acid.

True Iceland lichen, also known as Iceland moss (*Cetraria islandica*),

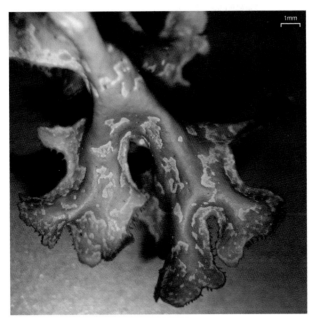

Cetraria islandica ssp. *islandica* (Iceland Moss)

and related species have been used as food and medicine for centuries. On a visit to Iceland a few years ago, I found the lichen available in every supermarket. There it is known as *fjallagros*. One of the first written laws of the country, in 1280 CE, banned the picking of this lichen on someone else's land.

Cetraria islandica is best collected in summer, when green and fully grown. An average yield of 700 kilograms (1540 pounds) per acre of air-dried lichen can be expected if solidly covered. It takes about forty kilograms of lichen to produce one kilogram of antibiotic material.

This lichen is symbolic of health and is associated with the birth date of January 16. Other lichens, such as *Cladonia* and *Ramalina*, symbolize dejection, and relate to the date of January 14.

Traditional Uses
Both shield lichen (*Cetraria crispa/C. ericetorum*) and curled shield lichen were traditionally used by Inuit as a fish or duck soup condiment (Wilson 1978).

The Dehcho of the Northwest Territories drank decoctions of this true Iceland lichen to treat tuberculosis. They would boil it until it turned red, and take one-third cup warm, three times daily (Lamont 1977).

The Chipewyan (Denesuline) call it *tsanju* and used it for both food and medicine. The Yup'ik in Alaska use this lichen, or related *Cetraria laevigata*, for flavor and thickening soups.

Historical Uses

Iceland moss lichen is sweet, cool, nutritive, and demulcent, and is of benefit in dry, irritated conditions of the digestive and respiratory systems. This includes peptic ulcers, hiatus hernia, and esophageal reflux, as well as unproductive, irritating coughs, croup, and pneumonia.

One of my favorite Eclectic physicians, Dr. John King, wrote his first dispensatory in 1870, and this was released as *King's American Dispensatory* by Harvey Wickes Felter and John Uri Lloyd in 1898.

Dr. King wrote that this lichen is "used as a demulcent in chronic catarrhs, chronic dysentery, and diarrhoea, and as a tonic in dyspepsia, convalescence, and exhausting diseases. Boiled with milk it forms an excellent nutritive and tonic in phthisis and general debility. It relieves the cough of chronic bronchitis." Its soothing demulcent properties make it useful for vaginal irritation, as a mild, cooled, and strained douche.

In 1840s Europe, this lichen was listed in fifty pharmacopeias or dispensatories.

Modern Uses

A recent review of Iceland moss by Sanchez et al. (2022) covers all aspects, including phytochemistry, traditional uses, and new pharmacological possibilities. Lichenins (water-soluble polysaccharides) comprise over 50% of this lichen's weight (lichenin 30–40%, isolichenin 10%).

The German Commission E approved Iceland moss to treat irritation of the oral and pharyngeal mucous membranes and accompanying dry cough, with loss of appetite. In an open trial, 100 patients with pharyngitis, laryngitis, or bronchial ailments were treated with lozenges containing 160 mg of an aqueous extract of Iceland moss. The results were determined to be positive in 86 cases, with good gastric tolerance and lack of side effects (European Scientific Cooperative, 2003).

A clinical trial involving sixty-one patients after nose surgery, with dryness and inflammation, was conducted by Kempe et al. (1997). They were given lozenges, and after five days their symptoms showed significant improvement.

Anna Rósa Róbertsdóttir (2016) is Iceland's preeminent herbalist and a good friend. She notes that *Cetraria islandica* contains both bitter and mucilage properties, somewhat rare in herbs. The mucilage soothes and protects, while the bitterness stimulates and strengthens digestion. *Helicobacter pylori*, for example, is a leading cause of gastritis and ulcers, and these ailments are reduced by drinking decoctions of the lichen. Protolichesterinic acid and aliphatic alpha-methylene-gamma-lactone were found by Ingólfsdóttir et al. (1997) to exhibit in vitro inhibition of *Helicobacter pylori*.

This lichen clears damp heat, due to the bitter protocetraric, cetraric, lichesterinic, and lichenostearic acids. In addition, lichenin shows activity against leukemia cell lines (Marquez 2019).

Brian Kie Weissbuch (2014) used this lichen in a formula for AIDS patients with *Mycobacterium avium intracellular* (MAI) complex. This close relative of *M. tuberculosis* is opportunistic in immune-compromised patients and is now seen in those without HIV or cancer. This pathogen was found in a majority of showerheads tested (Feazel et al. 2009).

The depsidone fumarprotocetraric acid (FUM) is a major secondary metabolite of this lichen. Work by Fernández-Moriano et al. (2017) induced oxidative stress (H_2O_2) and cytotoxicity on neurons and astrocyte cell (SH-SY5Y and U373-MG) lines. When FUM was used as pretreatment, the oxidative stress and cytotoxicity were met with significantly enhanced cell viability. FUM also had a protective role against oxidative damage in mitochondrial membrane, and it diminished apoptosis. This suggests FUM as a potential candidate for oxidative-stress-related diseases, including neurodegenerative disorders.

Water extracts of *Cetraria islandica* upregulate IL-10 and IL-12p40 in an arthritic rat study, suggesting anti-inflammatory activity (Freysdottir et al. 2008). Other extracts of this lichen also have effects: Protolichesterinic acid, when isolated from an ether extract, exhibits antiproliferative activity on several cancer cell lines, including breast (Bessadóttir et al. 2014). Protolichesterinic acid, isolated from the same lichen, shows significant activity against the protozoal parasite *Trypanosoma brucei brucei*. Carried by the tsetse fly in sub-Saharan Africa, the parasite is a leading cause of livestock infection. This variety rarely transmits to humans, but two related variants cause sleeping sickness, a condition recognized in Egypt for several millennia (Igoli et al. 2014).

The extract component protolichesterinic acid is cytotoxic against T-47D and ZR-75-1 (breast) and K-562 (erythro-leukemia) cancer cell lines, an effect possibly related to 5-lipoxygenase inhibition (Ogmundsdóttir et al. 1998).

The lichen also contains a melanin compound, allomelanin. Work by Malo et al. (2022) on mice models suggests allomelanin may be an easily sourced, cost-effective countermeasure to accidental radiation exposure. The compound suppresses tumor cell growth in vitro and in vivo and is cytotoxic to HCt-15 (colorectal) cancer cell lines by blockage of the S phase (Kamei et al. 1997).

Water extracts of *Cetraria islandica* may be useful for early intervention in risk reduction of type 1 diabetes, based on a study of normal and diabetic rats (Colak et al. 2016). Also, this lichen contains traces of iodine, making it useful to support thyroid health. Taken as a cooled decoction, the lichen helps increase breast milk production. In Switzerland, this lichen is an additive in luncheon meats and pastries.

In homeopathy, Iceland moss is used for acute and chronic bronchitis, asthma, and chest pain while coughing. The dose is 10–20 drops of tincture as needed. The mother tincture is prepared from the dried lichen at 1:10 in 40% alcohol.

Iceland moss may aggravate gastric or duodenal ulcers and is contraindicated in cases of excessive catarrh or mucus congestion. It works well for dry, hot, irritated coughs. Do not use during fever states. It may relieve night sweats, but should be taken during the day.

In the opinion of Dr. Gordon Ross (1970), both *Cetraria islandica* and the homeopathic Sticta Pulmonaria (based on *Sticta* lichens) "should be thought of in cystic fibrosis of children." He suggests to think of it in cases of diverticulitis, because one of the characteristic *Cetraria* symptoms was "chronic diarrhea with slimy taste in the mouth" which are "the usual symptoms of diverticulitis" (see *Lobaria pulmonaria*, pages 132–38).

Striped Iceland lichen (*Cetraria laevigata*) ranges from Alaska to Newfoundland and south to northeastern North America. The Yup'ik of Alaska used the dried lichen to thicken and flavor soups. (*Yuk* means "person," and *pik* "real," hence "real person.")

Polysaccharides from this lichen may inhibit the growth of sarcoma 180, Ehrlich ascitic tumor, and cervical carcinoma (U14) in mice. The reticuloendothelial system phagocytic function was increased with its application (Wang et al. 1991). The striped Iceland lichen contains graciliformin, a weak cytotoxin acting against human lung (A549) carcinoma, as well as fumarprotocetraric, protolichesterinic, and lichesterinic acids.

CETRELIA

Sea Storm Lichens

Geographic Range: eastern North America from Nova Scotia to
Great Lakes and south to Appalachia

Habitat: wood and rocks in shaded humid forest

Medicinal Applications: preventing cancer cell migration, inhibits MRSA

Notable Chemicals: alectoronic, alpha-collatolic mbricaric, olivetoric,
and perlatolic acids; atranorin, lecanorine, orcinol depsides

Sea storm lichen (*Cetrelia monachorum*) is found around the Appalachian Range
and Great Lakes region. The species name derives from the Latin, meaning "of
the monks." The term *Icoa* or *Joca monachorum* means "monk's pastimes" or
"monk's jokes." Oh, the frivolity in the monastery! The Old Testament was a
favored source of riddle popularity, with rib-ticklers such as "Who died but was
not born?" Why, Adam of course.

Which reminds me of a joke that is not very popular with my wife, or polit-
ically correct, as follows: Adam was all alone in the Garden of Eden and asked
God for a companion. "Please send me someone to care for, love, and share our
lives together," he pleaded. God thought for a moment and then replied that
this would cost him an arm or a leg. To which Adam responded, "What could
you give me for a rib?" Not sure the monks would have enjoyed it either.

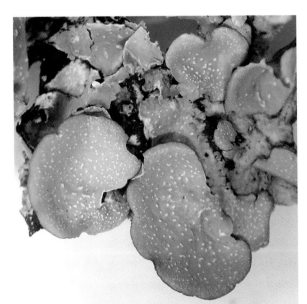

Cetrelia monachorum
(Sea Storm Lichen)

This also led to the best known, and world's shortest sentence palindrome, *Madam, I'm Adam.*

Sea storm lichen contains the secondary metabolite imbricaric acid, which reduces inflammation (Oettl et al. 2013). The related *Cetrelia alaskana* syn. *Cetraria alaskana* grows on tundra on the west coast of Alaska and contains imbricaric acid.

This lichen also contains perlatolic acid, which appears to inhibit acetylcholinesterase, suggestive of benefit in neurological and brain-related dysfunction (Reddy et al. 2016). *Cetrelia chicitae* syn. *Cetraria chicitae* also contains perlatolic acid, as does the related *Cetrelia cetrarioides*. Perlatolic acid inhibits methicillin-resistant *Staphylococcus aureus* (MRSA) and appears synergistic with gentamicin, but antagonistic with levofloxacin (Bellio et al. 2015).

In the United States, the Centers for Disease Control and Prevention (CDC) estimated 108,000 cases and nearly 20,000 deaths from MRSA in 2006. The worldwide death rate from MRSA in 2019 rose to 100,000 patients. MRSA has killed more people than HIV every year since 2006, often attacking young, healthy babies and adults.

One sea storm lichen, *Cetrelia olivetorum*, is found on wood and rocks in shaded forest from the Great Lakes to Nova Scotia and south to northern Georgia (Ceker et al. 2018).

Sea storm lichen also contains olivetoric acid, which displays potent anti-angiogenic activity, suggesting possible benefit in preventing cancer cell migration (Koparai et al. 2010).

CHAENOTHECA
Stubble Lichens

There are sixteen species of stubble lichens in North America.

Brown-head stubble lichen (*Chaenotheca brunneola*) is found on wet or rotten wood. It contains baeomycesic and squamatic acid.

Sulfur stubble lichen (*Chaenotheca furfuracea* syn. *Coniocybe furfuracea*) is found on tree stumps in shaded woods. It contains vulpinic acid.

Polypore stubble or pin lichen (*Chaenotheca obscura* syn. *Calicium obscurum*) is a very small lichen, less than 1/8" (4mm) high, growing on violet-pored bracket fungus (*Trichaptum abietinum*) in the boreal forest. Its sexual

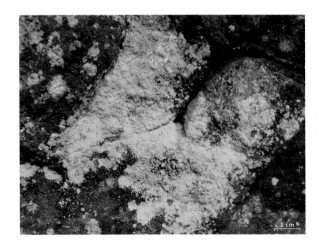

Chaenotheca furfuracea
(Sulfur Stubble Lichen)

ascospores rest in a cup-shaped exciple on a tiny stalk, looking like a dress-maker's pin (mazaedium).

The polypore lichen was utilized by the Thompson (Nlaka'pamux) of British Columbia, who called it owl wood, or *kalulaa'iuk*. The ascospore powder was used as a rub to give strength to young men. The lichen is overlooked by many people, but not by an intrepid lichen enthusiast such as Lawrence Millman.

CHRYSOTHRIX

Gold Dust Lichen   Sulfur Dust Lichen

Gold dust lichen (*Chrysothrix candelaris* syn. *Lepraria candelaris* syn. *L. flava*) contains the yellow pigment calycin, as well as pinastric acid, leprapinic acid,

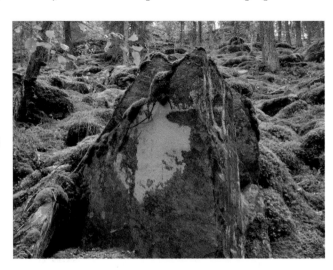

Chrysothrix chlorina

and leprapinic acid methyl ether. There may or not be vulpinic acid present. Its sister sulfur dust lichen (*Chrysothrix chlorina*) contains both vulpinic acid and calycin. These are mainly found on shaded rocks, not trees.

CIRCINARIA
Crustose Lichen

Crustose lichen *Circinaria calcarea* (syn. *Aspicilia calcarea*) grows on dolomite or carbonate-rich rocks. The biodeterioration of rocks by this lichen produces only calcium oxalate monohydrate (whewellite). Other genera, such as *Dirina*, on the other hand, produce calcium oxalate dihydrate (weddellite) (Edwards et al. 2003). The former is named in honor of Cambridge professor William Whewell (1794–1866).

Both oxalates are common in oxalate kidney stones found in humans and dogs. French and English juvenile bulldogs are more prone to urolithiasis than other breeds (Saver et al. 2021). Dogs with whewellite (WH) stones are significantly older than dogs with weddellite (WE) stones.

Breeds more prone to whewellite stones are the Norwich terrier, keeshond, Norfolk terrier, fox terrier, and sheltie, while weddellite stones are more common in the Pomeranian, borzoi, Japanese spitz, Finnish lapphund, and bichon frise (Hesse et al. 2018).

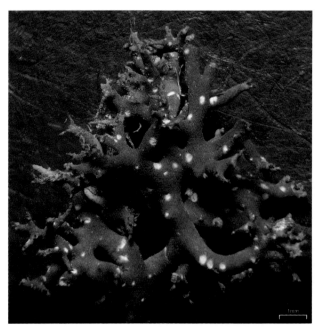

Circinaria hispida

Relatedly, the fungal sclerotia chaga (*Inonotus obliquus*) has become faddish as a coffee substitute. Kidney disease, stones, and even death have been implicated in cases of chronic consumption.

CLADINA

Geographic Range: the arctic, mainly northern North America

Habitat: grass, rocks, thin acidic soil, moss, heath

Practical Use: food

Medicinal Applications: respiratory disease, tuberculosis, drug-resistant bacteria, antiviral, lung damage

Notable Chemicals: norrangiformic, rangiformic, and usnic acids

In early taxonomy there was considerable confusion between the *Cladina* and *Cladonia* genera. Thus, unspecified *Cladina* species were widely used by Indigenous people of Alaska.

Work by Smith (1973) reported hunters chewed the lichen when climbing hills to maintain their wind. In this context, air pollution and particulates are a serious health concern, especially in terms of respiratory disease and lung damage.

Caribou benefit from eating lichen, processed with lichenase, an enzyme found in their rumen. Snail livers also contain lichenase. Unfortunately, the caribou also concentrate strontium and cesium in lichens into their fat and meat. Climate change is affecting the arctic snow, causing ice formation on the surface and restricting access to the buried reindeer lichen, for both caribou and people.

Shrubby or northern reindeer lichen (*Cladina/Cladonia arbuscula*) is rare in the Pacific Northwest and the American Southwest, but plentiful in arctic regions and on the eastern side of the North America continent. This lichen was recently named the unofficial provincial lichen of Newfoundland. *Arbuscula* derives from the Latin meaning "tree-like shrub." Unlikely but interesting is a connection to *Arbuscula*, a first-century BCE woman and pantomine actor in Rome. Cicero mentions her giving him much pleasure.

Cladina/Cladonia arbuscula contains (+)-usnic acid, which inhibited the growth and proliferation of breast (T47D) and pancreatic (Capan-2) cancer cell lines (Einarsdóttir et al. 2010).

Northern reindeer lichen (*Cladina arbuscula*) exhibits activity against *Mycobacterium tuberculosis* (Gordien et al. 2009). It is used in China for the same purpose, and is known as *lin shi ruî*, "forest stone bud."

Green reindeer lichen (*Cladina mitis*) is sometimes confused, even among lichenologists, with northern reindeer lichen (already described). They are often found growing together on grass, rocks, thin soil, moss, and heath. It contains usnic, norrangiformic and rangiformic acid. *Mitis* derives from the Latin, meaning "mild." This lichen shows activity against *Staphylococcus aureus* and *Bacillus subtilis*. Early work by Burkholder and Evans (1945) found activity against *Staphylococcus aureus, Diplococcus pneumoniae, Streptococcus hemolyticus, S. viridans, Bacillus mycoides,* and *Sarcina lutea. Streptococcus viridans* is implicated in 40% of acute adult heart valve endocarditis, and on rare occasions causes meningitis. Relatedly, Viridans Group Streptococci Shock Syndrome is uncommon, but has a high mortality rate in children with relapsed acute lymphoblastic leukemia.

A study by Grudzinska et al. (2022) tested acetone extracts for their usnic acid content, and then tested their activity on three melanoma cell lines. No relationship was found between usnic acid content and activity of extracts. Rather low anti-tyrosinase activity was noted. More study is required before the lichen extracts could be used as an adjuvant external treatment for skin melanoma.

Green reindeer lichen essence is used for transmutation, according to Findhorn Flower Essences.

Traditional Uses

The Den'ina call it *k'udyi* and decocted the lichen for diarrhea (Kari 1987). Known by the Sugpiaq/Aleut as *kinadam aiyukax*, the lichen was used as a tea for chest pain (Bank 1953). It was also reported that a "liquor" prepared from the lichen was drunk for colds (McKenna 1959).

Various Indigenous peoples have used this lichen for colds, fever, arthritis (both internal and external), jaundice, constipation, convulsions, coughs, and tuberculosis. The Anishinabee (Ojibwe/Chippewa) of Minnesota and Wisconsin call this lichen *asa' gunink*. It was boiled and the water was used to wash a newborn baby (Smith 1932).

In Quebec, the Whapmagoostui Cree use two names for this lichen, *whapskukmuk* and *epshatuk*. Work by Fraser (2006) recorded its use by residents to treat inflammation associated with diabetes. The tribal name Whapmagoostui means "place of the beluga," describing a community on Great Whale River in northern Quebec.

Cladina lichen is said to taste like sweet bran. When boiled for an hour and then fried, it was said to be like eating cornflakes. The Woods Cree of Saskatchewan call it *wapis-kastaskamih*, or *atikomiciwin*. The Aleut (Sugpiaq/Alutiiq) of Alaska drank infusions for chest pain, while the Tanaina (Dena'ina) boiled and consumed it for diarrhea. The Northern Tutchone of Yukon boiled it for medicine.

The Gwich'in reside in an area that straddles the Yukon and Northwest Territories. They refer to reindeer lichen as *Uhdeezhù'* or *Uudeezhu'*, meaning "white moss." The lichen makes a stimulating tea that is good for stomach and chest pain. Lazarus Sittichininli notes in *Gwich'in Ethnobotany* by Andre and Fehr (2001) "that if you eat animals that eat willow, like moose, you will get hungry more quickly than eating animals that eat lichen, like caribou." Children were not allowed to play on the lichen. Drinking the boiled tea has been considered good for stomach and chest pains. Annie Norbert, the elder mentioned in *Gwich'in Ethnobotany*, said that men used to drink this tea before going to the mountains because it helped them keep their wind for walking and climbing.

Northern hemisphere Indigenous people have also used reindeer lichen in tea to treat colds, arthritis, and fever (Perez-Llano 1944). In another approach, this lichen was separated from grass in rumen contents and stirred with oil. The word *teniyash* (increase) was repeated while stirring, to help the mixture rise and become light.

This lichen produces a clear, colorless jelly, whereas black-footed reindeer lichen (*Cladina stygia*) gives a pinkish jelly.

Star-tipped reindeer lichen (*Cladina stellaris*) is a yellow-green ground-cover over large areas of northern Canada. As the name suggests, it is a major source of nutrition for caribou. The lichen was recently proclaimed Canada's unofficial national lichen. The Nihithawak or Saāwithiniwak of east-central Saskatchewan know it as *wäpiskastastkamihk* or *atikömïciwin*. Either it was decocted, or the dried powder was added to water in order to expel intestinal parasites (Leighton 1985).

The contents of the caribou rumen, which the Chipewyan (Denesuline) call *ebúrti*, was boiled using heated rocks in the cut-out rumen or large intestine, with added fat, meat, and blood. They know the lichen itself as *tsanju*. *Ebíe hechélh*, or caribou bowel soup, was easily digestible due to initial fermentation. Other lichens, plants, and berries may also be present.

When separated from grass in caribou stomachs, star-tipped reindeer lichen was stirred with fish oil by the Aleut people of Alaska. The word *teniyash*, meaning "increase," was sung while doing so, to make the mixture light.

Historical Uses

True reindeer lichen (*Cladina rangiferina* syn. *Cladonia rangiferina*) has been used for more than five centuries for respiratory conditions. It is slow-growing, averaging 3–4 mm per year. After grazing by caribou, it requires up to fifteen years to recover. And since each caribou eats about three kilograms daily, a large herd can require a vast rangeland. It is Quebec's unofficial lichen.

Cooke (1893) wrote, "But after swallowing it there remained in the throat, and upon the palate, a gentle heat or sense of burning, as if a small quantity of pepper had been mixed with the lichen . . . Cooling and juicy as it was to the palate, it nevertheless warmed the stomach when swallowed, and cannot fail of

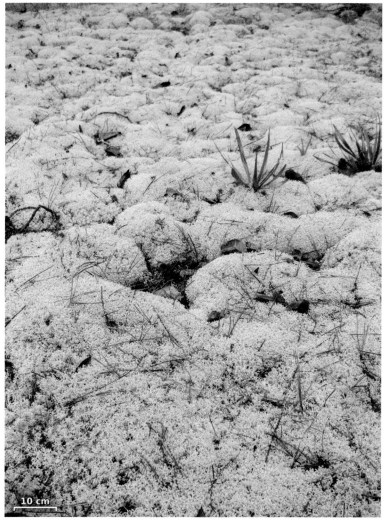

Cladina rangiferina (True Reindeer Lichen)

proving a gratifying article of food to man or beast during the dry winter of the frigid zone."

Modern Uses

Work by Bustinza (1952) and Ingólfsdóttir et al. (1985) identified activity by this lichen against *Staphylococcus aureus*, *Bacillus subtilis*, and *Candida albicans*. Water-soluble polysaccharides showed antitumor activity (Nishikawa et al. 1974). Methanol extracts exhibited tyrosine inhibition and activity against various gram-positive bacteria, including *Bacillus subtilis*, *Propionibacterium acnes*, and *Staphylococcus aureus* (Yamamoto et al. 1998).

Hanagokenols A and B and other previously identified compounds show activity against MRSA (methicillin-resistant *Staphylococcus aureus*) and against vancomycin-resistant *Enterococci* species (Yoshikawa et al. 2008). Relatedly, a hot-water extract of alpha-glucan polysaccharides shows antioxidative benefit and protects alveolar epithelial cells from lead-induced injury to A549 lung cells (Huang et al. 2018).

An ethanol extract proved useful in treatment of alcohol-induced hepatoxicity and oxidative stress in lab animals. Depsidone may be the compound most responsible for the antioxidant, anti-inflammatory, and antiapoptotic activities (Shukla et al. 2020). Another study found an extract may be more effective on chronic inflammation rather than on acute inflammation (Süleyman et al. 2002). Methanol extracts of this lichen exert significant antiproliferative effects and induce apoptosis on MCF-7 (breast) cancer cell lines (Coskun et al. 2015).

This lichen exhibits antiviral activity. Work by Kurskaya et al. (2022) found an extract significantly reduced the infectivity of the influenza H3N2 virus, in vitro. The related so-called swine flu virus (H1N1) was responsible for the pandemic of 1968. The honey mushroom (*Armillaria luteo-virens*) also showed antiviral activity in the same study.

A homeopathic proving of *Cladina rangiferina* was conducted by Misha Norland in 2002. A complete synopsis of the proving is found in Vermeulen (2007, 688–698). Here are a few of the themes: brittle and small, anxiety and anticipation, feeling of being used, duped, or trapped; dirt and bathing, cleaning and organizing; fragmentation, scattered and disorganized, issues around money and material value; jealousy, suspicion, and curiosity; and prevalent dreams of crime, evil, guns, murder, war, fights, and robbery. Also, headaches and sinus issues are prominent.

Mushroom Essences: Vibrational Healing from the Kingdom Fungi (Rogers 2016) introduces the vibrational benefits of 48 mushrooms and lichen essences. Flower essences, such as the Bach flower remedies, are produced in sunlight, bringing light to areas of darkness, whereas mushroom essences are produced under lunar influence and relate to our shadow side. They are popular in Jungian psychology, examining the parts of ourselves that many humans do not wish to explore, but rather suppress. True reindeer lichen, or reindeer moss, is for those individuals feeling coerced or beginning to take on the personas of those around them. They are easily swayed by the opinions of others. Stuttering may be helped (pp. 218–221).

Reindeer lichen contains significant amounts of vitamin D (87 μg/100 g) (Benedik, 2022). This vitamin is extremely important everywhere, but especially in the far north, where the sun may not make much of an appearance for 4–5 months. Reindeer lichen contains ergosterol, common to many fungi. In the presence of ultraviolet (UV) radiation, ergosterol is converted to D2. Ergosterol enhances the activity of antibiotics (Andrade et al. 2018). The PubMed search engine lists more than 6,000 studies on this compound.

As already mentioned, the Gwich'in of the Mackenzie River delta know this lichen as white moss or *uhdeezhù*. The boiled tea was good for stomach and chest pain. It was also boiled for an hour or more and then fried into a crispy treat. When removed from the caribou rumen it is known as *it'rik*. It is said that the best *it'rik* is from caribou shot early in the morning before it has begun to eat.

This lichen can also be mixed with dog food or grass from muskrat push-ups to rid dogs of tapeworms (Andre and Fehr, 2001). What is a muskrat push-up, you may ask? In order for muskrat to have a hole kept open in the ice, it would fill the opening with frozen vegetation to ensure an easier escape from the water. Muskrat or rat root (*Acorus calamus* and *Acorus americanus*) is a favorite food, and the "meat" retains a hot, spicy flavor. This is used to make a soup or is added to other meat to tenderize it or add flavor. Sometimes the muskrat meat was hung for a week to age, then mixed with fat, marrow, and berries.

The Inuit/Inuk of Nunavut collect *nirnait* lichen and prepare a broth for sickness and eye infections. It is decocted until the liquid turns black (Black et al. 2008). The Inuktitut word *inuit*, as mentioned earlier, means "human being" or "the people."

Early work by Gordien et al. (2009) identified activity of this lichen against *Mycobacterium tuberculosis*.

CLADONIA

Cup Lichen

Deformed Cladonia

Dragon Lichen

Felt Cladonia

Fishnet Cladonia

Lung Cladonia

Many-Forked Cladonia

Olive Cladonia Lichen

Organ Pipe Lichen

Peg Lichen

Pixie Cup Lichen

Powder-Foot British Soldiers Lichen

Reindeer Lichen

Reindeer Moss Lichen

Slender Ladder Lichen

Smooth or Black-Foot Cladonia Lichen

Soldiers Lichen

Split-peg Lichen

Thorn Cladonia Lichen

Trumpet Lichen

Wand Lichen

Geographic Range: United States and Canada

Habitat: on soil and rocks in sun, rotting wood

Practical Use: dye

Medicinal Applications: cancer, central nervous system pathologies, cough, digestive enzyme dysregulation, eye disease, inflammation, insect bites, labor induction, lung carcinoma, melanoma, sores, staph, strep throat, whooping cough

Notable Chemicals: atranorin; and baeomycesic, divaricatic, fumarprotocetraric, gyrophoric, lecanoric, lobaric, perlatolic, protocetraric, psoromic, squamatic, siphulellic, and usnic acids; zeorin

Cladonia species number about 128 in North America. Over the years *Cladina* and *Cladonia* species have been taxonomically confused, and this issue persists today.

Carbonero et al. (2002) more than twenty years ago isolated *Cladonia* and *Cladina* polysaccharide structure and found no difference. She suggested the DNA studies support the idea that *Cladina* be reduced to a synonym under *Cladonia*. Good idea!

Cladonia species have been found to photosynthesize at –24°C. Zonca (2023) reminds us of the artwork of Escher, the famous Dutch lithographer: In *Waterfall* (1961) are found several large *Cladonia* on the bottom left, alongside a foliose lichen.

It is a lichen day. Not a bit of rotten wood lies on the dead leaves, but it is covered with fresh, green cup lichens . . . All the world seems a great lichen.

HENRY DAVID THOREAU

Toy soldiers lichen (*Cladonia bellidiflora*) is so named for its prominent red fruiting pods. *Bellido* derives from the Spanish, meaning "handsome," with *flora*, meaning "flower." Technically this lichen does not flower, but the bright red apothecia makes it appear to be flowering.

The Tlingit of Alaska mix the powdered lichen with breast milk to treat eye disease (Garibaldi 1999). The Indigenous people of Haida Gwaii dipped the red tips of this lichen in breast milk for a similar purpose (Turner 2004). The Indigenous name may be *xil tl'a.āang* (Newcombe 1897).

Boreal pixie cup lichen (*Cladonia borealis*) is widespread throughout most of Canada and is found in elevated regions of the Rocky Mountains, south to Colorado. It grows in full sun on soil and rocks, and contains usnic, barbatic and 4-O-demethylbarbatic acids. An extract of this lichen inhibited all five bacterial species tested (Micheletti et al. 2021).

Fishnet Cladonia (*Cladonia boryi*) contains the red pigment boryquinone and usnic acid. Crowning pixie cup lichen (*Cladonia carneola*) contains zeorin, and usnic and barbatic acids. Granite thorn (*Cladonia caroliniana* syn. *Pycnothelia cladinoides*), as the name suggests, is found on granite rocks in Appalachia. It contains usnic acid and traces of squamatic acid.

Fuzzy reindeer lichen (*Cladonia confusa*) and four other lichens were tested

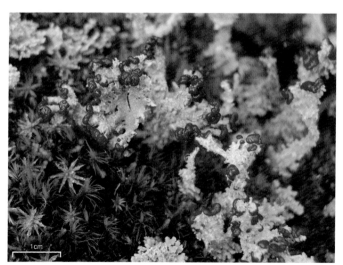

Cladonia bellidiflora (Toy Soldiers Lichen)

for cytotoxicity against UACC-62 melanoma cell lines. Protocetraric acid was highly selective and may be best suited, as both divaricatic and perlatolic acids were also cytotoxic to normal fibroblast 3T3 cells (Brandão et al. 2013).

Mealy pixie cup lichen (*Cladonia chlorophaea*) is widespread, from Alaska to Florida, on wood, bark, rocks, and soil in full to partial sun. Mealy pixie cup lichen was decocted as a wash for indolent sores by the Okanagan (Syilx) of British Columbia. It is known as *pen'pen'emekxisxn'*, which means "liver on rock" (Turner et al. 1980). This lichen was used as a traditional cough remedy in Europe, usually boiled in milk. In Wales, it was boiled in milk for whooping cough and known as *cwpanau pas*.

Recent work by Torres-Benítez et al. (2022a) looked at the antioxidant and anti-inflammatory properties of this lichen. Inhibition of both cholinesterase enzymes (acetylcholinesterase and butyrylcholinesterase) and digestive enzymes (alpha-glucosidase and pancreatic lipase) was noted. These authors suggest *Cladonia* species show promise in the treatment of central nervous system pathologies, inflammatory disorders, and digestive enzyme dysregulation.

Mealy pixie cup lichen was found active against *Staphylococcus albus*, *Diplococcus pneumoniae* (*Streptococcus pneumoniae*), *Bacillus subtilis*, *B. mycoides*, and *Sarcina lutea* in early work (Burkholder and Evans 1945). This matters because *Streptococcus pneumoniae* is the leading cause of community-spread pneumonia, and of meningitis in children and the elderly. This bacterium is also complicit in various pneumococcal infections including bronchitis, rhinitis, acute sinusitis, otitis media, sepsis, osteomyelitis, endocarditis, cellulitis, and peritonitis. Atromentin from this lichen, and also isolated from various macrofungi such as *Hydnellum peckii*, inhibits the enzyme necessary for production of fatty acids by the bacterium. Mealy pixie cup also contains hyperhomosekikaic acid.

Madame's cup lichen is common in North America. It was listed in the 1846 *Pharmacopoeia Universalis* as an important medicinal (Vartia 1973). Elf cup or madame's cup (*Cladonia coccifera*) lichen essence is helpful in issues around liberation, according to Findhorn Flower Essences.

Organ pipe lichen (*Cladonia crispata*) is widespread from Alaska and throughout all of Canada, and in the east extending down into the Mid-Atlantic states. It is found on soil and rocks in open areas, frequently in or near bogs. This lichen is a pioneer species growing after forest fires. It contains squamatic and thamnolic acids. Water-soluble polysaccharides found in this lichen show antitumor activity (Nishikawa et al. 1974).

British soldiers lichen (*Cladonia cristatella*) is an Eastern species, following the Canadian Shield from northern Saskatchewan to Newfoundland and down the East Coast to Florida. *Cristatella* means "crested." In the 1970s, Vernon Ahmadjian separated the fungal and algae parts of this lichen, and then cultured them and induced them to reconnect. This lichen contains usnic, didymic, barbatic, and rhodocladonic acids, as well as cristazarin and 6-methylcristazarin. The related *Cladonia cryptochlorophea* contains cryptochlorophaeic acid.

Ahmadjian also cultured and explored the widespread red-fruited pixie cup lichen (*Cladonia pleurota*) and thorn Cladonia lichen (*Cladonia uncialis*).

Work by Jeong et al. (2021) investigated cristazarin in *Cladonia* species. The cancer cell lines AGS (gastric), CT26 (colon), and B16F1 (melanoma) were found to be sensitive to cristazarin.

Deformed cladonia (*Cladonia deformis*) contains graciliformin, an iron-rich compound that exhibits weak inhibition of human lung (A549) carcinoma. This lichen also contains usnic acid and zeorin. The lichen is used in Finland traditional medicine for tuberculosis and coughs.

Southern soldiers lichens (*Cladonia didyma*) are restricted to the northeastern and southeastern United States, and west to Indiana and Texas. There are two variations, *didyma* and *volanica*. The former is richer in barbatic acid, while the latter contains barbatic, didymic, isodidymic, and thamnolic acids. Both prefer living on sandy soil or rotting wood.

Finger pixie cup lichen (*Cladonia digitata*) is found from Alaska south to northern Idaho, as well as from northern Ontario east to Newfoundland and south to Appalachia. It grows mainly on rotten logs, or among the mossy bases of trees. It contains the secondary metabolites bellidiflorin, thamnolic acid, and decarboxythamnolic acid and the red pigment rhodocladonic acid.

Powder puff lichen, also known as deer moss or reindeer moss lichen (*Cladonia evansii* syn. *Cladina evansii*), is restricted to the extreme southeastern United States, usually on sandy soils. This species is named in honor of lichenologist Alexander William Evans (1868–1959), who specialized in *Cladonia* species.

Lecythophora sp. FL1031 is an endolichenic fungus found living within this lichen. Oxaspirol B, found in this fungus, as well as in the endolichenic fungus in *Parmotrema tinctorum*, shows moderate p97 ATPase (enzymes that catalyze the hydrolysis of adenosine triphosphate) inhibition. Work by Wijeratne et al. (2016) found this compound was a reversible non-ATP competitive and specific inhibitor of p97. This work should be followed up, as p97 or

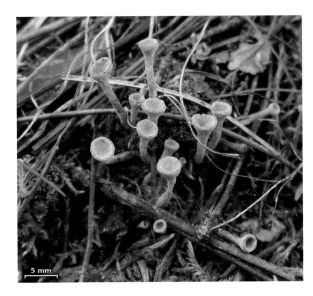

Cladonia fimbriata
(Trumpet Lichen)

valosin-containing protein ATPase inhibitors play a role in three human neuron diseases: Paget's disease of the bone, frontotemporal dementia, and familial amyotrophic lateral sclerosis (ALS) (Wang et al. 2022).

Trumpet lichen (*Cladonia fimbriata* syn. *Cladonia major* syn. *Scyphophorus fimbriatus*) is found on soil or rotting wood throughout Canada and northern states. *Fimbriatus* is from the Latin, meaning "fibrous" or "fringed." Work by Goncu et al. (2020) found this lichen had no antiproliferative effect on PC-3 (human prostate) cancer cell lines. It contains atranoric, fimbriatic, and fumaroprotocetraric acids, as well as carotenoids, which led to its former use as a red dye for wool.

Ethanol extracts of trumpet lichen exhibit activity against *Bacillus subtilis*, *Candida albicans*, and *Trichophyton mentagrophyte*s, and cytotoxicity against murine leukemia cells and slow-growing BS-C-1 cells (African green monkey kidney, ATCC CCL 26) (Perry et al. 1999).

Gritty British soldiers lichen (*Cladonia floerkeana*) is found on rocks and rotten logs from Newfoundland, around the Great Lakes, and south to northern Florida. It contains barbatic, usnic, didymic, rhodocladonic, and condidymic acids.

Many-forked Cladonia (*Cladonia furcata* syn. *Cladonia sub-rangiformis*) is found on the Pacific Coast from Alaska to California, on the Atlantic Coast from Newfoundland to Georgia, and inland to the Great Lakes and south. The branched or forked lichen is found in shaded forests. Work by Rankovic et al. (2011) found extracts of many-forked Cladonia to be active against

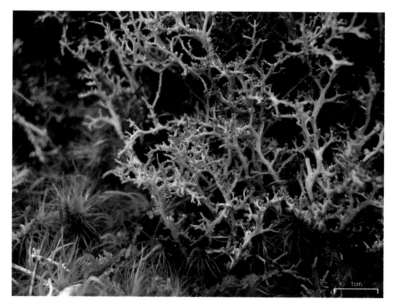

Cladonia furcata
(Many-Forked Cladonia)

bacteria and to have strong anticancer activity against both FemX (human melanoma) and LS174 (human colon) cell lines. Later, Rankovic (2018) looked at five *Cladonia* lichens and their biological compounds. The highest cytotoxic effect on HeLa (cervical/epithelial) cell lines was observed from this lichen.

Water-soluble polysaccharides derived from many-forked Cladonia induced apoptosis in human leukemia (K562) cancer cell lines (Lin et al. 2001). Methanol extract also exhibited cancer chemopropreventative and cytotoxic activity (Ingólfsdóttir et al. 2000)

A few years later, Lin et al. (2003) took a deeper look at these polysaccharides. Their induction of apoptosis in HL-60 and K562 (leukemia) cancer cells was accompanied by a decreased telomerase activity, compared to untreated control cells.

Smooth or black-foot Cladonia lichen (*Cladonia gracilis*) is found as four subspecies. The first subspecies *elongata*, formerly subspecies *nigripes,* and another subspecies *vulnerata* are found in the boreal arctic. *Cladonia gracilis* subsp. *gracilis* is found in eastern North America. It contains graciliformin.

This lichen shows a significant effect on estrogen formation, due to containing the enzyme sulfatase (Rogers 2011). Sulfatase regulates the formation of estrone, suggesting this lichen be avoided by women with hormone-dependent breast cancer.

When dried and mixed with ash, this lichen produces a green dye for wool.

Gray's pixie cup lichen (*Cladonia grayi*) contains grayanic acid (orcinol depsidone), first identified in 1963. It also contains the secondary metabolites 4-O-demethylgrayanic acid, colensoic acid, confumarprotocetraric acid, divaronic acid, fumarprotocetraric acid, protocetraric acid, 4-O-demethylgrayanic acid, and stenosporonic acid. The grayanic acid shows a beautiful white-mauve color under UV light.

Humble pixie cup lichen (*Cladonia humilis*) is widespread throughout North America. When originating from the Sonoran Desert it contains atranorin, while one specimen in Arizona yields bourgeanic acid (fatty acid). Monoacetylgraciliformin is also present. An in vivo study examined the antidiabetic effects of a humble pixie cup lichen extract (Zhang et al. 2012). An extract of the cultured tissue and natural thalli exhibits superoxide dismutase (SOD) content, exhibiting antioxidant potential (Yamamoto et al. 1998).

Powder-foot British soldiers lichen (*Cladonia incrassata*) is found on well-rotted logs and stumps, from the Great Lakes and New England, south to northern Florida. This lichen contains (–)-usnic acid, didymic acid, condidymic acid, squamatic acid, thamnolic acid, and prasinic acid. The first three compounds exhibit activity against *Staphylococcus aureus* (Dieu et al. 2014). Prasinic acid exhibits moderate activity against various cancer cell lines (Chakor et al. 2012).

Lipstick powderhorn or pin lichen (*Cladonia macilenta*) is widespread on old wood, soil, and rocks. It comes in two forms: one containing thamnolic acid, and the other, rich in barbatic acid, which is known as *Cladonia macilenta* var. *bacillaris*. An acetylcholinesterase (AChE) inhibitor, biruloquinone, was extracted from this lichen. It was found to be a mixed-II inhibitor of acetylcholinesterase (AChE), and it improved the viability of PC12 cells injured by hydrogen peroxide and beta-amyloid, due to its potent antioxidant activity (Luo et al. 2013).

Cladonia merochlorophaea contains merochlorphaeic acid, 4-O-methylcryptchlorophaeic acid, 4-O-methylnorcryptochlorophaeic acid, and submerochlorophaeic acid.

Reptilian pixie cup lichen (*Cladonia metacorallifera* syn. *C. straminea*) is found in both the arctic and Antarctica. It contains orsellinic acid, ethyl 4-carboxyorsellinate, psoromic acid isomer, and succinprotocetraric, siphulellic, connorstictic, cryptostictic, lecanoric, lobaric, gyrophoric rhodocladonic, thamnolic, usnic, squamatic, and didymic acids, and fumarprotocetraric acid derivatives. When it was cultured in 1% fructose, both cristazarin and 6-methylcristazarin were produced. In turn, cristazarin shows activity against

AGS (gastric), CT26 (colorectal), and B16F1 (melanoma) cancer cell lines (Jeong et al. 2021a).

Nancy Turner (2004) mentions a reindeer lichen (*Cladonia pacifica*) identified on Haida Gwaii called *k'al.aa skusaang.u*, literally meaning "muskeg (special)-roots." This may be *Cladonia portentosa* subsp. *pacifica*.

Perforate reindeer lichen (*Cladonia perforata*) is an endangered species in Florida and was declared as such by the United States in 1993. When rarely found, it is on open sandy soil. The Red List of Threatened Species now exceeds one thousand, many of them fungi.

Felt Cladonia (*Cladonia phyllophora*) is widespread on soil, from Alaska down the Rocky Mountains to Colorado, and from Labrador to the eastern United States. It contains fumarprotocetraric and confumarprotocetraric acids.

Lung Cladonia (*Cladonia pleurota*) contains iso-usnic acid.

Rosette or carpet pixie cup lichen (*Cladonia pocillum*) extracts increased apoptosis in MCF-7 (breast) cancer cells (Ersoz et al. 2017). Antimicrobial and antifungal activity was noted from various extracts. The lichen is widespread on thin, lime-containing soil over rocks.

Peg lichen (*Cladonia polycarpoides* syn. *C. subcariosa*) is widespread from the Great Lakes to the southeastern United States and parts of the Midwest. It is usually found on sandy soil in open areas. It contains norstictic acid and homoheveadride.

Cream cup lichen (*Cladonia portentosa*) acetone extracts exhibit antifungal activity against *Botrytis cinerea*, *Colletotrichum lindemuthianum*, *Fusarium solani*, *Pythium ultimum*, *Phytophthora infestans*, *Rhizoctonia solani*, *Stagonospora nodorum*, and *Ustilago maydis* (Halama and Van Haluwin 2004).

The latter fungus is responsible for the creation of huitlacoche, a delicious corn smut. It starts its life as a saprobic yeast in the ground and then infects the leaves, turning into hyphae that enter the corn silk and kernels. In Mexico, it has been "cultivated" since the time of Aztecs. Huitlacoche is rich in the essential amino acid lysine, adding a smoky, unami-like flavor to tacos. The fresh product is amazing, and the canned form just okay. The Zuni of Arizona gave the fungus to pregnant women to hasten their delivery by making labor more severe and robust. After birthing, it was given to stop hemorrhage or any abnormal lochial discharge, ensuring the placenta was totally discharged. A pinch of ustilago powder was infused in warm or cold water and taken as required (Vogel 1970).

The homeopathic *Ustilago maydis* relieves several menstrual issues involving ovarian pain, excessive bleeding between periods, or a cervix that bleeds

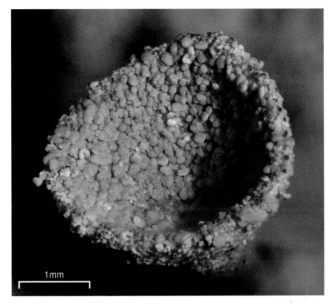

Cladonia pyxidata (Pebbled Cup or Chin Cup Lichen)

1mm

easily. It may bring relief to men with an obsessive need to masturbate. *Ustilago*, in fact, means "burning."

Pebbled cup or chin cup lichen (*Cladonia pyxidata*) has been used traditionally for its demulcent, antitussive, and expectorant properties in treating bronchitis, tuberculosis, and whooping cough. The name "chin cup" derives from its use in whooping cough or chin cough, as it was then known. *Pyxidata* derives from the Latin *pyxis,* meaning "a box." This lichen was mentioned in the *Pharmacopoeia Universalis* of 1846 (Vartia 1973).

Cladonia pyxidata contains atranorin, and fumaroprotocetraric, barbatic, parellic, protofumarcetraric, and psoromic acids. It is rich in minerals, mucilage, and the enzyme emulsin. The latter compound is present in almonds. Early work by Burkholder and Evans (1945) found Brown pixie cup lichen exhibited activity against *Staphylococcus aureus* and *Bacillus subtilis.*

Work by Thuan et al. (2022) found that usnic acid and fumaroprotocetraric acid, isolated from the lichen, effectively inhibited *Mycobacterium tuberculosis* H37Ra and six multiple-drug-resistant strains. This is significant because the increased resistance to standard antibiotic treatment is a growing concern for those who are infected, and for overall community health. The WHO estimated 450,000 cases of drug-resistant disease in 2021, resulting in over 190,000 deaths.

An interesting double-blind, randomized study of beta-oligosaccharides derived from *Cladonia* species was conducted by Kershengolts et al. (2015) on type two diabetic patients. One hundred patients received one capsule three times daily of the extract for three months, while fifty patients received a placebo. At three months, blood glucose was reduced and glycosylated hemoglobin was reduced (from 9.8–11.4% to 7.6%). Low-density lipoprotein (LDL) also fell by 1.3% across six months.

Homeopathy is a form of medicine based on a principle of "similar cures similar." What produces symptoms in material doses, relieves them when taken in small amounts. Biomedicine constantly denigrates its effectiveness, but in twenty years of clinical practice I empirically saw significant benefits from homeopathy for my clients.

A small homeopathic treatment proving of nine people (three male, six female) was conducted in 1994 by Izzie Azgad and Rosalind Floyd with 6c and 30c potencies of pebbled cup lichen. Symptoms that resulted included a hurried feeling, being anxious and nervous, bursting headache, stomach and intestinal gas, disorientation, and uncertainty. Dryness of tongue, lips, throat, and shin was also noted. Energy was low among these people, with a desire for open air, with breathing difficult in hot rooms. The symptoms appeared on the right side of body and then moved to the left (Vermeulen 2007).

Slender ladder lichen (*Cladonia rappii*) is found on acidic soil along the east coast of North America, south to northern Florida, and along the Gulf Coast. It contains psoromic acid and rappiidic acid (*o*-orsellinic acid derivative). In free radical scavenging tests, it showed twice as much power as resveratrol but was less efficient than (+)-usnic acid (Lage et al. 2016).

Wand lichen (*Cladonia rei*) is found on wood and soil, ranging from Alaska to the Mid-Atlantic states. Work by Valadbeigi and Shaddel (2016) found that this lichen inhibits alpha-amylase, involved in the breakdown of starch in the digestive system. This inhibition reduces serum blood sugar levels.

Cladonia rangiformis lichen extracts show strong cytotoxicity toward MCF-7 breast cancer cell lines (Acikgöz et al. 2013). This lichen contains atranorin, and usnic and fumarprotocetraric acids. Earlier work by Bézivin et al. (2003) found in vitro cytotoxicity against murine and human cell cultures. The bacterium *Escherichia coli* was found particularly sensitive to both water and methanol extracts of this lichen (Rafika and Monia 2018).

Dragon funnel or dragon Cladonia lichen (*Cladonia squamosa* syn. *C. squamosa* var. *subsquamosa*) is widespread throughout forested areas of northern, western, and eastern North America. It contains either squamatic or thamnolic acid.

Dixie reindeer lichen (*Cladina/Cladonia subtenuis*) is confined to the southeastern quadrant of the United States, from Florida up to the Great Lakes. The Keetoowah (Tsalaqi, Cherokee) of North Carolina applied the wet, chewed lichen to insect stings, sometimes combined with tobacco (Garrett 2003). (The name "Cherokee" may derive from the Creek word "people of different speech.")

Olive Cladonia lichen (*Cladonia strepsilis*) is found from Newfoundland south along the East Coast, and around the Great Lakes south to Louisiana, usually on dry, exposed soils, but is also found in Ozark glades. It contains baeomycesic, squamatic, barbatic, and subdidymic acids and strepsilin.

Greater sulfur cup lichen (*Cladonia sulphurina* syn. *C. gonecha*) is widespread. It is the tallest of the yellow, sorediate, red-capped cup lichens. It contains usnic and squamatic acids. Very common in North America, it has been declared endangered in Iceland.

Split-peg or greater thatch soldiers lichen (*Cladonia symphycarpa*) is common in open areas on thin and sandy soil, especially in limestone (calcium-rich) areas. It is widespread from Alaska to Labrador and south to the Great Lakes and beyond. It may contain atranorin, as well as norstictic and, perhaps, psoromic acids. The lichen *Diploschistes muscorum* often starts its life as a parasite on split-peg lichen and then develops an independent lichen thallus (Wedin et al. 2016).

The endogenous fungus, *Diaporthe mahothocarpus*, living within Split-peg has been studied for medicinal benefit. Work by Jeong et al. (2021) found various compounds in this fungus to be potent and selective inhibitors of human monoamine oxidase A (hMAO-A). These are alternariol, 5'-hydroxy-alternariol, and mycoepoxydiene. They are reversible competitive inhibitors of hMAO-A, with better binding than for hMAO-B. They are highly absorbable through the gastrointestinal tract, without violating the therapeutic concept called Lipinski's rule of five. Only mycoepoxydiene showed a high probability of crossing the blood–brain barrier. This work suggests possible benefit in neuropsychiatric disorders including depression and possibly in cardiovascular disease.

Lipinski's rule of five is also known as Pfizer's rule of five. It describes molecular properties important to pharmacokinetics in the human body, including absorption, distribution, metabolism, and excretion. It does not, however, determine whether a compound is active. Only about 50% of new molecules taken orally obey this odd rule, including natural products.

However, Greta Thunburg, the Swedish environmental activist, reminds us that we can no longer save the world by playing by the rules.

Thorn Cladonia lichen (*Cladonia uncialis*) is active against several bacteria already mentioned in this section, as well as against several *Streptococcus* species, including *Streptococcus pyogenes* and *Streptococcus viridans*. More than 700 million people acquire group A *Streptococcus* infections annually. Generally, *Streptococcus* creates pharyngitis (strep throat) or impetigo, which has a characteristic strawberry-like rash. In about 650,000 people the bacterium creates severe health issues, with about 25% mortality. Work by Ceker et al. (2018) identified antimutagenic and antioxidant potency against *Escherichia coli* and *Salmonella* strains (see the earlier description of *Cetraria aculeata*, p. 45).

Water and methanol extracts of thorn Cladonia lichen possess antioxidant activity and do not negatively affect human peripheral lymphocytes. The phenolic compounds found in this lichen, as well as in leather lichen (*Dermatocarpon miniatum*) and crottle (*Parmelia saxatilis*), may be of interest for food, natural supplements, and pharmaceutical application (Emsen and Kolukisa 2020).

Thorn Cladonia lichen (*Cladonia uncialis*) extracts and isolated usnic acid were tested against various clinical strains of bacteria. The extract, containing (–)-usnic acid and squamatic acid, was more active than usnic acid alone in its pure form. *Staphylococcus epidermidis* and *Enterococcus faecium* showed similar inhibition by usnic acid, but no activity was demonstrated against fungal strains (Studzinska-Sroka et al. 2019).

This lichen extract activity is significant because drug-resistant strains of *Enterococci* are becoming problematic. In hospital settings, both *E. faecium*

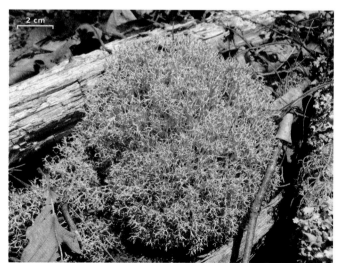

Cladonia uncialis (Thorn Cladonia Lichen)

and *E. faecalis* spread through central lines, urinary catheters, and ventilators. The former is less common (5–10%) than the latter (85–90%), because it is more virulent. The problem begins when broad-spectrum antibiotics are used and the normal enterococci population, which helps control *Escherichia coli*, is eliminated. This causes a decrease in the thickness of the gastrointestinal mucosa, leading to further problems. Enterococcal infections are the third most common hospital-acquired infections, with a mortality rate of 25–50%. The bacterium is becoming more alcohol tolerant, suggesting a need for different disinfecting protocols.

Earlier work by Studzinska-Sroka et al. (2015) examined various solvents and found thorn Cladonia methanol extracts exhibited the strongest activity against *Staphylococcus aureus* (SA) and methicillin-resistant SA (MRSA). No activity against *Escherichia coli* and *Candida albicans* was observed.

Huovinen and Ahti (1986) examined the contents of forty-two species of *Cladonia* for chemistry and aromatic substances. Usnic acid was present in all, averaging about 3.0% of dry weight. Other medullary substances are the beta-orcinol depsides barbatic acid (0.5%), squamatic acid (2.3%), and thamnolic acid (1.2%).

A *Streptomyces* species associated with thorn Cladonia lichen contains the unique compound uncialamycin (Parrot et al. 2016). Uncialamycin exhibits potent activity against gram-positive and gram-negative bacteria, including *Burkholderia cepacian*, which is a major cause of concern and mortality in patients with cystic fibrosis (Davies et al. 2005). A patent for this use has been applied for and granted (U.S. Patent # 10,233,192 B2) to Rice University for uncialamycin's antitumor activity (March 19, 2019).

The same *Streptomyces uncialis* also produces the alkaloids cladoniamides A–G, which show cytotoxicity against MCF-7 (breast) cancer cell lines (Williams et al. 2008). Synthesis of cladoniamide G was later accomplished by Loosely et al. (2013).

Cladonia verticillaris, ladder lichen, is somewhat rare, or, more accurately, newly identified in North America. It has been found in the Targhee National Forest in Wyoming, and in Blue Ridge Mountains of North Carolina. It contains fumarprotocetraric acid. A mice study by de Barros Alves et al. (2014) found oral administration of an extract of this lichen produced expectorant and antioxidant activity in lung tissue. At eight days after application, fumarprotocetraric acid shows 100% termiticidal activity against worker termites (Martins et al. 2018).

COCCOCARPIA
Salted Shell Lichen

Salted shell lichen (*Coccocarpia palmicola* syn. *Pannaria molybdaea* var. *cronia*) is widespread in parts of North America but is Red Listed as vulnerable in Wisconsin, Minnesota, and a few other regions. Extracts of this lichen show cytotoxicity against murine leukemia cells and slow-growing BS-C-1 cells (Perry et al. 1999).

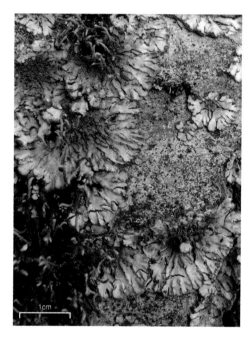

Coccocarpia palmicola
(Salted Shell Lichen)

COLLEMA
Fingered Jelly Lichen

Collema was once a larger genus in North America, with about thirty-five species. Over the past twenty years, they have been reclassified down to about fifteen species, as a result of DNA and other taxonomic studies.

Fingered jelly lichen (*Collema cristatum/Lathagrium cristatum*) is not widespread but is found in southern British Columbia and parts of western Colorado, growing on limestone or limy soil among mosses.

A novel photoprotective mycosporine was isolated from this lichen by Torres et al. (2004). When applied to the skin tissue prior to irradiation, the

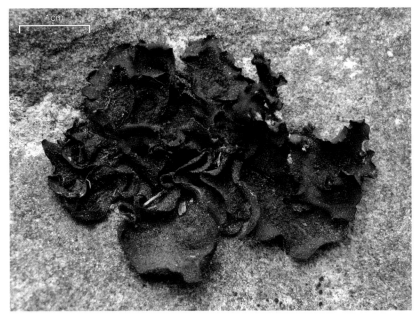

Collema subflaccidum

isolated compound prevented UV-B-induced erythema on cultured keratino-cytes, prevented pyrimidine dimer formation, and completely prevented UV-B induced erythema. This is exciting news, as skin destruction is common in patients undergoing radiation treatment. Relatedly, in clinical practice I found that a 5% dilution of Niaouli essential oil from *Melaleuca viridiflora*, applied before and after radiation, prevented and alleviated skin burns.

Ironically, when fingered jelly lichen was exposed to full sunlight, its content of zeaxanthin (carotenoid) was completely absent. On the other hand, with increased exposure to sunlight, levels of zeaxanthin increased in the lichen *Peltigera rufescens* (Adams et al. 1993).

Flaccid jelly lichen (*Collema flaccidum* syn. *Synechoblastus ruprestris*) contains colleflaccinosides A and B, with the latter showing significant antitumor activity (Rezanka and Dembitsky 2006).

CRYPTOTHECIA

Christmas Lichen

Christmas lichen (*Cryptothecia rubrocincta* syn. *C. sanguineum* syn. *Herpothallon rubricinctum*) is named for its green and red appearance. The species name means "red wreath."

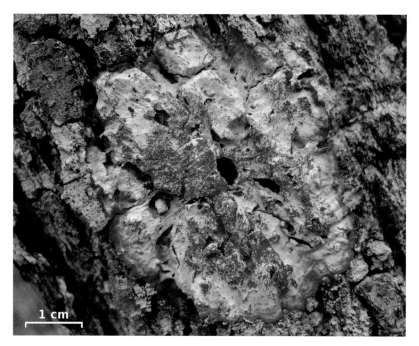

Cryptothecia rubrocincta
(Christmas Lichen)

This astoundingly beautiful lichen is found in subtropical regions of Florida, west to Louisiana, and slightly northward to South Carolina. It is found on bald cypress and oak trees in swamps and hummocks. It contains chiodectonic acid. A yeast, *Fellomyces mexicana*, isolated from this lichen contains CoQ_{10} in the mitochondrial membrane (Lopandic et al. 2005). This is significant because CoQ_{10} is widely present in humans when young, and its levels decline as we age. Lower levels have been found in patients with diseases of the heart and brain, diabetes, and cancer. Whether the change in enzyme is caused by the condition or the condition is worsened by its deficiency is uncertain. It is widely available as a supplement in health food stores.

DACTYLINA

Arctic Finger   Dead Man's Fingers

Arctic finger or dead man's fingers lichen (*Dactylina arctica* syn. *Cetraria arctica*) contains gyrophoric and lecanoric acid. In an oxidative stress model using the neuroblastoma cell line SH-SY5Y, pretreatment with an extract from this lichen prevented cell death and morphological changes. It also increased superoxide dismutase (SOD) and catalase activities, as well as glutathione levels. These changes suggest possible use in treatment for oxidative stress-related neurodegenerative diseases (Urena-Vacas et al. 2022a).

The same research team (Urena-Vacas et al. 2022) sampled fourteen lichens and found this one stands out for its higher antioxidant capacity (see the earlier description of *Asahinea scholanderi*, pages 25–26).

The only other member of this genus, frosted finger lichen (*Dactylina ramulosa* syn. *Cetraria ramulosa*), is found on calcium-rich soils and contains physodalic and physodic acids.

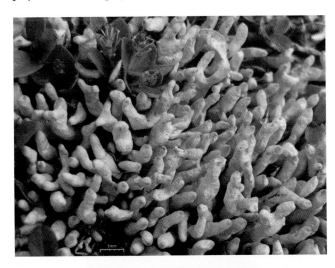

Dactylina arctica
(Arctic Finger or
Dead Man's Fingers
Lichen)

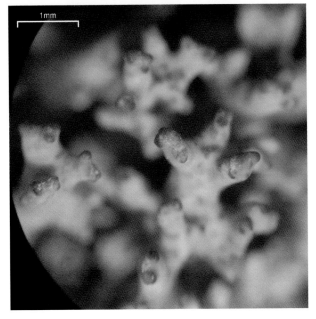

Dactylina ramulosa
(Frosted Finger Lichen)

DERMATOCARPON

Leather Lichen   Stippleback Lichens

Stippleback lichen (*Dermatocarpon moulinsii*) is mainly a western species in North America but has been found as far east as Fundy National Park in New Brunswick, Canada. It is often found growing on gravel, and when wet turns green and translucent. When soaked in water it can be chewed, or it can be boiled for fifteen minutes with some salt, resulting in a flavor reminiscent of mushrooms. This makes it a good addition to thicken and flavor rock soup. Crude extracts inhibit the growth of *Staphylococcus aureus* (Burkholder and Evans 1945). The genus name is derived from the Greek *derma,* meaning "skin," and *carpo,* for "fruit." (Carpo or Karpo was a Greek goddess associated with the fruits of the Earth.)

Leather lichen or common stippleback lichen (*Dermatocarpon miniatum* syn. *Endocarpon miniatum*) is common in most of the United States, as well as in the western Northwest Territories. Polysaccharides in this lichen scavenge oxygen radicals and inhibit lipid peroxidation (Jin et al. 2001). Methanol extracts of this lichen show strong antioxidant and significant antimicrobial activity (Aslan et al. 2006).

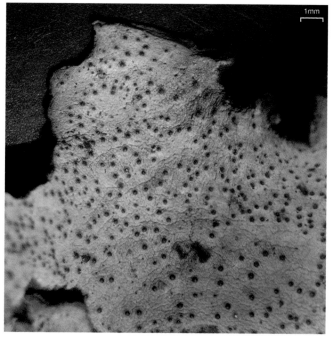

Dermatocarpon muhlenbergii

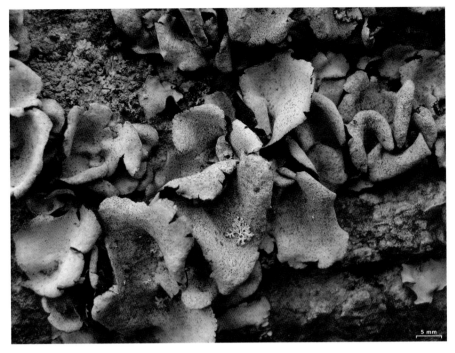

Dermatocarpon moulinsii
(Stippleback Lichen)

DIMELAENA
Moonglow Lichens

Geographic Range: North America

Habitat: siliceous soil and full sun

Medicinal Applications: potentially anticancer, sunscreen, and synergistic with gentamicin against *Staphylococcus*

Notable Chemicals: pannarin; norstictic, perlatolic, stictic, and usnic acids

Six *Dimelaena* species have been identified in North America to date, but this genus is slowly losing members due to taxonomic reclassification, with several moved to *Rinodina* genus.

California moonglow lichen (*Dimelaena californica/Monerolechia californica*) contains stictic, norstictic, 3-chloroperlatolic, and 3-chlorostenosporic acids.

Golden moonglow lichen (*Dimelaena oreina* syn. *Rinodina oreina*) is found in the Yukon and Northwest Territories on siliceous soil, and throughout most of southern Canada and large parts of the United States. It contains usnic, fumaroprotocetraric, hyperlatolic, gyrophoric, norstictic and/or stictic, 3-chloroisosubdivaricatic, 3-chlorolecanoric, and isosphaeric acids and pannarin. The latter depsidone, pannarin, inhibits cell growth and induces cell death of DU-145 (human prostate carcinoma) cells (Russo et al. 2006).

Pannarin inhibits the growth of melanoma cells, inducing apoptosis, and increases caspase-3 activity (Russo et al. 2008). Pannarin shows a protective effect on plasmid DNA and exhibits a superoxide dismutase (SOD)-like effect. It also protects from skin cancer due to inhibition of reactive oxygen and reactive nitrogen species from UVA and UVB radiation. Pannarin appears synergistic with the antibiotic gentamicin, but antagonistic with levofloxacin in the treatment of methicillin-resistant *Staphylococcus aureus* (MRSA) (Celenza et al. 2012).

Silver moonglow lichen (*Dimelaena radiata* syn. *Buellia radiata* syn. *Rinodina radiata*) is confined to coastal ridges and canyons in mountains of California. The reference to silver is because this is the only white species of genus. It contains 3-chlorolecanoric, 3-chloronordivaricatic, 5-chlorodivaricatic, and 3-chloroisosubdivaricatic acids.

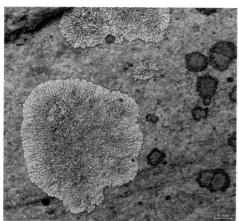
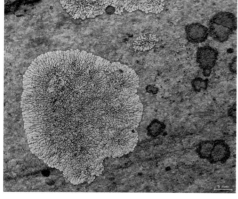

Dimelaena oreina
(Golden Moonglow Lichen)

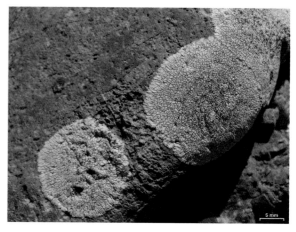

Dimelaena radiata
(Silver Moonglow Lichen)

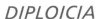

DIPLOICIA
White Pleated Lichen

Geographic Range: coasts of California and Florida

Habitat: wood, calcareous or siliceous rocks where birds perch

Medicinal Applications: antibacterial, antifungal, cancer, drug-resistant bacteria, sunscreen

Notable Chemicals: atranorin, chloroatranorin, diploicin, and secalonic acid

White pleated lichen (*Diploicia canescens* syn. *Buellia canescens*) is isolated to wood and rocks perched on by birds, and isolated to the California and Florida coasts, often within reach of saltwater spray. This is the only species in North America.

Diploicia is derived from the Greek *diploos*, meaning "twofold," in reference to this lichen's two-celled ascospores. Diplopia means "double vision" to optometrists. The name *Buellia* honors Esperanzo Buelli, chosen by his friend Giuseppe De Notarius. *Canescens* is derived from the Latin meaning "gray-haired" or "white with old age."

The lichen contains canesolide, buellolide, atranorin, scensidin, diploicin,

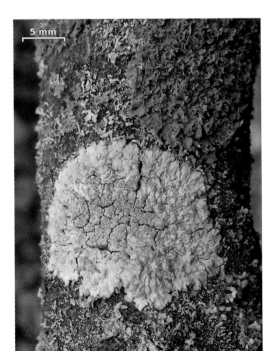

Diploicia canescens
(White Pleated Lichen)

chloroatranorin, 3-dechlorodiploicin, 3-dechloro-4-O-methyldiploicin, 3-O-demethylscensidin, issofulgidin, and secalonic acids B, D, and F. Secalonic acids B and D, as well as other compounds, were found to be cytotoxic against the B16 murine melanoma and HaCaT human keratinocyte cell lines (Millot et al. 2009). Secalonic acid D (SAD) exhibits cytotoxicity against pancreatic carcinoma PANC-1 cells (Tang et al. 2020). SAD also inhibits cell growth in multi-drug-resistant cells, by upregulating c-Jun expression. Work by Zhang et al. (2019) looked at cytotoxicity in H460 (non-small lung), MCF-7 (breast), MCF-7/ADR (multi-drug-resistant), and other cell lines.

SAD also shows potent cytotoxicity to HL60 and K562 (promyelocytic and myelogenous leukemia) cancer cell lines, by inducing apoptosis (Zhang et al. 2009). The compound may be useful as an antitumor pituitary treatment, based on in vitro cytotoxic effects on the GH3 cell line (Liao et al. 2010). SAD shows potential as a biofilm inhibitor against *Staphylococcus aureus*, and shows synergistic activity with antibiotics (Wang et al. 2017).

Secalonic acid F (SAF) represses the progression of HepG2 and Hep3B (hepatocarcinoma cells) by targeting MARCH1 (Xie et al. 2019). In fact, SAF inhibits hepatocellular carcinoma more effectively than 5-fluorouracil, which has nasty, predictable side effects (Gao et al. 2017). SAF induces cell death in multiple myeloma cells (Özenver et al. 2020).

Derivatives of diploicin exhibit activity, in vitro, against *Mycobacterium smegmatis*, *M. tuberculosis*, and *Corynebacterium diphtheriae* (Barry and Twomey 1950).

This lichen contains twelve metabolites that may play a role in UVA or UVB protection. The wavelengths and oscillator strengths are similar to UVA referent sunscreens (Millot et al. 2012).

Extracts of this lichen test positive against gram-positive bacteria and dermatophyte fungi (Taylor and Fourie 2019).

DIPLOSCHISTES

Cowpie Lichen   Crater Lichens

Crater lichen (*Diploschistes scruposus* syn. *Urceolaria scruposa*) is a very aggressive crust lichen that overgrows noncalcareous rocks. It contains up to 9.34% organic zinc. The species means "sharp" or "rugged stone." The term *scruposa* in turn refers to the uncomfortable pain from a sharp stone in a shoe. It has come to refer, in its form "scrupulous," to someone of high morals or integrity.

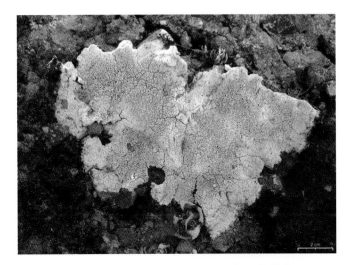

Diploschistes scruposus
(Crater Lichen)

Diploschistes diacapsis
(Desert Crater Lichen)

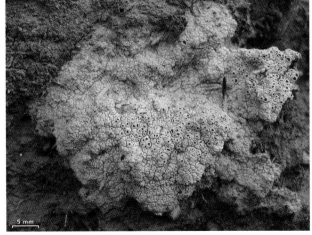

This lichen contains the unusual diploschistesic acid. Acetone extracts at an elevated level show activity against *Bacillus cereus*, *B. megaterium*, *Staphylococcus aureus*, and *Klebsiella pneumoniae* (Saenz et al. 2006).

The related cowpie lichen (*Diploschistes muscorum*) is well named, as it is found on soil, moss, and other lichens throughout the entire continent. It generally is parasitic on other lichens, often *Cladonia* species, helping itself to the host's algae, and then later finding its own home on soil or moss. The thick, round lichen looks somewhat like old dog poop, or cow pies, especially when found on lawns. It contains diploschistesic acid, as well as atranorin and lecanoric acid.

Desert crater lichen (*Diploschistes diacapsis* syn. *Urceolaria albissima*) is found on rocks in arid parts of the southwestern United States. It contains lecanoric and diploschisteric acids.

DIRINA

Dirina catalinariae lichen is found from Monterey, California, to the Baja peninsula of California and Mexico. The species name comes from its discovery on Catalina Island in 1911. *Dirina* may originate from an Old English term meaning "gift of god."

This lichen contains erythrin, which is found to work better than three clinically recommended antidiabetic compounds, namely, metformin, repaglinide, and sitagliptin (Rao and Hariprasad 2021).

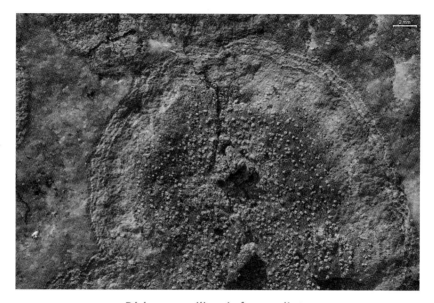

Dirina massiliensis f. *sorediata*

DIRINARIA

Grainy Medallion Lichen

North America has ten species of *Dirinaria* lichens.

Grainy medallion lichen (*Dirinaria aegialita* syn. *Physcia aspera*) grows on hickory, oak, and other hardwood trees in the southeastern United States. The endolichenic *Bacillus gibsonii* syn. *Alkalihalobacillus gibsonii* was isolated from this lichen by Dawoud et al. (2020). Its yellow pigment shows antifungal activity against pathogens of economic importance. Alkaline protease from this gram-positive bacterium demonstrates efficient blood stain removal for detergents and other industrial applications.

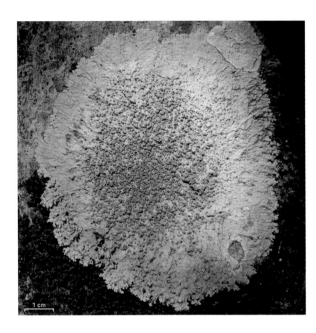

Dirinaria aegialita
(Grainy Medallion Lichen)

The lichen contains divaricatic acid which exhibits activity against B16-F10 melanoma cancer cell lines and are most cytotoxic to 3T3 normal cells (Brandão et al. 2013).

The medallion lichen (*Dirinaria applanata*) is found on the U.S. Gulf of Mexico coastal plain and is very similar looking to *Dirinaria picta*, described

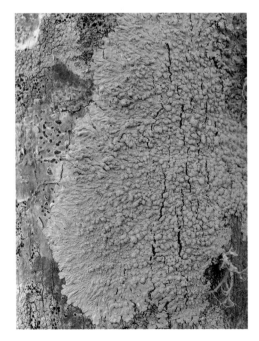

Dirinaria applanata
(Medallion Lichen)

below. This lichen contains hopane derivatives, as well as divaricatinic acid, methyl divaricatinate, methyl-beta-orcinolcarboxylate, methyl haematommate, divarinol, ramalinic acid, lichenxanthone, and 4,5-dichlorolichenxanthone (Nguyen et al. 2021).

Powdery medallion lichen (*Dirinaria picta* syn. *Physcia picta*) and purple-eyed medallion lichen (*Dirinaria purpurascens* syn. *Physcia purpurascens*) are found on bark in the Gulf Coast region, and contain divaricatic acid.

ENDOCARPON

Scaly Stippled Lichen

Scaly stippled lichen (*Endocarpon pusillum*) is found mainly on limestone rocks, and rarely at the bases of elms. It ranges from southeastern British Columbia and southwestern Alberta to the northeastern United States and south to Arizona and beyond.

Extracts of this lichen isolated by Yang et al. (2018) show selective cytotoxicity against AGS human gastric cancer cells and CT26 mouse colon cancer cell lines. A pure compound, myC, isolated from this lichen's mycelium in liquid

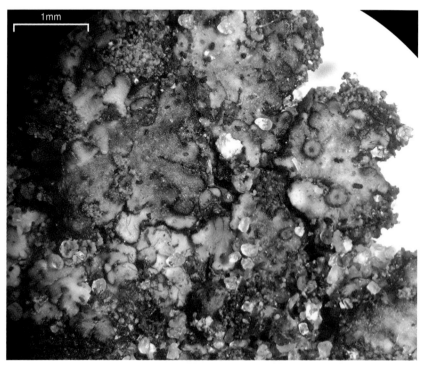

1mm

Endocarpon pusillum (Scaly Stippled Lichen)

culture showed more potent activity against the AGS line, including apoptosis. In vivo skin and xenograft tumors were significantly smaller than found in a control group. The extract showed a synergistic effect with docetaxel (chemotherapy drug) on both cancer cell lines.

ERIODERMA
Mouse Ears Lichen

The spruce and cedar on its shores, hung with gray lichens, looked at a distance like the ghosts of trees.

HENRY DAVID THOREAU

Mouse ears lichen (*Erioderma sorediatum*) is very rare and is an indicator of unpolluted woods. It is a coastal species found from northern British Columbia to northern Oregon. It contains the unusual depsidone, eriodermin.

EVERNIA
Oakmoss Lichens

Geographic Range: North America
Habitat: usually on trees, both hardwood and conifers
Practical Use: perfume base
Medicinal Applications: antibacterial, anticancer, snow blindness
Notable Chemicals: divaricatic, evernic, physodic, and usnic acids; lupeol, taraxerol

Evernia lichen species in North America number only four. *Evernia* may derive from the Old Latin version of the Greek *euernês*, meaning "sprouting well."

Mountain oakmoss lichen (*Evernia divaricata*) extracts show both antiproliferative and apoptotic effects on PC-3 (prostate) cancer cell lines. Apoptosis (cell death) was induced by both intrinsic and extrinsic pathways (Goncu et al. 2020). The lichen is rich in divaricatic acid.

Methanol extracts of this lichen are not antioxidative but have significant antimicrobial activity (Aslan et al. 2006).

Boreal oakmoss lichen (*Evernia mesomorpha*) is found from Alaska to eastern Canada and some northern states but is not common to most of British Columbia.

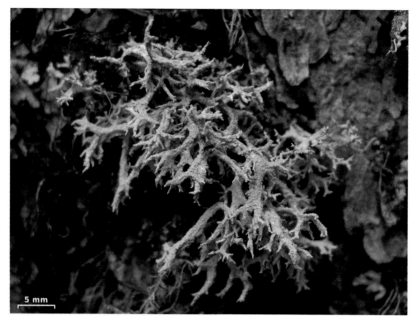

Evernia mesomorpha (Boreal Oakmoss Lichen)

My good friend and ethnobotanist Dr. Robin Marles (in 1984) studied with the *Chipewyan* (*Denesuline*) of northern Saskatchewan. They call this "birch lichen" or *k'i tsa"ju*. After harvest, it was decocted, then cooled, and a few drops were applied to snow-blinded eyes. Further south, the Cree squeezed juice from the white snowberry (*Symphylocarpus albus*) into eyes for the same purpose.

Divaricatic acid, derived from the boreal or spruce oakmoss (*E. mesomorpha*), shows activity against gram-positive bacteria such as *Bacillus subtilis*, *Staphylococcus epidermidis*, *Streptococcus mutans*, and *Enterococcus faecium*. Divaricatic acid potency was higher than for the pharmaceutical vancomycin against *S. epidermidis* and *E. faecium*, and the acid was as active as vancomycin against MRSA 3A048 (Oh et al. 2018).

Oakmoss lichen (*Evernia prunastri*) is widely overharvested in Europe to make an "absolute" used for perfume. Up to 10,000 tons are harvested annually, then stored for fermentation before extraction. The odor is earthy, woody, musky, and sharp. There is skin sensitivity to the absolute for up to 3% of wearers. However, the absolute is found at about 0.1% in a number of famous French perfumes. The European *Pseudevernia furfuracea* is used as the base note in Chanel No. 5 and in Miss Dior. The European Commission banned oakmoss lichen use in perfumes in 2017. This was due to the skin-sensitizing compounds

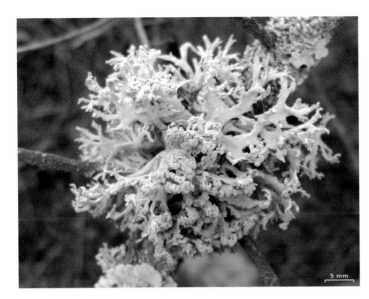

Evernia prunasatri (Oakmoss Lichen)

atranol and chloroatranol. Recent work by Avonto et al. (2021) suggests orcinol, ethyl orsellinate, and usnic acid are also candidate sensitizers to skin.

> *Down deep in the hollows, so damp and so cold*
> *Where oaks are by ivy overgrown,*
> *The gray moss and lichen creep over the mould,*
> *Lying loose on a ponderouse stone.*
>
> REBECCA S. NICHOLS

Today, nearly all perfumes are synthetically based, with small amounts of essential oils required to round out or smooth the scent. India also uses large quantities of lichens to produce ottos and attars (essential oils), with the harvest estimated in 1980 to be approximately 1,000 tons.

My wife, Laurie, and I began to sell essential oils under the name "Scents of Wonder," more than 30 years ago. At the time, beautifully scented oakmoss absolute was readily available, but today, most of the products on the market are significantly inferior.

In North America, oakmoss lichen is confined to the Pacific Northwest, from British Columbia to California. Early work by Bustinza (1952) found that it had activity against various bacteria and fungi, including *Staphylococcus aureus, Bacillus mycoides, B. licheniformis, Mycobacterium phlei, Actinomyces sulfuroides, Tricophyton farineculatum, T. interdigitalis,* and *Epidermophyton inguinale.*

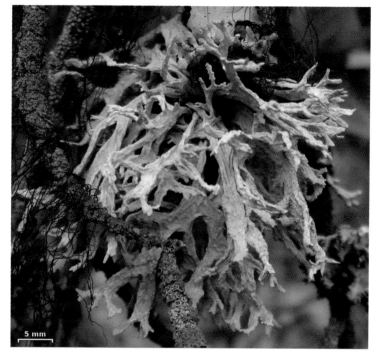

Evernia prunasatri (Oakmoss Lichen)

Medical Uses

Methanol extracts of oakmoss lichen cultured tissue exhibit activity against *B. subtilis*, *Staphylococcus aureus*, and *Propionibacterium acnes* (Yamamoto et al. 1998). Antioxidant activity was noted by Racine et al. (1980), and methanol extract of oakmoss lichen showed significant antimicrobial activity (Aslan et al. 2006).

Unlike many other lichens, oakmoss lichen produces nitric oxide in response to mercury contamination. The NO was released from the lichen donor sodium nitroprusside (Kovácik et al. 2023). The pharmaceutical sodium nitroprusside was first identified in 1849 and approved by the Food and Drug Administration in 1974 as a fast-acting intravenous intervention for acute hypertension and associated acute pulmonary edema. It acts as a rapid and potent vasodilator of arterial and venous systems.

Oakmoss lichen (*Evernia prunastri*) water extracts were found to lower systolic, diastolic, and mean arterial blood pressure and heart rate in hypertensive rats, but not in those with normal blood pressure. A vasorelaxant effect was identified in the isolated thoracic aorta (Amssayef et al. 2021).

Water extracts were also orally tested in rats that had induced diabetes, and produced significant reductions in blood glucose, triglycerides, and very-low-density lipoprotein (VLDL) levels. Repeated oral administration for a week ameliorated the liver function by increasing its glycogen content (Amssayef et al. 2022).

Kosanic et al. (2013) found physodic acid, which is present in both this lichen and *Pseudoevernia furfuracea*, to possess significant antioxidant activity. Anticancer activity was tested against FemX (human melanoma) and LS174 (human colon carcinoma) cell lines. In other effects of this acid, strong cytotoxic and antiproliferative activity was found against HeLa (human epithelial cervical) cancer (Kizil et al. 2014), and a decrease in proliferation of A549 (lung) cancer cells was observed (Kizil et al. 2015).

Evernic acid from oakmoss lichen shows mild cytotoxicity against glioblastoma multiforme cell lines (Studzinska-Sroka et al. 2021). Evernic acid is neuroprotective in vitro, and in a mouse model it attenuated motor dysfunction, with a reduction in dopaminergic neuronal death and astroglial activation (Lee et al. 2021). This is suggestive of potential benefit in patients with Parkinson's disease.

Methanol extracts showed in vitro activity against *Staphylococcus aureus* (Rafika and Monia 2018). Work by Shcherbakova et al. (2021) also found activity against *Staphylococcus aureus*, as well as against the gram-negative bacteria *Pseudomonas aeruginosa* and *Escherichia coli* and the fungus *Candida albicans*. Strong activity against *Candida albicans* biofilm was found by Girardot et al. (2021).

Earlier work by Sökmen et al. (2012) found that acetone extracts of *Evernia palustris* possess antioxidant and antimicrobial activity. The lichen contains 4,2'-di-O-methylgyrophic acid, evernic acid, lanosterol, taraxerol, evernine, 2'-O-methylevernic acid, methyl 3'-methyllecanorate, methyl everninate, moretenone, friedelin, lupeol, atraric acid, ursolic acid, and 29-nor-21α-hopane-3,22-dione.

Taraxerol has been the subject of numerous scientific papers, at last count numbering 165 on PubMed. Herbalists will quickly recognize the compound. as it is found in dandelion root, a valuable medicinal plant, and it is present in *Evernia palustris*. Taraxerol has shown beneficial effects in reducing cancer, blood sugar dysregulation, and neurodegenerative disease. Taraxerol induced cell apoptosis in HeLa (cervical/epilethial) cancer cells (Yaoi et al. 2017); exhibits an in vivo benefit in diabetic neuropathy (Khanra et al. 2017), and inhibition of acetylcholinesterase in an animal hippocampus (Berté et al. 2018).

Oakmoss lichen (*Evernia prunastri*) contains atraric acid, which gives the resinous extract its unique scent. The compound, at 3% dilution, inhibited melanin and tyrosinase activity on skin, with almost no side effects. Work by Li et al. (2022) found that atraric acid suppresses melanin formation by downregulating the PKA/CREB/MITF signaling pathway. This suggests possible use as an ingredient in skin-lightening cosmetics and inhibition of hyperpigmentation.

I pause to reflect here that lichen growth is admittedly slow and steady, but also tenacious. It is only our human cultural linear time/space and anthropocentric view of our place in the universe that interprets a lichen's life in this manner. The movement of slow food versus fast food is one example of a worldwide return to a gentler, respectful and more thoughtful, ecological approach to living.

My father used to say, "The hurrier I am, the behinder I get."

FLAVOCETRARIA

Crinkled Snow Lichen   Curled Snow Lichen

Geographic Range: Northern Canada
Habitat: on ground, amongst mosses and heath species on tundra soil
Practical Uses: soup flavor and thickener
Medicinal Applications: cancer
Notable Chemicals: lupeol; baeomycesic, protolichesterinic, salazinic, squamatic, and usnic acid

Curled snow lichen (*Flavocetraria cucullata* syn. *Cetraria cucullata*) is found in northern Canada, from Newfoundland across through British Columbia. Indigenous people used it in northern Canada as a complement, or as a thickener for fish/duck soup. The Yup'ik of Yukon and Alaska know it as *ninguujug*, meaning "would like to be stretched," perhaps in reference to its belly-filling capacity.

Work by Urena-Vacas et al. (2022) found the lichen inhibits both acetylcholinesterase and butyrylcholinesterase. This suggests possible application in various neurodegenerative diseases. Protolichesterinic acid may be involved.

Among 17 lichens tested for anticancer activity by Nguyen et al. (2014), this lichen exhibited the most potent cytotoxicity against several human cancer cell lines. The extract, which contains usnic acid but also salazinic, squamatic, baeomycesic, and D-protolichesterinic acids, is more potent than when usnic acid was tested alone. The lichen also contains the unique 7-demethylcristazarin.

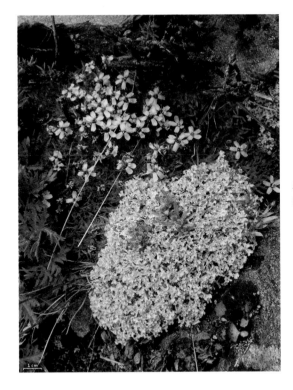

Flavocetraria cucullata
(Curled Snow Lichen)

The extract decreased cancer cell motility, and specifically activated the apoptotic signaling pathway. Inhibition of epithelial-mesenchymal transition was noted.

The related crinkled snow lichen (*Flavocetraria nivalis* syn. *Cetraria nivalis*) is found on heath-related grounds near the tree line, or on tundra soil.

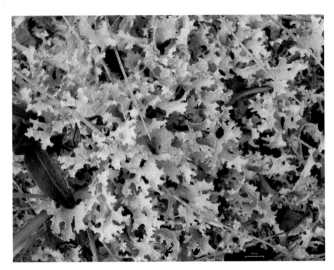

Flavocetraria nivalis
(Crinkled Snow Lichen)

The Qollahuaya (Callawaya) Andean people of Bolivia brew this lichen as a tonic for altitude sickness, motion sickness, heart problems, and heart attacks (Bastien 1983). I have purchased it in the street markets of La Paz. *Nivalis* means "snow." It contains the unusual compound 22a-hydroxystictane-3-one.

According to the *Pharmacopoeia Universalis* of 1846, this lichen has benefits similar to those of Iceland moss.

Crinkled snow lichen contains friedelan-3ß-ol (epifriedelinol), friedelin, and lupeol. Lupeol helps rejuvenate antioxidant, anti-inflammatory, and anti-apoptotic pathways. Research has found benefits in diabetes, obesity, cardiovascular, liver and kidney disease, skin problems, and neurological disorders (Sohag et al. 2022). Lupeol induces autophagy in triple-negative breast cancer, due to antiproliferative and antimetastatic action both in vitro and in vivo (Zhang et al. 2022a). Lupeol is synergistic with doxorubicin, a common chemotherapy drug. In work by Malekinejad et al. (2022), lupeol synergistically enhanced the antiproliferative effect on MCF-7 and MDA-MB-231 (breast) and HFF (foreskin fibroblast) cancer cell lines. The combination synergized three- to four-fold downregulation of MMP-9 expression in cell lines.

FLAVOPARMELIA
Greenshield Lichens

Geographic Range: eastern North America and southwestern deserts
Habitat: on trees and rocks in sun or shade
Medicinal Applications: burn treatment; reduced cancer cell migration and inhibited the pro-inflammatory activation of leukocytes; potential in treating dementia, bone health.
Notable Chemicals: atranorin, and caperatic, protocetraric, protolichesterinic, and usnic acids

There are only four *Flavoparmelia* lichens in North America. The name derives from the Latin *flavus,* "yellow," and *parmelia,* meaning "little shield," hence shield lichens.

Rock greenshield lichen (*Flavoparmelia baltimorensis* syn. *Pseudoparmelia baltimorensis*) contains protocetraric and (occasionally) gyrophoric acids, and a polysaccharide fraction, PB-2, with potential for treating senile dementia, by promoting synaptic plasticity in the hippocampus (Hirano et al. 2003). Previous work with common greenshield lichen, another species, investigated

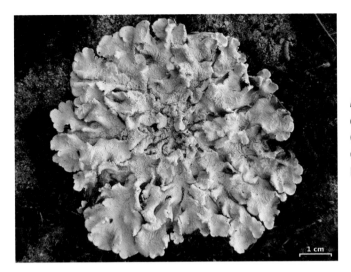

Flavoparmelia caperata (Common Greenshield Lichen)

PC-2 for similar induction of long-term potentiation in a rat dentate gyrus in vivo.

Common greenshield lichen (*Flavoparmelia caperata* syn. *Parmelia caperata*) was traditionally powdered and applied to burns by the Tarahumara (Rarámuri) of Mexico, who know it as *reté* (Pennington 1963). *Caperata* is derived from the Latin for "wrinkled." I have found it on walks in isolated parts of northern Alberta.

Common greenshield lichen contain atranorin, and caperatic, protocetraric, and usnic acids, which show activity against *Staphylococcus aureus* (Dieu et al. 2020). The water-soluble polysaccharide glucans enhanced hippocampal plasticity and behavior in a rat study by Smriga and Saito (2000). This lichen induced Ca^{2+} signaling, reduced cancer cell migration, and inhibited the pro-inflammatory activation of leukocytes (Ingelfinger et al. 2020).

None of the *Flavoparmelia* lichens showed any detrimental influence on the viability of endothelial cells. The pro-inflammatory activation of leukocytes was inhibited by both oakmoss and common greenshield lichens. Work by Bézivin et al. (2003) and Manojlovic et al. (2012) showed cytotoxicity to various cancer cell lines.

The *Flavoparmelia caperata* exhibit alpha-amylase inhibition, suggestive of benefit in reducing digestive assimilation of sugars, and thus for blood sugar control (Shivanna et al. 2015; Valadbeigi and Shaddel 2016). An extract of *Flavoparmelia* species inhibits osteoblast formation, suggesting potential benefit in osteoporosis and other bone disease (Kim et al. 2019).

Early work by Burkholder and Evans (1945) with *Flavoparmelia caperata* found activity against *Staphylococcus aureus, Diplococcus pneumoniae, Streptococcus hemolyticus, S. viridans, Bacillus subtilis, B. mycoides,* and *Sarcina lutea.* Usnic acid, extracted from these lichens, showed antibacterial activity comparable to that of streptomycin. Furthermore, ethanol extracts exhibit activity against the virulent strain of *Mycobacterium tuberculosis* $H_{37}R_v$ (Gupta et al. 2007). For more information on greenshield lichens, (see *Parmelia caperata* on page 157).

FLAVOPUNCTELIA
Greenshield Lichens

Speckled greenshield lichen (*Flavopunctelia flaventior* syn. *Parmelia flaventior*) is found on various tree barks in open woods and along roadways. It ranges from Alberta to New England, as well as in California and the Rockies from Wyoming to Mexico.

Powder-edged speckled greenshield lichen (*Flavopunctelia soredica* syn. *Parmelia ulophyllodes* syn. *Punctelia soredica*) is found on tree bark from northern Saskatchewan to New Mexico. The Navajo of the region used the lichen to make a colored dye.

Colloidal silver has long been used for antimicrobial benefit, usually in wound dressing, but also internally. Relatedly, silver nanoparticles (AgNPs) have been joined with methanol extracts of this lichen, in work by

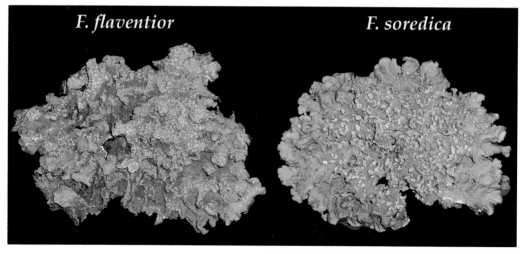

Flavopunctelia flaventior (left)
(Speckled Greenshield Lichen),
Flavopunctelia soredica (right)
(Powder-Edged Speckled Greenshield Lichen)

Alqahtani et al. (2020), and were tested against various pathogens. The highest antibacterial activity in that work was noted against *Pseudomonas aeruginosa*, MRSA (methicillin-resistant *Staphylococcus aureus*), VRE (vancomycin-resistant *Enterococcus*), and *Escherichia coli*. Cytotoxicity was noted against FaDu (pharynx) and HCT 116 (colorectal) cancer cell lines.

This activity suggests a possible new avenue to address the increasing population of multi-drug-resistant organisms and various cancer cells.

GRAPHINA
Script Lichens

There are 23 *Graphina* species in North America, most of them on hardwood trees and shrubs in subtropical regions, such as Louisiana and Florida. They contain stictic, norstictic, constictic, protocetraric, or psoromic acids.

Script lichen (*Graphina perstriatula*), like a number of these species, inhibits tyrosinase and xanthine oxidase, suggesting possible benefit in removing uric acid to relieve gouty conditions (Behera et al 2004).

GRAPHIS
Common Script Lichens

Common script lichen (*Graphis scripta*) is an eastern species named for the slender, elongated fruiting bodies, which form "scribbles" on the bark. On birch bark there are linear apothecia that follow, like worms, giving the bark texture. It is also known as secret writing lichen. I have also found the script on trees near the Pacific Coast from Alaska to Northern California. *Graphis* derives from *graphein* "to write." *Scripta* is obvious. One can spend an afternoon trying to transcribe what messages the lichen is expressing in its own language. Some authors have imagined Hebrew letters or Chinese script.

Work by Yamamoto et al. (1993) identified antioxidant activity and inhibition of tyrosinase and xanthine oxidase from extracts of the common script lichen. The latter enzyme is present in rheumatic conditions, especially gout, due to uric acid excess, and inhibition via the enzyme can provide relief. It also contains graphislactones A and B.

Later work by Yamamoto et al. (1998) found activity against various gram-positive bacteria such as *Bacillus subtilis*, *Propionibacterium acnes*, and *Staphylococcus aureus*. Superoxide dismutase activity and inhibition of

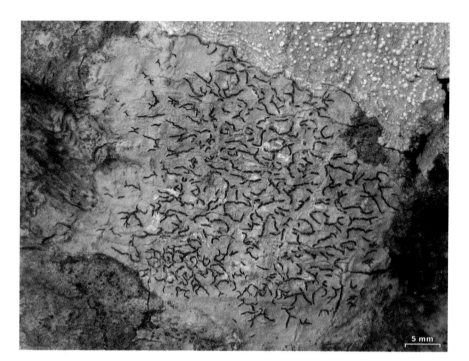

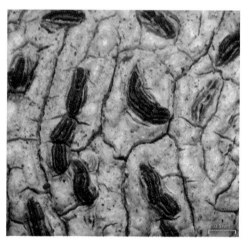

Graphis elegans

Epstein–Barr virus activation induced teleocidin B-4 (showing anticancer potential).

The related *Graphis desquamescens* also contains graphislactones, and pigment, graphisquinone. The latter compound exhibits cytotoxicity against SW620, FADU, and MDA-MB-231 (breast) cancer cell lines (Miyagawa et al. 1994).

Both *Graphis persicina* and *Graphis pyrrhochelloides* exhibit inhibition of tyrosinase and xanthine oxidase (Behera et al. 2004).

GYMNODERMA
Rock Gnome Lichen

Rock gnome lichen (*Gymnoderma lineare* syn. *Cetradonia linearis*) is rare and endangered. It prefers hanging cliffs with running water in deep forests of Appalachia. It contains atranorin and protolichesterinic acid. Obviously, it should be viewed, maybe photographed, and left in place.

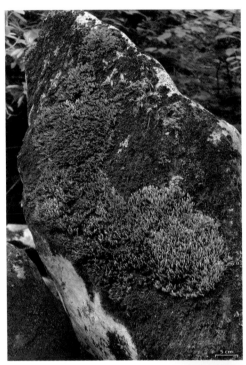

Gymnoderma lineare
(Rock Gnome Lichen)

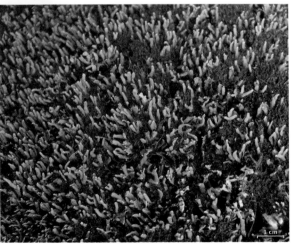

GYPSOPLACA
Changing Earthscale Lichen

Changing earthscale lichen (*Gypsoplaca macrophylla* syn. *Lecidea macrophylla*) is restricted to gypsum (calcium sulfate) soil in arid areas of Utah and Colorado. It contains gypmacrophin A (pentacyclic sesterterpenoid), and brialmontins 1–3. Gypmacrophin A shows weak inhibition of acetylcholinesterase (Zhou et al. 2017).

HAEMATOMMA
Bloodspot Lichens

Rock bloodspot lichen (*Haematomma fenzlianum* syn. *H. subpuniceum*) is found on siliceous rocks in southern Arizona and southwestern Texas. It contains atranorin, sphaerophorin, isosphaeric acid, and russulone; rarely with psoromic acid.

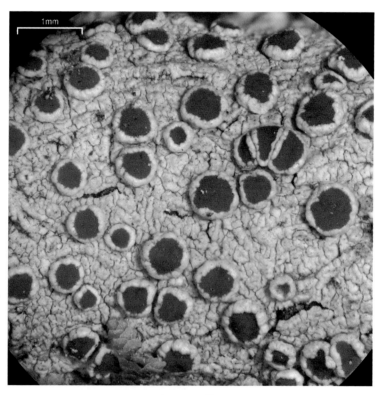

Haematomma flexuosum
(Flexible Bloodspot Lichen)

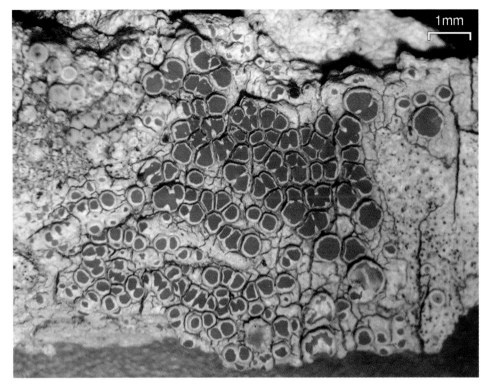

Haematomma persoonii
(Sunken Bloodspot Lichen)

Flexible bloodspot lichen (*Haematomma flexuosum*) is also found on the southeastern coast of North America. It contains haematommone, isoplacodiolic acid, and isopseudoplacodiolic acid.

Bloodspot lichen (*Haematomma lapponicum* syn. *Ophiopharma lapponica*) contains porphyrillic acid, which exhibits antibiotic activity, as well as the secondary metabolites usnic and divaricatic acids.

The very rare yellow bloodspot lichen (*Haematomma ochroleucum*) is found near oceanside terrain in the Pacific Northwest. It contains zeorin, methyl barbatate, and porphyrilic acid.

Sunken bloodspot lichen (*Haematomma persoonii*) is usually found on the bark of deciduous trees in subtropical regions of the Gulf Coast and coastal Southern California. It contains atranorin, sphaerophorin, russulone, and haematommone. Russulone is a bright red pigment that gives many *Russula* mushroom species their distinct color. Tree bloodspot (*Haematomma accolens*) contains atranorin and placodiolic acid, *Haematomma americanum* contains sphaerophorin. *Haematomma rufidulum* contains placodiolic acid.

HETERODERMIA
Fringe Lichens

Geographic Range: southern eastern Canada and United States; many are coastal

Habitat: oak and hardwood bark, junipers, rock faces, mossy bases of trees

Medicinal Applications: androgenic alopecia of the scalp; anti-inflammatory, cancer, healing cuts and wounds, pain relief

Notable Chemicals: atranorin, atraric acid, chloroatranorin, emodin, norstictic and salazinic acid and lobaric acids; zeorin

Fringe lichens, the *Heterodermia* species, number 25 in North America. The genus name is derived from the Greek *hetero*, meaning "other" or "different," and *dermia*, related to our dermis, or inner skin.

Cupped fringe lichen (*Heterodermia diademata* syn. *Anaptychia diademata*) is found in the extreme Southwest, usually on oak bark. In Sikkim, the lichen is used to heal cuts and wounds. In Nepal the lichen is known as *Dhungo ku seto jhau'* (Saklani and Upreti 1992). This lichen contains atranorin, chloroatranorin, zeorin, and norstictic, salazinic, and lobaric acids. Methanol extracts exhibit activity against seven fungal species (Tiwari et al. 2011).

Another cupped fringe lichen *Heterodermia hypoleuca*, is found in the eastern United States on hardwood bark. It contains atraric acid, which exerts an anti-inflammatory effect, possibly due to the inactivation of the ERK/NF_kB signaling pathway. This suggests potential use in treating inflammatory conditions (Mun et al. 2020). Atraric acid is also present in *Evernia prunastri* and various *Stereocaulon* and *Parmotrema* species. Also, atraric acid induces cellular senescence and inhibits prostate tumor growth, via a different pathway than clinically used androgen receptor drugs (Ehsani et al. 2022).

A topical formula for androgenic alopecia of the scalp has been developed, and in mice trials it compared favorably with minoxidil and oral finasteride. It is composed of atraric acid, ethanol, oleic acid, and water (Pulat et al. 2023).

The popular Pygeum bark products marketed in health food stores for prostate health contain both atranorin and atraric acid (Thompson et al. 2019). When atranorin is dissolved in methanol/ethanol it degrades to atraric acid. This suggests another potential use for the cupped fringe lichens.

Elegant fringe lichen (*Heterodermia leucomela* syn. *H. leucomelaena*,

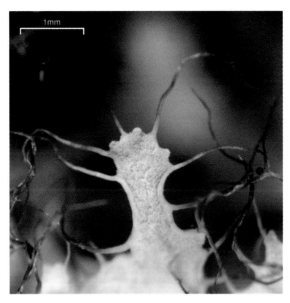

Heterodermia echinata

syn. *Physcia leucomela*) is commonly known as elegant centipede lichen. It is found on mossy hardwoods, or on rock faces in open woodlands. It is not all that common and contains salazinic acid. It is one of a few lichens hosting cystobasidiomycete yeasts (Lendemer et al. 2019).

The elegant fringe lichen inhibits alpha-amylase (Shivanna et al. 2015; Hengameh et al. 2016), suggestive of modifying blood sugar levels. Water extracts possess fungicidal activity against a wide range of dermatophytes (Furmanek et al. 2019). Work by Gupta et al. (2007) found an ethanol extract active against a virulent strain of tuberculosis. In addition, this lichen contains hydroxy-4-methoxybenzoic acid, which has exhibited activity against mosquito larvae (Kathirgamanathar et al. 2006).

Orange-tinted fringe lichen (*Heterodermia obscurata* syn. *Anaptychia obscurata* syn. *A. heterchroa*) contains the polysaccharide glucomannan. Cordova et al. (2013) studied the extract for effects on acute and chronic pain in mice. Levels of interleukin-1-beta were reduced with use of this extract in spinal cord and nerves in the partial sciatic nerve ligation model. The injection of various irritants, with the afforded relief, is suggestive of possible use in management of pain.

Orange-tinted fringe lichen also contains atranorin, chloroatranorin, zeorin, emodin, 5-chloroemodin and 7-chloroemodin, 5,7-dichloroemodin, AO1- and AO2-anthrone, and flav-obscurin A, B_1, and B_2.

In *The Fungal Pharmacy* (on page 468) I mentioned that Pierre Cohen studied this lichen and *Nephroma laevigatum* for his Ph.D. thesis at Berkeley, but the Ph.D. was actually from the University of British Columbia. He notes that this lichen is not found on the West Coast but is abundant in the southeastern United States. In fact, orange-tinted fringe lichen (*Heterodermia obscurata*) is found to range from Nova Scotia to Florida and west to Texas.

Kang et al. (2022) investigated this lichen, as well as *Parmotrema tinctorum* and *Usnea articulata*, for potential macrofilaricidal activity. Such activity might relate to onchocerciasis, for example, a parasitic infection that affects cattle. Ivermectin and moxidectin are efficacious against microfilaricidal species, as in onchocerciasis, but show no activity against adult worms. *Parmotrema tinctorum* and *Usnea articulata* were more active against the adult worms than was orange-tinted fringe lichen.

Orange-tinted fringe lichen contains highly branched glucomannans. Intraperitoneal administration of water and alkaline extractions of this lichen reduced visceral pain and inhibition by 88%. It also reduced leukocyte migration by 58%, suggesting potential for pain relief and anti-inflammatory utilization (Pereira et al. 2010).

Fringe footed lichen (*Heterodermia podocarpa*) was cultured and then extracted with methanol by Verma et al. (2008). It exhibited lipid peroxidation and tyrosinase enzyme activity, and zeorin, isolated from the same culture, exhibited antioxidant activity.

Centipede lichen (*Heterodermia speciosa* syn. *Anaptychia pseudospeciosa* var. *tremulans* syn. *A. speciosa*) contains atranorin, and norstictic, salazinic, and lobaric acids, as well as hopane, hopan-6a,22-diol (zeorin), and hopane-6a,16ß 22-triol.

Work by Jha et al. (2017) found moderate antioxidant activity, and antimicrobial activity against *Staphylococcus aureus*.

HYPERPHYSCIA

Grainy Shadow Crust Lichens

Grainy shadow crust lichen (*Hyperphyscia adglutinata*) is found on hardwood bark in mid-west and eastern states.

Alpha-amylase inhibition, suggesting blood sugar control, was discovered in work by Valadbeigi and Shaddel (2016).

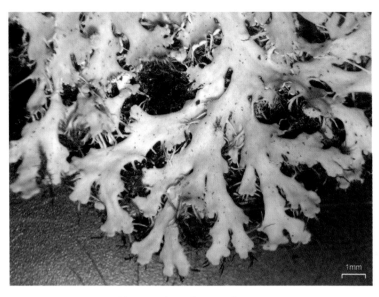

Heterodermia speciosa
(Centipede Lichen)

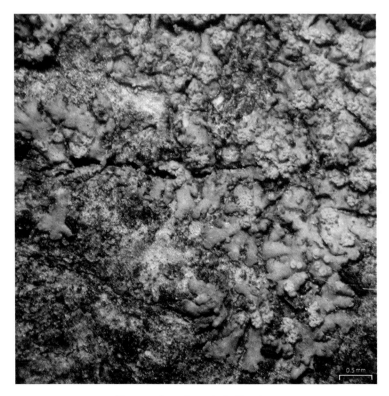

Hyperphyscia adglutinata
(Grainy Shadow Crust Lichen)

HYPOCENOMYCE

Clam Lichens

Common clam lichen (*Hypocenomyce scalaris* syn. *Psora scalaris*) is widespread from Yukon across to New Brunswick and south to Arizona, growing on burnt wood as well as conifer and acidic barks.

Lecanoric acid, derived from clam lichen, shows moderate cytotoxicity against HCT116 and DLD-1 (colorectal) cancer cell lines (Paluszczak et al. 2018). Lecanoric acid also showed moderate cytotoxicity against HCT116 (colorectal) cancer cell lines in another study (Roser et al. 2022).

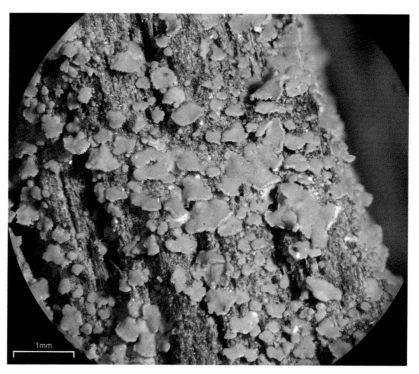

1mm

Hypocenomyce scalaris
(Common Clam Lichen)

HYPOGYMNIA

Beaded Tube Lichen   Hooded Bone Lichen   Powder-headed Tube Lichen

Budding Tube Lichen   Monk's Hood Lichens

Geographic Range: cooler climates or higher elevations in North
   America
Habitat: on conifer bark and wood, occasionally on mossy soil or rocks
Medicinal Applications: antibiotic, antibacterial, antifungal, arsenic
   remediation, potentially anticancer; protocetraric acid
Notable Chemicals: atranorin, chloroatranorin; diffractaic,
   gyrophoric, physodic, physodalic, and protocetraric acids

Hypogymnia derives from the Greek *hypo* for "under" and *gymnia*, meaning
"naked" or "bare."

Beaded tube lichen (*Hypogymnia apinnata*) grows along the Pacific
Coast from Alaska to Northern California, southwestern Alberta, and
south into Idaho and Montana. It grows on conifers in protected areas and
contains atranorin. I found it growing on a spruce tree outside my cabin
in Waterton National Park many years ago when I was presenting at the
Wildflower Festival.

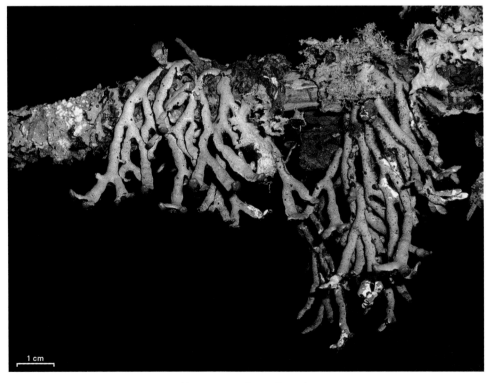

Hypogymnia apinnata
(Beaded Tube Lichen)

Medical Uses

Beaded tube lichen, as well as *Letharia columbiana* showed significant antibiotic activity against *Micrococcus luteus,* and moderate effect against *Staphylococcus aureus* and *Salmonella gallinarum.* The same study found *Usnea filipendula* showed a promising effect on *Serratia marcescens* (Crockett et al. 2003).

The latter is an opportunistic drug-resistant pathogen that causes 1.4% of hospital-acquired infections, from contaminated catheters and so on. *Serratia* is named to honor the Italian physicist Serfino Serrati. *Marcescens* is from the Latin, meaning "decaying." This pathogen is especially problematic for patients with cystic fibrosis, due to its respiratory issues.

Serratia marcescens is found on grout in shower stalls and tiles, exhibiting an orange pink to red color. The bacterium produces a red dye, prodigiosin, which can grow on bread. The Eucharist celebrates bread and wine as the body and blood of Jesus Christ in the Roman Catholic tradition. In 1263, a contaminated facial sculpture wept red from the eyes, and when the red was wiped away, continued to bleed, due to this contamination. "The Miracle of Bolsena" is still celebrated in some quarters.

Budding tube or gut lichen (*Hypogymnia enteromorpha* syn. *Parmelia physodes* var. *enteromorpha*) grows on conifer bark or dry wood, in full or partial shade, on the Pacific Coast and in the Rocky Mountain temperate rainforest from British Columbia into Idaho. This substantial-size lichen contains protocetraric, physodalic, physodic, and diffractaic acids.

Physodic acid appears to inhibit the formation of reactive metabolites by blocking the hepatic microsomal oxidation systems. Physodic and physodalic acid both inhibit mutagenicity of indirect mutagens associated with *Salmonella typhimurium* TA98 (Osawa et al. 1991). Salmonella is a major foodborne pathogen, with *S. typhimurium* one of the leading causes of salmonellosis worldwide. Multi-drug-resistant strains have emerged in cattle, pigs, and chickens, including chicken eggs (Wang et al. 2019).

Methanol extracts of cultured budding tube lichen tissue exhibited inhibition of tyrosinase and superoxide dismutase-like activity (Yamamoto et al. 1998).

Hooded bone or monk's hood lichen (*Hypogymnia physodes* syn. *Parmelia physodes* syn. *P. oregana*) is one of the most widespread tree lichens of the north, found mainly on Douglas fir and other conifer bark. *Physodes* derives from the Greek meaning "like a bellows," or "bladder-like," in reference to the

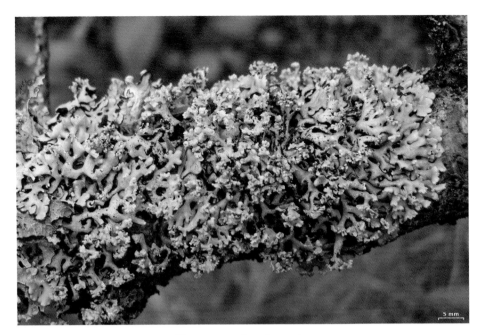

Hypogymnia physodes
(Hooded Bone, Monk's Hood Lichen)

bursting lobe tips. The Neshnabé/Nishabek (Potawatomi) of Wisconsin call it *wa'kwunuk*, "egg bush." For constipation it was eaten raw, but it was also added to hot soups (Smith 1933).

As an aside, the tribal name Potawatomihk was given to this group of people by the Ojibwe, meaning "people of the place of fire." Nishabek, their preferred name, means "people."

In fifteenth-century Europe, hooded bone lichen was combined with *Evernia prunastri* and *E. furfuracea* to create *lichen quercinus virides*. Early work by Burkholder and Evans (1945), and Mordraksi (1956) reported antimicrobial activity for hooded bone lichen. Later work by Yamamoto et al. (1998) and Rankovic (2007; 2008) found extracts of lichen, cultured tissue, and gyrophoric acid active against 10 bacteria and a dozen fungal species.

Several interesting studies that relate to *Hypogymnia* lichens have been conducted in the past decade. For instance, Ari et al. (2014) studied the antigrowth effect of an extract of this lichen on two different breast cancer cell lines (MCF-7 and MDA-MB-231). The extracts exhibited an antigrowth effect at relatively low concentrations, while higher amounts were required for genotoxic activity.

In the same year, Stojanovic et al. (2014) examined the activity of physodalic acid, physodic acid, and 3-hydroxy-physodic acid on HeLa (cervical/ epidermal) cell viability and growth. The latter two compounds exhibited higher activity. The cytotoxicity of physodic acid was also assessed against three breast cancer cell lines, the already-mentioned MCF-7 and MDA-MB-231 as well as T-47D (Studzinska-Sroka et al. 2016). The compound was inactive against the nontumor MCF-10A but showed strong cytotoxicity against all three lines. Extracts of *Hypogymnia* lichens possess high antioxidant activity and show cytotoxicity against the human HL-60/MX2 acute CKL-22 (CRL-2257) promyelocytic leukemia tumor cell line (Hawry et al. 2022).

The latest research on this lichen and physodic acid looked at both anticancer activity and a neuroprotective aspect (Studzinska-Sroka et al. 2021). Strong inhibition of glioblastoma cell proliferation and hyaluronidase activity was noted, as well as COX-2 and tyrosinase. The glioblastoma cell lines used were A-172, T98G, and U-138. The acetylcholinesterase and butyrylcholinesterase inhibition by an extract of this lichen and physodic acid were mild. However, physodic acid does cross the blood–brain barrier and may be protective against central nervous system conditions. Physodic acid, 3-hydroxyphysodic acid, physodalic acid, and atranorin have been isolated from this lichen. Work by Elecko et al. (2022) found 3-hydroxyphysodic acid to be the strongest free radical scavenger (antioxidant) of the group. Physodic acid at 6–12 µg/mL inhibits *Mycobacterium tuberculosis* (Rogers 2011).

Hypogymnia lichens exhibit activity against bacteria, including staphylococci, enterococci, and *Stenotrophomonas maltophilia* strains (Tapalsky et al. 2017).

Hypogymnia physodes exhibits antifungal activity against *Aspergillus niger* (Furmanek et al. 2021). This black mold is found on grapes, dates, peanuts and apricots, but is also used to produce digestive enzymes. Pu-erh, a pricey Chinese tea, is fermented aerobically with this fungus, together with *Blastobotrys adeninivorans*, a yeast-like fungus. The bacterium was commercialized over a century ago, by Pfizer, to produce citric acid. However, this hyphal fungus can cause severe lung infections, which can be treated in the early stages.

Hooded bone lichen appears to remediate arsenic, both by arsenite excretion and by methylation of the toxic mineral (Rogers 2011).

Powder-headed tube lichen (*Hypogymnia tubulosa* syn. *Parmelia tubulosa*) is found on conifer and birch trees in the boreal forest, but also in the

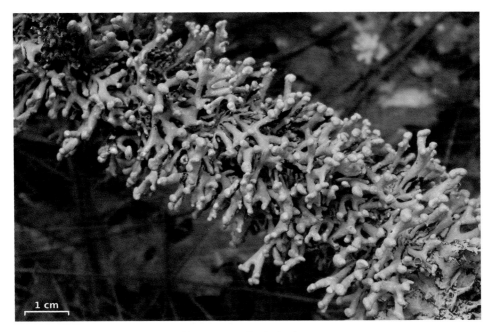

Hypogymnia tubulosa
(Powder-Headed Tube Lichen)

northeastern United States and in the Atlantic provinces of Canada. Its activity against numerous bacteria has been noted. Work by Stojanovic et al. (2018) determined its activity against two gram-positive and three gram-negative bacteria, as well as its antioxidant activity. The team identified depsidones, 3-hydroxyphysodic, 4-O-methylphysodic acid, physodic, physodalic acid, atranorin, chloroatranorin, atranol, chloroatranol, atraric acid, olivetol, olivetonide, and 3-hydroxyolivetonide.

Yilmaz et al. (2005) looked at extracts of powder-headed tube lichen, and the specific 3-hydroxyphysodic acid constituent. They found the lichen extract and specific constituent active against *Aeromonas hydrophila*, *Bacillus cereus*, *B. subtilis*, *Escherichia coli*, *Klebsiella pneumoniae*, *Listeria monocytogenes*, *Proteus vulgaris*, *Salmonella typhimurium*, *Staphylococcus aureus*, *Enterococcus faecalis*. The last in this list is a drug-resistant pathogenic gram-negative bacterium, common in hospitals, and is associated with sink drains, shower heads, and faucets. It also is found on hand soap and in contaminated disinfectants and hospital suction tubing.

Brownish monk's hood lichen (*Hypogymnia vittata*) is found on northern coasts, generally in conifer forests, but also on mossy, damp soil or on rocks. It contains physodic, vittatolic, and 3-hydroxyphysodic acids.

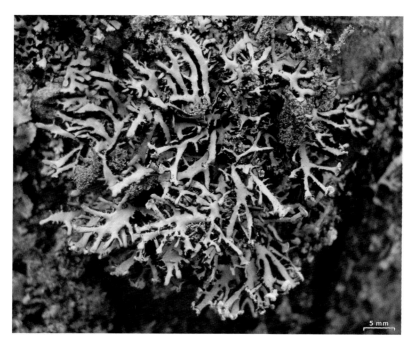

Hypogymnia vittata
(Brownish Monk's Hood Lichen)

HYPOTRACHYNA

Loop Lichens

Geographic Range: North America

Habitat: trees

Medicinal Applications: antibacterial, neurodegenerative diseases, cancer, potential inhibitor of topoisomerases

Notable Chemicals: anziaic acid, atranorin, lividic, physodic, stictic, and usnic acid

There are more than 40 identified species of loop lichen (*Hypotrachyna* sp.) in North America. The genus name derives from the Greek *hypo*, means "under," and *trachys*, "rough."

Bristly loop lichen (*Hypotrachyna horrescens* syn. *Parmelia horrescens*) contains 5-O-methylhiascic acid.

Wrinkled loop lichen (*Hypotrachyna livida* syn. *Parmelia livida*) is very common on trees in the eastern United States, and south to northern Florida and west to Texas. It contains atranorin, lividic acid complex, 4-O-methylphysodic acid, and 3-methoxycolensoic acid. Lividic acid is a major secondary metabolite in this genus. Work by Seiteiglesias et al. (2019) found lividic acid exhibits high antioxidant activity and may be a promising compound for treatment of neurodegenerative diseases such as Alzheimer's and Parkinson's.

The related grainy loop lichen (*Hypotrachyna osseoalba* syn. *Parmelia formosana*) contains lichexanthone and lividic and 2-hydroxycolensoic acids. Work by Sieteiglesias et al. (2019) found that an extract of this lichen improved cell viability in the Fenton reagent-treated SH-SYSY (human neuroblastoma cell) line, suggesting promising multi-targeted neuroprotection, mediated by the reduction of ROS and lipid peroxidation.

Powdered loop lichen (*Hypotrachyna revoluta* syn. *Parmelia revolta*) is found on trees, rocks, and soil in New England/New Brunswick, the Appalachian Mountains, and higher elevations of Wyoming and Colorado. Compounds identified include 8'-methylstictic acid, 8'-methylmenegazziaic acid, stictic acid, 8'-ethylstictic acid, atranorin, hypotrachynic acid, deoxystictic acid (stictinolide), cryptostictinolide, and 8'-methylstictic acid (Papadopoulou et al. 2007).

Green loop lichen (*Hypotrachyna sinuosa*) is the only member of this genus reported to contain usnic acid.

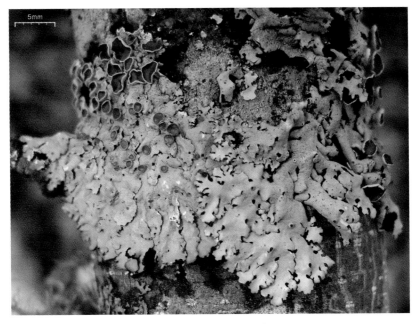

Hypotrachyna livida
(Wrinkled Loop Lichen)

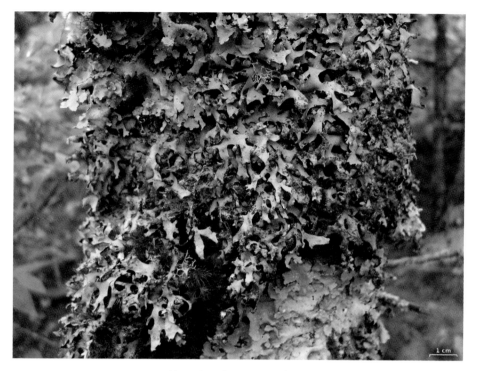

Hypotrachyna revoluta
(Powdered Loop Lichen)

Anziaic acid, from an unidentified species in this group of lichens, is a topoisomerase poison inhibitor. This compound effectively acts as an antibacterial and anticancer agent, due to an accumulation of intermediate DNA cleavage complexes formed by topoisomerase enzymes, which trigger cell death.

This is also significant because anziaic acid (depside) is an inhibitor of both *Yersinia pestis* and *Escherichia coli* topoisomerase I. *In vitro* studies found anziaic acid active against *Bacillus subtilis* and a membrane-permeable strain of *Escherichia coli*. It was found to inhibit human topoisomerase II but had little effect on topoisomerase I (Cheng et al. 2013). (Topoisomerases are DNA processing enzymes necessary for normal cell division. Type I is overexpressed in cancer tumors and a target for chemotherapy.) *Yersinia pestis* is a chemoheterotroph bacteria carried by fleas riding on rats and was responsible for the Black Plague or Death. Up to 200 million people died in Europe and parts of Africa during 1346–1353 CE. Swollen lymph nodes are a common sign of contagion. The disease is still a health concern in parts of Africa and Asia, with a few cases annually in parts of the western United States. It can be treated with antibiotics if administered promptly.

ICMADOPHILA

Candy or Spray Paint Lichen

To study lichens is to get a taste of earth and health.

HENRY DAVID THOREAU

Spray paint or candy lichen (*Icmadophila ericetorum* syn. *Baeomyces aeruginosa*) is the unofficial provincial lichen of Alberta. The genus name derives from the Greek *icmado*, for "moisture," and *phila*, "loving." The species name means "of the heath lands," and peat is certainly one of its favorite habitats. It is a beautiful lichen, but I am probably biased as I live in the province.

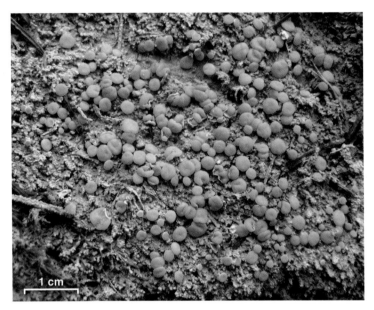

Icmadophila ericetorum
(Spray Paint, Candy Lichen)

LASALLIA

Toadskin Lichens

Geographic Range: colder and elevated regions of North America

Habitat: noncalcareous boulders and cliffs, in sun or shade

Medicinal Applications: cancer, antimicrobial, wound healing

Notable Chemicals: gyrophoric and usnic acid

Common toadskin lichen (*Lasallia papulosa* syn. *Umbilicaria papulosa*) was collected by the Innu of Ekuanitshit in northern Quebec. (*Ekuanitshit* means "where things run aground.") Known as *uakuanapishku* or "rock ear," a tea was prepared with this lichen for those with urinary troubles (Clément 1990; Uprety et al. 2012).

Usually gray, common toadskin lichen is sometimes covered with rusty-red pruina (anthraquinone pigments). Constituents include gyrophoric acid, valsarin (papulosin), 5-chloro-1-O-methylitreorosein, and 5-chloro-1-O-methylemodin. There are polysaccharides among these, significant because polysaccharides show antitumor activity on implanted sarcoma 180 in mice (Shibata et al. 1968).

Pustular toadskin lichen (*Lasallia pustulata* syn. *Umbilicaria pustulata*) has been reported from North America and Europe. Methanol, acetone, and water extracts of this lichen show strong antioxidant activity, and strong anticancer activity against FemX (human melanoma) and LS174 (human colon carcinoma) cell lines (Kosanic et al. 2011; Kosanic et al. 2016). Antiproliferation of MM98 (mesothelioma) and A431 (vulvar carcinoma) cell lines was also noted in work by Burlando et al. (2009). They found wound healing was better when gyrophoric acid and usnic acid were combined.

Ilbäck and Källman (1999) tested the effect of 30% supplementation with this lichen on growth, metabolism, and immune function in mice. After three weeks the growth rate in the lichen group was higher than for the control. Spleen

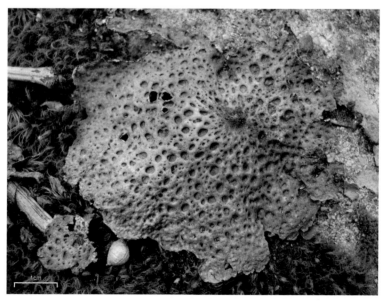

Underside of *Lasallia papulosa* (Common Toadskin Lichen)

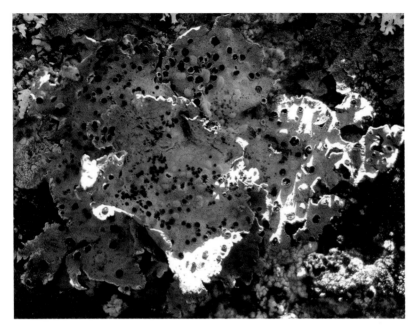

Lasallia papulosa (Common Toadskin Lichen)

B-lymphocyte activity increased by 40%, showing an immune-modulating effect. The lichen as a food could be used in survival settings without adverse effects on metabolism.

Acetone and methanol extracts of this lichen show activity against gram-positive bacteria but resistance against *Escherichia coli*. The largest zone of inhibition by the acetone extract was for *Klebsiella pneumoniae*. Nine of 11 fungi species treated with the extracts were susceptible. Among the fungi, the largest zone of inhibition was for the fungus/mold *Paecilomyces variotii*, which is an emerging opportunistic pathogen. Immune-compromised individuals, especially diabetics and those on long-term corticosteroids, are more susceptible to the fungus. Its presence is related to sinusitis, endophthalmitis, onychomycosis, osteomyelitis, and otitis media, as well as peritonitis in dialysis patients. Water-damaged flooring and carpeting create the perfect environment for contamination with the fungus.

Pustular toadskin lichen was tested for antimicrobial activity and the minimal inhibitory concentration was lowest against *Bacillus mycoides* (Rankovic et al. 2007). This gram-positive bacterium affects fish. One incident where the bacterium caused necrotic lesions in channel catfish was reported in Alabama.

Pustular toadskin lichen exhibits a sun protection factor (SPF) of higher than 5, and better than the SPF 4 of homosalate (Lohézic-Le Dévéhat et al. 2013). Homosalate is a UVB blocker found in 45% of sunscreens sold in the United States. In vitro trials found that homosalate increased breast cancer cell growth by a factor of 3.5. It is an endocrine disruptor and an antagonist affecting estrogen, progesterone, and androgen. Pregnant women would be advised to avoid any products containing this chemical. Sunlight breaks it down into toxic chemicals, and it appears to increase absorption of pesticides. Thus, replacing homosalate in sunscreens could reduce potential health risks. In addition, the lichen showed anti-aging effects on dermal fibroblasts, suggesting protection from UVA radiation as well (Shim 2020).

LECANORA

Rim Lichens

Geographic Range: widespread throughout North America
Habitat: tree bark, rocks, and other substrates
Medicinal Applications: cancer, tea for treating colic
Notable Chemicals: atranorin, epanorin, pannarin, zeorin; psoromic, usnic, lecanoric, and norstictic acids; xanthones

> *To the wall of the old green garden*
> *A butterfly quivering came;*
> *His wings on the sombre lichens*
> *Played like a yellow flame.*
>
> HELEN GRAY CONE

There are more than 180 species, at last count, of *Lecanora* lichens in North America. The genus name derives from the Greek *lekanon,* meaning "a small bowl," and *ora,* "form" or "beauty." Indeed, they are beautiful!

Brown-eyed rim lichen (*Lecanora allophana*) is common on maple and other hardwoods in eastern North America. I have found it on aspen poplar in southwestern Alberta. It contains atranorin.

Varying rim lichen (*Lecanora argopholis*) is found on exposed rocks. One population is found in Alaska, Yukon, Baffin Island and other arctic regions, while another is found in southern Alberta and British Columbia south into west Texas, and across the northern plains to the Great Lakes. It contains epanorin, atranorin, zeorin, and gangaleoidin. The latter compound is also found in the related *Lecanora argentea*, which is found on rocks in northern forests. Epanorin inhibits proliferation of MCF-7 breast cancer cell lines but is not cytotoxic to normal HEK-293 and human fibroblasts in vitro (Palacios-Moreno et al. 2019).

California rim lichen (*Lecanora californica*) contains didechlorolecideoidin, norgangaleoidin, and nephrosteranic acid. The related red Caesar or frosted rim lichen (*L. caesiorubella ssp. caesiorubella*) found on hardwood bark in southeastern North America contains virensic acid, which shows stronger inhibition of alpha-glucosidase than the drug acarbose (Broda et al. 2001).

There are a number of subspecies, including ssp. *merillii*, found in southern California on oak and containing norstictic acid.

Smoky rim lichen (*Lecanora cenisia*) is found on weathered wood or rocks throughout much of North America. It contains atranorin, roccellic acid, and occasionally gangaleoidin.

Brown rim lichen (*Lecanora chlarotera*) is commonly found on tree bark. *Tremella macrobasidiata* was found present in all studied specimens (Tuovinen et al. 2021). The macrofungi *Tremella* species are an important commercial food and medicinal mushrooms (Rogers 2011).

Bearded rim lichen (*Lecanora cinereofusca*) is found in the Pacific Northwest and on the East Coast from Newfoundland south to South Carolina, on hardwoods. It contains pannarin, roccellic acid, and placodiolic acid.

Black-eyed rim lichen (*Lecanora circumborealis*) is widespread on alder, birch, willow, and conifer barks. It contains atranorin and roccellic acid. The related *L. conizaeoides* is yellow to yellow-green and commonly appears on urban trees in eastern North America. Its resistance to pollution allows it to live where there is poor environmental air quality, making it an indicator species.

Cypress rim lichen (*Lecanora cupressi*) is found along the East Coast south to Florida and across the Gulf States. It is a beautiful, bright yellow-orange color, frequently found on bald cypress, hence its common name. It contains usnic acid and zeorin.

Mortar rim lichen (*Lecanora dispersa* syn. *Myriolecis dispersa*) is found on calcareous rocks, but also lives on concrete and mortar in cities. The calcium in rocks helps reduce acid rain and sulfur dioxide effects, so that this lichen can survive pollution in major cities, such as New York. It contains xanthones, pannarin, isonorpannarin, nordechloropannarin, and 2,7-dichloronorlichexanthone.

Rim lichen (*Lecanora epanora*) contains pyxinol, and *L. chlarotera* contains norgangaleoidin.

The lichen *Lecanora epibryon* is rich in 5,7-dichloro-3-O-methylnorlichexanthone, 5,7-dichloro-6-O-methylnorlichexanthone, and 2,5-, 4,7-, and 5,7-dichloronorlichexanthones.

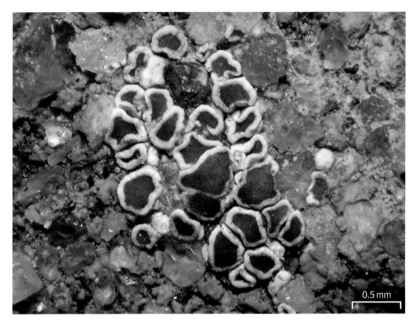

Lecanora dispersa (Mortar Rim Lichen)

Lecanora gangaleoides contains gangaleoidin and leoidin.

Bumpy rim lichen (*Lecanora hybocarpa*) is found on hardwood bark (occasionally conifer) from Nova Scotia south to Florida. It contains atranorin, arthothelin, 6-O-methyl arthothelin, roccellic acid, desmethylhybocarpone, and hybocarpone. The last of these compounds is a cytotoxic, antitumor naphthazarin derivative (Dragana et al. 2014). Work by Ernst-Russell et al. (1999) found hybocarpone to be a potent cytotoxin against the murine P815 mastocytoma cell line, which is often used in mice studies to determine treatment possibilities for melanoma.

Lecanora intumescens contains methyl 2'-O-demethylpsoromate. The related *L. leprosa* contains chlorolecideoidin.

Stonewall rim lichen (*Lecanora muralis* syn. *Protoparmeliopsis muralis*) was prepared as a tea for colic by the Nishinam (Nisenan) living near modern-day Sacramento, California (Powers 1877). The Yuman of northern Mexico know it as *Uja' tebiyauup*, or *Flor de Piedra*. It contains murolic acid, the optical antipode of protoconstipatic acid, as well as neodihydromurolic acid. This lichen shows activity against *Bacillus subtilis* (Rogers 2011), and against *B. cereus*, *B. megaterium*, *Staphylococcus aureus*, and *Klebsiella pneumoniae* (Saenz et al. 2006). It exhibits strong anticancer activity against FemX (melanoma) and LS174 (colon) cell lines (Rankovic et al. 2011). When combined with nanoparticles, its antibacterial activity was observed against *Staphylococcus aureus*, *Escherichia coli*, *Pseudomonas* spp., and *Candida* spp. (Abdullah et al. 2020).

New Mexico rim lichen (*Lecanora novomexicana* syn. *Rhizoplaca novomexicana*) ranges from southwestern Alberta south to New Mexico, growing on rocks in dry, elevated locales. It contains usnic, psoromic, lecanoric, and hypopsoromic acids.

Granite-speck rim lichen (*Lecanora polytropa*) lives on all seven continents. Work by Zhang et al. (2022) revealed up to 103 species in the clade, with 75 corresponding to the nominal taxon *L. polytropa*. The authors suggest this lichen likely ranks as one of the largest species complexes of lichen-forming fungi known to date.

The related seaside sulfur rim lichen (*Lecanora pinguis*) contains zeorin, usnic acid, and thiphanic acid. *Lecanora pseudistera* contains 2'-O-methylhyperlatolic acid.

The lichen *Lecanora rupicola* (syn. *Glaucomaria rupicola* syn. *G. sordida*) contains eugenitin, sordidone, theophanic acid, atranorin, roccellic acid, and eugenitol. The last of these, eugenitol, ameliorates memory impairment in 5XFAD mice by reducing amyloid beta plaques and neuroinflammation. It also ameliorated hippocampal long-term potentiation impairment. This suggests promise in the treatment or alleviation of Alzheimer's disease (Cho et al. 2022).

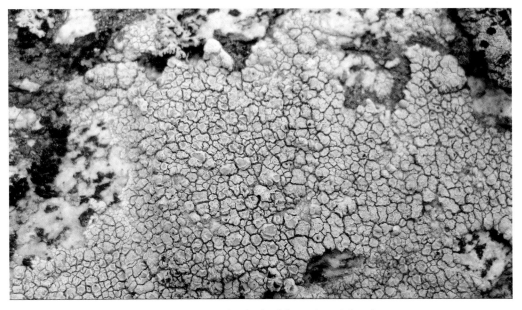

Lecanora rupicola (White Rim Lichen)

Other rim lichens, such as *Lecanora contractula* (syn. *Myriolecis contractula*), contain 5-chloro-6-O-methylnorlichexanthone and 5- and 7-chlorolichexanthone. Both *Lecanora populicola* and *Lecanora salina* contain 2-chloronorlichexanthone. The lichen *Lecanora straminea* (syn. *Myriolecis straminea*) contains 4-, 5-, and 7-chloronorlichexanthone, as well as 2,4- and 4,5-dichloronorlichexanthones. The torrid rim lichen (*Lecanora torrida* syn. *Myriolecis torrida*) contains isonorpannarin, and *Lecanora stenotropa* contains isorangiformic acid. Shrubby rim lichen (*Lecanora phryganitis*) contains usnic acid, zeorin, and thiophanic acid.

Lecanora sulphurea syn. *Lecidia sulphurea* contains leoidin. Work by Taylor and Fourie (2019) found this lichen's extract active against gram-positive bacteria. Leoidin inhibits forkhead box protein M1 (FOXM1). Work by Lee et al. (2021) found cell proliferation of FOXM1 overexpressed cell lines in the breast cancer cell lines MCF-7 and MDA-MB-231.

Maple dust lichen (*Lecanora thysanophora*) is common on maple, beech, basswood, oak, and other hardwoods in eastern North America. As it spreads, it releases alkaline, nitrogen-rich compounds that promote a large community of lichens. It contains usnic acid, atranorin, zeorin, and often porphyrilic acid.

Driftwood rim lichen (*Lecanora xylophila* syn. *L. grantii* syn. *L. riparia*) is found near the coastline of British Columbia, the Atlantic provinces of Canada, and a little farther south. As the name suggests, it frequents shoreline driftwood logs. It contains atranorin.

LECIDEA

Rose Tile Lichen

Art's finest pencil could but rudely mock
The rich grey lichens broider'd on a rock.

JOHN ELLOR TAYLOR (1879)

There are approximately 136 North American *Lecidea* species. They mainly grow on rocks, looking like black dots. More taxonomic research is required.

Rose tile lichen (*Lecidea roseotincta*) from the Appalachian Mountains hosts cystobasidiomycete yeasts (Lendemer et al. 2019). *Lecidia plana* contains 4-O-methylplanaic acid. The related lichen *Lecidea diducens* contains 2'-O-methylanziaic acid. *Lecidea leucophaea*, now known as *Miriquidica leucophaea*, contains normiriquidic acid.

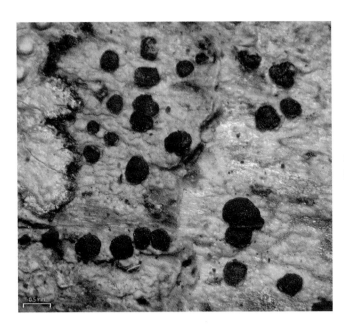

Lecidea roseotincta
(Rose Tile Lichen)

LECIDELLA
Disk Lichens

Twenty-six or so disk lichens (*Lecidella* spp.) live in North America, mainly on calcium-rich rocks, but also on soil, bark, and wood. *Lecidella granulosula* syn. *Lecidea granulate*, usually found on noncalcareous rocks, contains chodatin and demethylchodatin. The disk lichen *L. carpathica* contains 4,5-dichloro-3-O-methyl norlichexanthone, atranorin, diploicin,

Lecidella granulosula
(Disk Lichen)

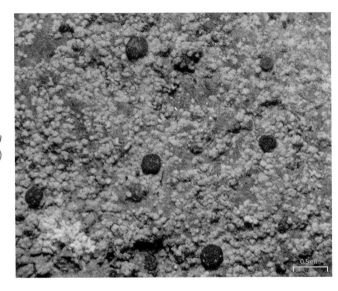

and thuringione. The related *Lecidella. asema* syn. *Lecidea catalinaria* contains 3-O-methylasemone, asemone, and theophanic acid. *Lecidella patavina* syn. *Lecidea spitsbergensis* contains zeorin and atranorin; its hymenium contains drops of oil. The Pacific Coast rock-hugging *Lecidella elaeochromoides* (*Lecidea asema*) contains arthothelin.

LEPRARIA
Dust Lichens

Dust lichens (*Lepraria* species) number about 34, at last count, in North America. As the name suggests, they cannot absorb rain from the sky, due to an inability to absorb water. They absorb their moisture from the air, explaining their need for humid environments.

The terms *Lepraria*, leprosy, leptin, and lepidoptera (butterflies) derive from the Greek, *lepein*, meaning "to peel."

Membranous dust lichen (*Lepraria membranacea* syn. *Leproloma membranaceum* syn. *Amphiloma lanuginosum* syn. *Pannaria lanuginosa*) contains pannaric and roccellic acids.

Zoned dust lichen (*Lepraria neglecta* syn. *Crocynia neglecta* syn. *L. zonata* syn. *L. alpina*) forms concentric "zones" or rings on granite rock. It may also

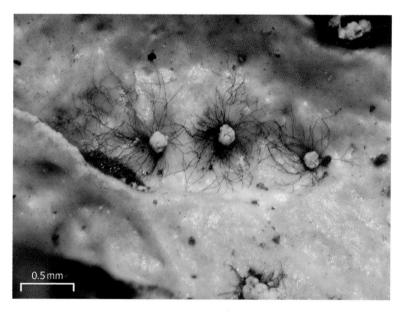

0.5 mm

Lepraria neglecta
(Zoned Dust Lichen)

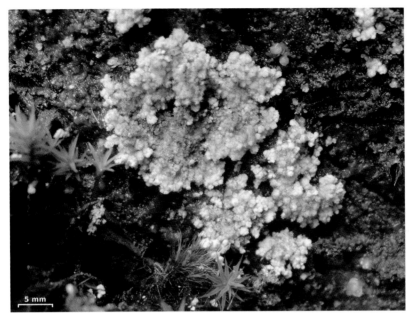

Lepraria lanata

be found associated with moss in the arctic and alpine regions. Its main range, however, is around the Great Lakes to New Brunswick and down Appalachia to South Carolina. The lichen contains psoromic, alectoralic, fumaroprotocetraric, and angardianic acids.

The related *Lepraria lanata* and *Lepraria elobata* are found in the Smoky Mountains and contain angardianic acid. Fluffy dust lichen (*Lepraria lobificans* syn. *L. finkii*) contains atranorin and stictic and constictic acids. Some species contain demethyleprapinic acid. *Lepraria jackii* contains jackinic, toensbergianic, and norjackinic acids. The related *Lepraria rigidula* contains nordechloropannarin.

LEPROCAULON
Sticky Mealy Lichen

Sticky mealy lichen (*Leprocaulon adhaerans* syn. *Lepraria adhaerens* contains pannarin, norpannarin, dechloropannarin, hypopannarin, atranorin and zeorin. The lichen was discovered in North America less than two decades ago, growing on mosses and other lichens.

Pannarin inhibits cell growth and induces apoptosis in DU-145 prostate cancer cells (Russo et al. 2006).

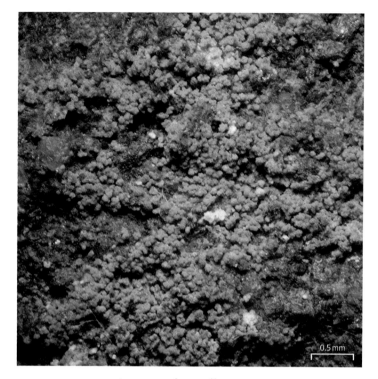

Leprocaulon adhaerens
(Sticky Mealy Lichen)

LEPTOGIUM

Jellyskin Lichens

Blue jellyskin or blue oilskin lichen (*Leptogium cyanescens*) is usually found on bark at the base of trees, and sometimes on fallen logs. It is mainly an eastern North American lichen, but I have found it in mountains of southeastern British Columbia. According to Brodo et al. (2001), this is the most common *Leptogium* of the 53 species on the continent. Ethanol extracts show cytotoxicity against murine leukemia cell lines (Perry et al. 1999).

Bearded jellyskin lichen (*Leptogium saturninum*) is widespread, growing on poplar and willow barks and sometimes on rocks. Its white hairs give the common name. Liers et al. (2011) found that it utilizes a heme peroxidase to help it be successful in extreme microenvironments. This compound may have commercial application for synthetic dyes.

Many of the *Leptogium* species were formerly classified in the genus *Scytinium*. Under the latter name, the Yuman of northern Mexico call this *Lama*.

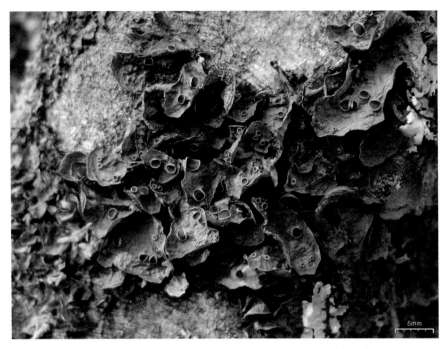

Leptogium corticola (Blistered Jellyskin Lichen)

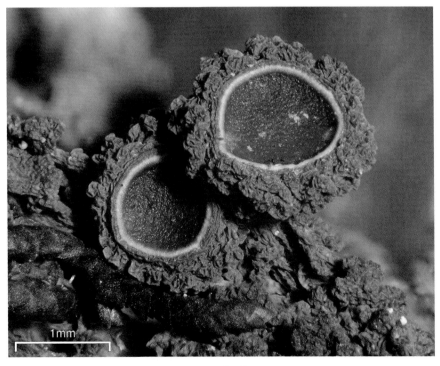

Leptogium phyllocarpum

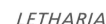

LETHARIA
Wolf Lichens

Geographic Range: North America

Habitat: tree branches, conifers and wood, rarely on rocks

Practical Uses: dyes, body painting, poison for combat

Medicinal Applications: treating skin conditions; soothing effects on the vagus nerve

Notable Chemicals: vulpinic acid

Wolf lichen (*Letharia vulpina* syn. *Evernia vulpina*) was used to kill wolves in Europe in late 1750s, but there is no record of such use on the North American continent. The Latin name literally means "deadly to foxes."

Mountain wolf lichen (*Letharia lupina*) looks similar and may differ only in having a different algae symbiont. Both are close cousins of the beautiful brown-eyed wolf lichen (*Letharia columbiana*), so named for its apothecia that appear eye-like.

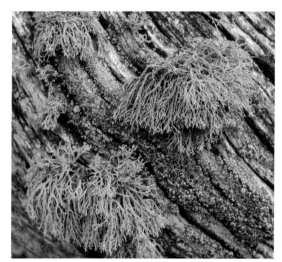

Letharia lupina
(Mountain Wolf Lichen)

Letharia columbiana

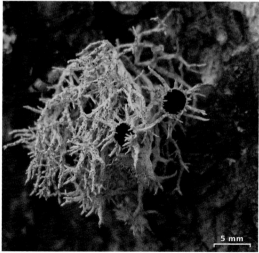

5 mm

Traditional Uses

The Nlaka'pamux (Thompson) of British Columbia know wolf lichen as yellow tree lichen, or /kʷ el'-m-éke?, meaning "light yellow branch." They used the bright yellow dye as face paint, or to color hides, horsehair for bridles, or wool (Turner et al. 1990). It may have been mixed with deer tallow and heated to make the color more fixed.

The Secwepemc (Shuswap) know this bright yellow lichen as *ta-kwul-a-muk'oo*. It was boiled in hot water and used as a hair dye and to color cloth.

The Chilkat Tlingit of Alaska traded fish oil for this lichen known as *sekhone*, using it to dye dancing blankets produced from yellow cedar bark and mountain goat wool. The blankets are still produced and worn today.

The Nuxalk obtained this lichen from the Ulkatcho Carrier, who then traded it to various coastal neighbors. "Wolf lichen was used by virtually all the interior people—the Ktunaxa, and the Salishan and Athapaskan peoples—as well as the Flathead Salish of Montana and the Blackfoot of Alberta" (Turner 1998). Turner notes that the Okanagan would add Oregon grape root bark to intensify the color. The Nlaka'pamux and perhaps others used this lichen to prepare a face and body paint.

The Dene know it as *tagha*, or *telax-tsugh*, "yellow on it," referring to a branch.

Wolf lichen is toxic to meat-eating mammals and insects, but is a source of food, and possibly medicine, for elk, deer, mice, rabbits, and other animals. Despite its toxicity to wolves, several Indigenous groups used this lichen for medicine.

The Cheyenne name is *he-ho-wa-ins'-tots*, and the Gros Ventre call the yellow dye *otsahaa*. Here are some further details on these tribal peoples: The Cheyenne (Suhtai) lived in Minnesota but were driven farther west by white settlers. The name Cheyenne was given them by the Sioux, meaning "a people of a different language." Tsitsistas, as one group prefer to be known, means "Like Hearted People." The Gros Ventre name is believed derived from the French for "big belly" but could be of Blackfoot origin. Today, the Indigenous people prefer to call themselves A'aninin or Haaninin meaning "white clay people."

The Inde (Apache) painted wolf lichen dye crosses on their feet to pass enemy territory unseen.

The Niitsitapii (Blackfoot) of Alberta call wolf lichen *e-simatch-sis*, meaning "yellow dye." This lichen makes an excellent yellow dye for porcupine quills.

Infusions of the lichen, combined with bone marrow, were taken for stomach complaints including ulcers (McClintock 1910).

The Káínawa (Blood) of southern Alberta know this lichen as *isimatsis*, meaning "wild owl cloves." They also used the yellow dye from it for porcupine quills, and as a decoction for constipation in children and to remedy chest pains (Kerik 1981). The lichen was also blackened over a fire and then rubbed on skin sores, rashes, eczema, and warts (Hellson and Gadd 1974).

The Okanagan (Syilx) of British Columbia know wolf lichen as *kware'uk* or *kwernikw*. Weak decoctions were taken for internal conditions, and a stronger decoction was used as a wash for external skin wounds and sores (Teit and Boas 1928; Turner et al. 1980).

The Stl'atl'imx along the Fraser River know this lichen as *kolmákst*, meaning "yellow/green on branch."

Further south, the Imatalamiáma (Umatilla) and Cayuse residing around the Columbia River call wolf lichen *laxpt* or *maqa'hl*. Poultices of the decocted lichen were applied to open sores, boils, bruises, swellings, arthritis, and eye issues. Internal hemorrhages were treated with internal consumption.

The Klamath of Oregon call it yellow moss or *shaw'wisäm*. Klamath tribes include the Klamath, Modoc, and Yahooskin-Paiute, known as *mukluks* and *numu* (the people). They used it to soothe saddle sores that resulted from chaffing on horses (Hunn 1990; 2005).

The Natinixwe or Hupa of Northern California used wolf lichen to dye bear grass (*Xerophyllum tenax*) leaves, and to add color to their woven baskets.

The neighboring Yuki (Yukiah) and Wailaki call wolf lichen *ol-gat'-i*. The lichen was used for inflammation (Chestnut 1902), and to dry up weeping skin sores (Mead 1972). Before settlers, the Yuki knew themselves as Ukomno'om, or "valley people." The name Yuki may derive from their neighbors the Wintu, meaning "enemy." The lichen may have been used as bedding, according to some authors.

Wolf lichen is used by Indigenous people of the Sierra Juarez region of Mexico, in cooled decoctions to wash their hair and remove vermin.

Brown-eyed wolf lichen was gathered in northeastern California by the Achomawi (river people) to poison arrows. An arrowhead would be packed in the wet lichen for up to a year, sometimes with rattlesnake venom added before use (Merriam 1966).

The Yuman of northern Mexico call brown-eyed wolf lichen, *Letharia columbiana*, by the names *toji de manzanita*, *flor de la manzanita*, or *brote de*

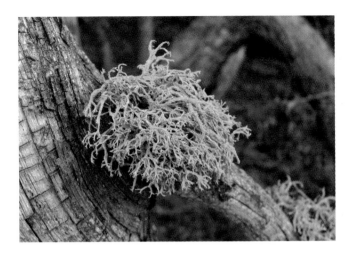

Letharia vulpina
(Wolf Lichen)

la manzanita. Some groups in the region consider it a parasitic plant, calling it *zacatito verde* (little green grass). Other people consider it a decoration on the tree and call it *toje, iwuil mushmá* (branch little root), *kook*, or *hongo de la manzanita*, as it grows on *Arctostaphylos pugens* trees.

Some people use this lichen and golden-eye lichen (*Teloschistes chrysophthalmus*) to decorate their homes, schools, and business. A branch of the tree is provided, on which to string jewelry. Various lichen from the genera *Acarospora*, *Caloplaca*, *Candelariella*, and *Protoparmeliopsis* are also used for home decoration, putting them on plates and watering them.

The bright yellow pigment of this lichen is vulpinic acid and functions as a strong blue-light screening mechanism for the lichen. The lichen also contains 4-hydroxyisovulpinic and 4-hydroxyvulpinic acids.

Wolf lichen (*Letharia vulpina*) essence helps move energy and improve connection between the solar plexus and heart chakras. It soothes and strengthens the vagus nerve, and may be useful in treating food addiction and bulimia. Between the solar plexus and the heart is a place called the alcoholic ocean. It is here that many of today's addictive behaviors begin their journey (Rogers 2016).

LETROUITIA
Spiral-Spored Wolf Lichen

Spiral-spored wolf lichen (*Letrouitia vulpina* syn. *Heterothecium vulpinum* is one of only three *Letrouitia* species found on tree bark in subtropical North America. It contains 8-chlorodioxocondidymic, 8-cholorodioxodidymic, letrouitic, oxodidymic, dioxocondidymic, and dioxodidymic acids.

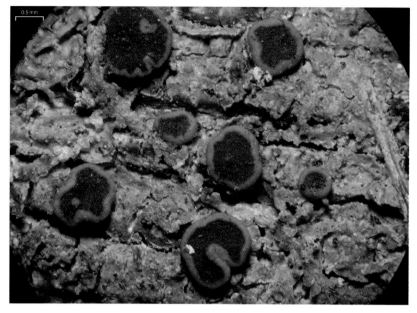

Letrouitia vulpina
(Spiral-Spored Wolf Lichen)

LOBARIA

Lungwort

Geographic Range: Alaska, Pacific Northwest, eastern North America

Habitat: trees

Practical Uses: fermentation, food, skincare

Medicinal Applications: arthritis, colds and flu, eye conditions, fever, fibromyalgia, hayfever, human milk production, intestinal issues, mucus membrane repair, respiratory conditions, skin conditions, stomach, sore throat, spongiform encephalopathy in animals, sheep health, tumors, yeast infections

Notable Chemicals: eumelanin, lichenin, rhizonaldehyde, rhizonyl alcohol; constictic, cryptostictic, fumaric, gyrophoric, methyl stictic, norstictic, oxalic, peristictic, stictic, thelophoric, and usnic acids

It is a lichen day, with a little moist snow falling. The great green lungwort shows now on the oaks.

HENRY DAVID THOREAU

In North America, there are two distinct gene pools for lungwort, one in the Pacific Northwest and the other in the eastern part of the continent. This may be due in part to the influence of the glaciation of the last ice age (Allen et al. 2021).

Lobaria species are widely used by Indigenous people of North America, yet there are only 11 species recorded. The genus name derives from Greek *lobos*, meaning lobe. (The word lobotomy is from the same source.)

That reminds me of a favorite joke I will occasionally pull out when drinking at a brewpub with friends: "I'd rather have a bottle in front of me, than a frontal lobotomy." It usually gets more laughs if told after consuming a few rounds of ale.

Lichens were used in Europe and Russia for brewing, before the Bavarian Beer Purity Law of 1516 allowed only hops, barley, and water be used, and fermentation was dependent on air-borne yeast. Wunderkammer Bier, a Vermont brewery, produces "a smoke beer with mixed culture, lichen, and mushrooms." I would like to try it!

Traditional Uses

The Gitksan (Gitxsan) near the Skeen River in northern British Columbia know the lungwort lichens as frog blankets, *gwilalh ganaaw*. Warm infusions were taken internally as a tonic for sore throats, or as a bath to ease arthritis. This was considered a spiritual and health-promoting spring bathing ritual or therapy (Johnson 1977). (Gitxsan means "people of the river mist.")

People of Haida Gwaii call these lichens *it kaya gysa'ad*, meaning "tree blanket." Lungwort was also called *hlk'inxa kwii'awaay* (forest cloud) or *xil kwii.awaa* (cloud leaves) (Turner 2004, 192–93).

The lungwort lichens *Lobaria pulmonaria* and *Lobaria oregana* and the dogtooth lichens (*Peltigera* spp.) were used as ingredients in Haida medicine.

The Nuxalk (Bella Coola) collected *Lobaria* species only from dogwood (*Cornus stolonifera*) or native crab apple (*Pyrus fusca*) for medicine. A decoction was made and drunk daily for stomach pain, but not for diarrhea, constipation, or vomiting. Also, a decoction was cooled and used as an eyewash. A poultice was applied on skin conditions (Smith 1929; Turner 1973).

The Gitga'at (Gitga'ata) of British Columbia use for *Lobaria oregana* the name *nagaganaw*, meaning "frog dress." They considered this lichen best for medicine when collected from an alpine fir (*Abies lasiocarpa*). It was boiled with juniper needles for a sore throat treatment (Turner and Thompson 2006).

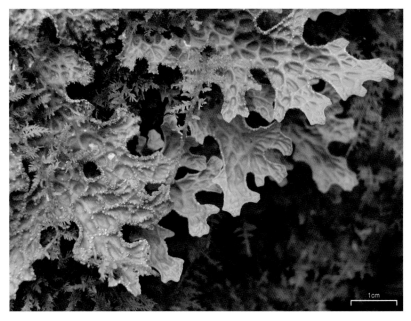

Lobaria pulmonaria
(Lungwort)

This lichen contains cryptostictic, stictic, constictic, norstictic, and methyl stictic acids.

The Nlaka'pamux (Thompson) know it as *tek /qᵂzém* or "yellowish frog moss."

The Tsimshian (Tsm'syen) used it for medicine in an unidentified manner. It is found on both hardwood and conifer trees.

The Hesquiat, from the West Coast, applied this lichen to the faces of children, when their skin was peeling. They also used it as a medicine for people coughing up blood (Turner and Efrat 1982).

The Saanich (WSÁNEC) of Vancouver Island may have used it like *Parmelia sulcata*, for birth control (Turner and Hebda 2012). Both lichens are called *smexdales* by the Saanich. Lung lichen grows on big leaf maple, while waxpaper lichen (*P. sulcata*) is abundant on Garry oak trees.

Smooth lungwort (*Lobaria quercizans* syn. *Ricasolia quercizans*) is found on the East Coast, from Newfoundland to South Carolina. It is commonly found on sugar maple tree bark, but occasionally on rocks.

Smooth lungwort lichen, or one closely related and known as *wakûn*, was used as a food and tonic by the Menomini of Wisconsin (Smith 1923; Brodo et al. 2001). According to one version of a Menomini legend (Smith 1923, 21),

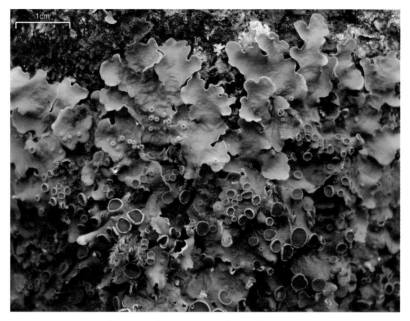

Lobaria quercizans syn. *Ricasolia quercizans*
(Smooth Lungwort)

lichens are the scabs from the head of Mâ'nâpus. He placed the scabs where they are, to keep his uncles and aunts from starving.

Herbalism

As an herbalist I find the word *alterative* interesting, as this means something that makes the eliminatory systems work more efficiently.

Lungwort (*Lobaria pulmonaria*) may be the most well-known medicinal lichen among herbalists and naturopaths. The name forms a rhyming pair, a taxonomic rarity. A few other such binomials are *Chrysanthemum leucanthemum* (ox-eye Daisy), and *Humulus lupulus* (hops).

Its resemblance to lungs is a true representation of the doctrine of signatures. English herbalists like Nicholas Culpeper (1616–1654) called it a kind of moss. He wrote *The English Physician*, later known as *Culpeper's Complete Herbal*, which was published after his passing.

Culpeper wrote,

Jupiter seems to own this herb. It is of great use to physicians to help the diseases of the lungs, and for coughs, wheezings, and shortness of breath, which it cures both in man and beast. It is very profitable to put into lotions that are taken to stay the moist humours that flow to ulcers, and hinder their healing, as also to wash all other ulcers in the privy parts of a man or woman. It is an excellent remedy boiled in beer for broken-winded horses.

As a side note: I have been researching my heritage, and now have determined over 70,000 relatives going back to Europe. One of them turns out to be this very Nicholas Culpeper, explaining in small part my fascination with medical astrology and plant medicine.

An English translation of *Hildegard von Bingen's Physica* by Priscilla Throop (1998) offers this insight in the lichen use.

Lungwort (lunckuwurcz) is cold and a bit dry and not much use to anyone. Nevertheless, one whose lung is swollen so that he coughs and can hardly draw a breath should cook lungwort in wine, and drink it frequently, on an empty stomach. He will become well.

If sheep eat lungwort often, they will become healthy and fat, and it does no harm to their milk. But if, as we said, one who has a swollen lung frequently drinks lungwort cooked in wine, his lungs will return to health, since the lung has the nature of a sheep.

Stehlow and Hertzka (1987) follow up this idea in their book *Hildegard of Bingen's Medicine*. They suggest drinking lungwort tea (with water) three times daily before and after meals, for those with breathing difficulties.

Lungwort is used today in herbal practice to treat various respiratory conditions, including hay fever, colds, and flu, as well as for intermittent fevers and night sweats. Its nourishing and blood-building nutrients are useful for those suffering chronic internal dryness, or for new mothers with scant breast milk.

It may be useful in treating gastric ulcers, as well as ulcerative colitis, combined with appropriate herbs in formula. It helps repair and regenerate mucus membranes and calm reactive mast cells. "Lungwort cough" is dry, wheezing, and persistent, often worse in dry, dusty summers.

Lungwort possesses antirheumatic and analgesic activity, useful in pain occurring between the scapula (shoulders) and occipital bone. Sometimes such pain extends into the chest and shoulders. Myalgia and arthralgia of the small joints may also benefit (Rogers 2011).

Lungwort is found in the homeopathic *Materia Medica*. Lungwort is described there as for a general feeling of dullness and malaise when a cold is coming on. The patient may feel as if floating in air and have a great desire to talk. This is accompanied by dull pressure in the forehead and the root of the nose, with an unsuccessful, constant desire to blow. There may be a dry, hacking cough during the night that is worse on inhalation. The extremities may be red and inflamed. Changes of weather affect the symptoms.

Several practitioners noted that lungwort helped maintain breast milk flow. It may be used in cases of dreams of flying, with the head feeling like it is floating off. The homeopathic *Materia Medica* also indicates it may help in baker's cysts, or fibromyalgia. The dosage is 6X, and the mother tincture is prepared from the fresh thallus.

Medical Uses

Work by Leal et al. (2018) found that methyl stictic acids possess optimal lipophilicity and permeability for skin penetration, suggesting benefit as an external ingredient for prevention of oxidative damage.

The lungwort lichen contains 2-5% lichenin, and stictic, norstictic, sticinic, constictic, peristictic, cryptostictic, methyl stictic, thelophoric, gyrophoric, fumaric and oxalic acids. It also contains essential fatty acids, trace minerals, ergosterol, fucosterol, and tannins.

Part of this lichen's fitness may be due to having more than 800 associated bacterial species (Chavarria-Pizarro et al. 2022). It is a relatively fast-growing lichen, with annual growth up to 4.8 millimeters.

Lungwort water extracts exhibited moderate anti-inflammatory and strong anti-ulcerogenic activity in a rat study (Süleyman et al. 2003). A methanol extract reduced indomethacin-induced gastric ulcers in rats. It increased levels of superoxide, glutathione peroxidase, and glutathione, and reduced lipid peroxidation levels (Karakus et al. 2009).

Eumelanin, derived from the lichen, protects rat livers from induced injury (Altindag et al. 2022). This compound is developed in the thalli from the precursor 3,4-L-dihydroxy-phenylalanine. During melanization, melanosome-like sacs move to the surface and are secreted into cell walls of the fungal hyphae. The melanization helps develop thicker cell walls and provides more protection from UV exposure (Daminova et al. 2022).

Two lichen metabolites, rhizonaldehyde and rhizonyl alcohol, have been identified. The former increased gastric lesions in a lab study, while the latter significantly reduced gastric ulcers, associated with indomethacin (Atalay et al. 2015).

A mixture of acetylated depsidones from lungwort showed moderate inhibition of acetylcholinesterase. This suggests a possible avenue for management of Alzheimer's disease and other neurological conditions (Pejin et al. 2012).

"Mad cow disease," in humans called Creutzfeldt–Jacob disease, a spongiform encephalopathy, is a neurodegenerative disease associated with misfolded prion protein. Three lichen extracts, including *Lobaria pulmonaria*, are the first treatments found to inactivate the proteins of transmissible spongiform encephalopathy (TSE) via lichen protease enzymes (Rodriquez et al. 2012). Tests performed upon infected hamsters, mice, and deer demonstrated clinical efficacy for *Lobaria* extracts (Johnson et al. 2011). It is the mycobiont that provides this prionicidal activity (Weissbuch 2014).

The *Stenotrophomonas* bacterium, found in *Lobaria pulmonaria* lichen, produces spermidine among its main bioactive compounds. This compound affects biofilm formation in various bacteria, including *Vibrio cholerae* (McGinnis et al. 2009). Dietary intake of spermidine improves the diastolic function or left ventricular elasticity in aging mice and probably humans (Eisenberg et al. 2016).

The false lungwort lichen *Lobaria pseudopulmonaria* tests positive for anti-tumor activity (Takahashi 1974).

The tree lichen was probably *Lobaria quercizans f. exsecta*, now known as *Ricasolia amplissima*. According to Smith (1923, 21), it was gathered only from hard maple or hemlock trees.

> It is in a sense a food, and yet a food eaten as a medicine to act as an alterative in run-down systems . . . When wanted for use it is put into soups, where it swells somewhat like Irish moss, and is eaten with a relish . . . it is highly esteemed by the Menomini for its tonic effect on the system and the blood.

This lichen accommodates the endolichenic fungus *Aspergillus versicolor*, which contains a number of interesting compounds. These include diorcinols F–H and 3-methyoxyviolaceol-II, eight bisabolene sesquiterpenoids, two tris(pyrogallol) ethers named sydowiols D and E, and 15 previously identified compounds.

Work by Li et al. (2015) found that some of these isolates inhibit *Candida albicans* and show cytotoxicity against human PC3 (prostate), A549 (lung), A2780 (ovarian), MDA-MB-231 (breast), and HePG2 (hepatic) cancer cell lines.

Reticulated lungwort, also known as smoker's lung lichen (*Lobaria retigera*), is found in British Columbia forests and elsewhere, where it is considered threatened. There are two variations, *retigera* and *subsidiosa*. The former contains retigeranic acids A–D and thelephoric acid. Thelephoric acid inhibits ß-secretase on the amyloid precursor protein that generates neurotoxic amyloid-ß. This suggests it may be useful for the prevention of neurodegenerative dysfunction, especially in Alzheimer's disease (Chon et al. 2016).

The latter variant lichen contains minor amounts of retigeric acids A and C, trace amounts of retigeric acid D, and major amounts of thelephoric acid. It also contains stictic, constictic, cryptostictic, and methyl stictic acids. Retigeric acid B (RAB), a major compound in this lichen, possesses antifungal and anticancer activity.

Candida albicans switches from a yeast to fungal form, creating chronic vaginal yeast infections. This can be more prevalent in women taking birth control pills, antibiotics, or cortisone. Retigeranic acid B, derived from variant *subsidiosa* inhibits adenyl cyclase activity via farnesol production, causing disruption and attenuating the virulence of *Candida albicans*. This includes a decrease in cAMP synthesis, leading to retarded yeast to hyphal transition (Chang et al. 2012).

The related *Candida auris* is an emerging drug-resistant fungal infection, first reported in the ear (hence *auris*) of an elderly Japanese patient. Since then, it has spread around the world and is both difficult to diagnose and resistant to standard antifungal medications, including azoles, echinocandins, and polyenes. The Centers for Disease Control and Prevention reported that cases tripled from 2020 to 2021, to a total of 4,041. According to the World Health Organization, the fungus has a death rate of 29% to 53%. It is found in hospital sinks and on bed rails, curtains, and floors, persisting for up to a month, according to the University of Minnesota's Centers for Infectious Disease Research and Policy. Diabetics, users of antibiotics and catheters, the immune compromised, and patients with organ transplants are especially susceptible to these infections (Sanyaolu et al. 2022).

Early work by Liu et al. (2013) reported retigeric acid B (RAB) as attenuating cell death (apoptosis) in human prostate cancer cells (PC3 and LNCaP), in vitro. The year before, Liu et al. (2012) isolated RAB from *Lobaria kurokawae*, and showed that it inhibited cell growth and induced apoptosis in androgen-independent prostate cancer cells. This work also showed inhibition of phosphorylation levels of l_kBa and the p65 subunit of NF-kappaB. When given to mice carrying RM-1 homografts, RAB inhibited tumor growth and triggered apoptosis by suppressing NF-kappaB activity in

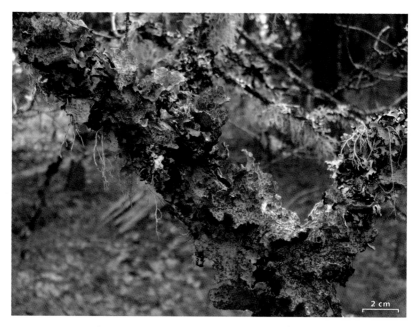

Lobaria scrobiculata (Textured Lungwort)

tumor tissue. More recent work by Liu et al. (2018) found that combining RAB with cisplatin produced significant synergistic cytotoxicity against prostate cancer cells. This works by inhibiting DNA damage repair and activating DR5 (protein death receptor 5).

It is hardly a surprise that this lichen is used in Traditional Chinese Medicine.

Textured lungwort (*Lobaria scrobiculata* syn. *Sticta scrobiculata*) is known to the Yup'ik of Alaska as *qelquaq*. It is generally found west of the continental divide, but also in parts of Newfoundland and Appalachia. This is the most common lungwort containing cyanobacteria, rather than algae, as a photobiont. It can be eaten raw by humans, right from the tree. It contains both *m*-scrobiculin and *p*-scrobiculin, as well as stictic, constictic, norstictic, and usnic acids.

Snails enjoy eating lungwort lichen but avoid the reproductive parts. This is due to a five times higher concentration of meta-scrobiculin there, compared to the somatic parts of this lichen (Asplund et al. 2010).

The cytotoxic metabolites exhibit activity against acute myeloid leukemia (HL-60) cancer cell lines (Schinkovitz et al. 2014).

LOBOTHALLIA

Variable Sunken Disk Lichen

To study lichens is to get a taste of earth and health, to go gnawing the rails and rocks.

Henry David Thoreau

Variable sunken disk lichen (*Lobothallia alphoplaca* syn. *Aspicilia alphoplaca*) is found from Yukon to Arizona, and east to the Great Lakes, growing on acidic granite and sandstone rocks. An acetone extract of this lichen arrests the MCF-7 breast cancer cell line in the G2 phase, whereas the DNA synthesis cell cycle (S) may be inhibited by the extract (Yeash et al. 2017). Work by Letwin (2017) also found activity against MCF-7 breast cancer cells with an IC_{50} of 87.0 µg mL^{-1}.

Methanol extracts of *Lobothallia* exhibit high ferric reducing antioxidant power, and high cytotoxicity against liver and colon cancer cell growth (Kumar et al. 2014).

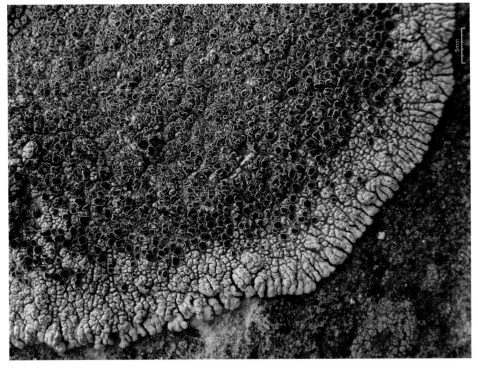

Lobothallia alphoplaca
(Variable Sunken Disk Lichen)

MASONHALEA
Arctic Tumbleweed

Arctic tumbleweed (*Masonhalea richardsonii* syn. *Cetraria richardsonii*) was traditionally used to prime wood fires by Indigenous people from Alaska to the Northwest Territories. This is the only member of the genus worldwide.

The Tlingit of Alaska and Yukon used it as a tea for inflammation of the lungs (Garibaldi 1999).

The neighboring Tutchone call it *hudzi ni* or caribou horn lichen. It was used for a variety of medical conditions and contains alectoronic acid (EDI 2005; Kwanlin Dün First Nation 2017; Na-Cho Nyak Dun First Nation 2015).

Masonhalea richardsonii was recently named the unofficial lichen of Yukon. The genus was named in honor of Mason Hale, an American lichenologist. The species may have been named to honor Sir John Richardson (1787–1865), a member of Sir John Franklin's ill-fated expedition to find the Northwest Passage through the arctic.

MEGALARIA
Dot Lichens

The variegated and fantastic lichens, white and blue, purple and red, all mellowed and mingled into a single garment of beauty.
JOHN RUSKIN (1819–1900),
THE ELEMENTS OF DRAWING

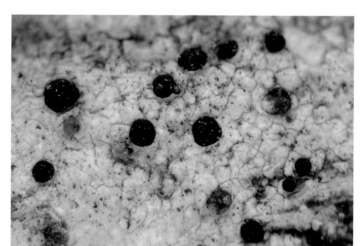

Megalaria laureri

The lichen *Megalaria pulverea* (syn. *Catillaria pulverea*) is found on both northwest and east coasts of North America. It is presently cited as endangered in Nova Scotia. The lichen contains atranorin, zeorin, fumaroprotocetraric acid, and succinsalazinic acid.

MELANELIA
Camouflage or Brown Lichens

Geographic Range: North America

Habitat: rocks, bark of trees

Medicinal Applications: antioxidant, antimicrobial, and anticancer activities; aromatase inhibition; certain species tea used for sore throats, colds, and tuberculosis

Notable Chemicals: 2'-O-methyl anziaic, caperatic, fumarprotocetraric, gyrophoric, lecanoric, perlatolic, and usnic acids

Mealy camouflage lichen (*Melanelia disjuncta* syn. *Montanelia disjuncta*) is widespread on exposed granite rocks. It contains perlatolic and stenosporic acids, with the latter didepside also found in southern strap lichen (*Ramalina stenospora*). Water extracts of mealy camouflage lichen show high nitric oxide scavenging capacity (Kumar et al. 2014). Methanol extracts exhibited high cytotoxicity against both HepG2 (hepatic) and RKO (colon) cancer cell lines.

Shiny camouflage lichen (*Melanelia fulginosa* syn. *M. glabratula*

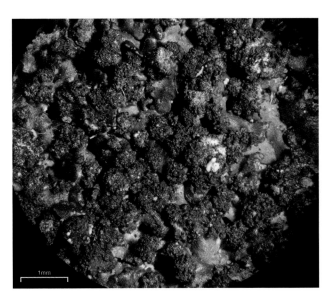

Melanelia disjuncta
(Mealy Camouflage
Lichen)

syn. *Melanelixia glabratula*) is found on bark of conifers and hardwood trees, on both the east and west coasts.

Its cousin abraded camouflage lichen (*Melanelia subaurifera* syn. *Melanelixia subaurifera*) is found from Yukon south to California and across the prairies to eastern provinces and states. It loves all kinds of bark, and is rarely found on rocks. Work by Ristic et al. (2016) looked at the antioxidant, antimicrobial, and anticancer activities of both lichens.

Lecanoric, gyrophoric, and anziaic acids, as well as atranorin, usnic acid, and 2'-O-methyl anziaic acid, were identified in these lichens. The latter compound showed the highest antimicrobial activity, and abraded camouflage lichen showed the highest cytotoxic activity against the tested cancer cell lines.

Rimmed camouflage lichen (*Melanelia hepatizon* syn. *Cetraria hepatizon* syn. *C. polyschiza*) grows on noncalcareous rocks in northern parts of the continent. Work by Ingolfsdottir et al. (2000) showed extracts prevented estrogen formation from estrogen precursors by inhibiting the enzymatic activities of aromatase. Aromatase inhibition is one avenue for preventing or treating hormone-sensitive cancers. As a clinical herbalist I found stinging nettle root, with its aromatase inhibition, useful in formulas for preventing and treating breast and prostate cancers.

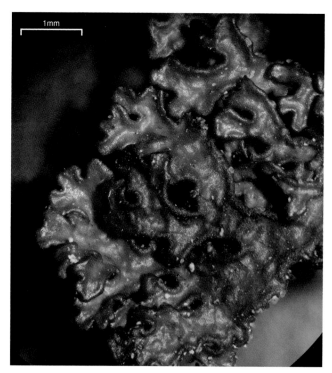

1mm

Melanelia hepatizon (Rimmed Camouflage Lichen)

Alpine camouflage lichen (*Melanelia stygia* syn. *Parmelia stygia*) is common on noncalcareous rocks at high elevation and in the arctic. It contains fumarprotocetraric, caperatic, and norcaperatic acids. The related *Melanelia substygia* may identify as *Montanelia tominii*, *M. saximontana*, or *M. secwepemc*. The lichen contains ovoic acid, which has been poorly studied. Work by Ureña-Vacas et al. (2023) suggests that many compounds such as ovoic, hiascic, lassalic, crustinic, and hypothamnolic acids require more in vivo exploration.

MENEGAZZIA
Tree Flute Lichen

Tree flute lichen (*Menegazzia terebrata* syn. *M. pertusa*) may be found on hardwood trees in damp forests of both coasts. It contains stictic, menegazziaic, and constictic acids.

An endolichenic fungus isolated from this lichen has been found to reverse damage caused by UVB radiation and inhibit melanin synthesis. This suggests UV-protectant properties for avoiding acute and chronic skin diseases, as well as natural sunscreen activity (Zhao et al. 2022).

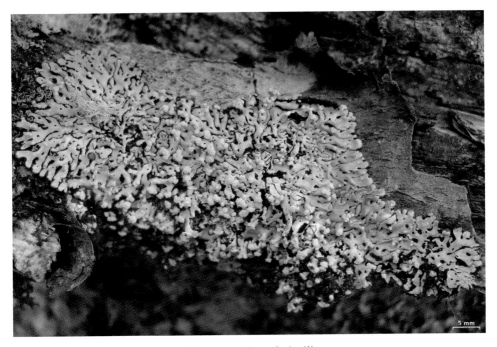

Menegazzia subsimilis
(Tree Flute Lichen)

MICAREA

Dot Lichens

The lichen genus *Micarea*, also named "dot lichens," contains at least 53 species in North America, mainly rich in gyrophoric acid (see the Lichen Chemistry chapter). *Micarea lignaria* syn. *Bacidia lignaria* syn. *Biatora milliaria* contains argopsin. Argopsin (1-chloropannarin) was first isolated from the lichen *Argopsis friesiana*. The compound exhibits in vitro effect on *Leishmania* at 50 μg/ml (Fournet et al. 1997).

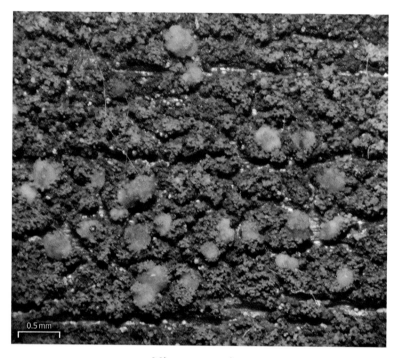

0.5 mm

Micarea prasina

MULTICLAVULA

Club Mushroom

Club mushroom (lichen) (*Multiclavula* sp.) does not strictly meet the definition of a lichen, because its association with algae does not produce a thallus. There are five species in North America, growing on rotting logs, sandy soil, or peat. *Multiclavula mucida* is an eastern boreal club mushroom on shaded rotten logs.

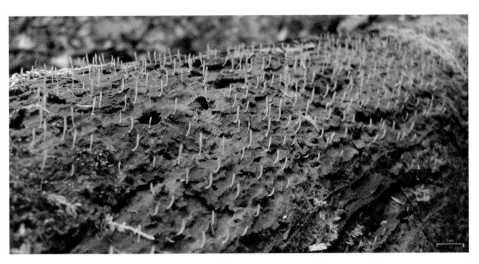

Multiclavula mucida (White Green-Algae Coral)

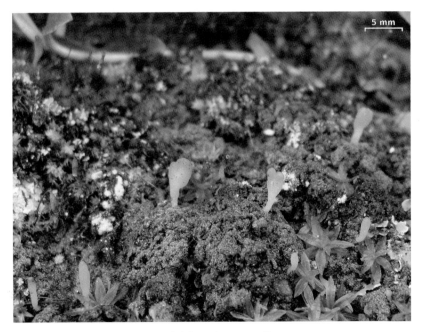

Multiclavula vernalis

One club mushroom is inhabited by an endophytic fungal *Pestalotiopsis* species, which contains seven ambuic acids and derivatives, as well as a torreyanic acid analogue. Ambuic acid and derivative 2 display activity against gram-positive *Staphylococcus aureus* (Ding et al. 2009).

Ambuic acid (AA) exerts anti-inflammatory activity by blocking the ERK/ JNK MAPK signaling pathway, without involving the p38 MAPK or NF-$_k$B signaling route (Zhang et al. 2018). AA inhibits the biosynthesis of the cyclic peptide quromones of gram-positive *Staphylococcus aureus* and *Listeria innocua* (Nakayama et al. 2009). This gram-positive *Listeria* species is innocuous, hence the species name. AA reduced MRSA-induced abscess formation in a mouse model. Further work by Todd et al. (2017) found activity against other *Staphylococcus* species, including *S. epidermis, S. saprophyticus,* and *S. lugdenensis,* as well as *Enterococcus faecalis* and *Listeria monocytogenes.*

The latter *Listeria* species is, however, a virulent pathogen that can remain active in the fridge at 0°C. Each year in the United States about 1,600 people become ill and 260 people die. It can be the cause of meningitis in newborns, killing about 80% of those infected. That is the reasoning behind informing pregnant women to avoid raw milk and soft cheese such as brie, camembert, feta, and queso blanco fresco.

MYELOCHROA

Axil-Bristle Lichens

Powdery axil-bristle lichen (*Myelochroa aurulenta* syn. *Parmelina aurulenta*) is confined to eastern North America, and is found on maple and oak tree bark, in moderately shaded forests.

Powdery axil-bristle lichen (*Myelochroa aurulenta* syn. *Parmelina aurulenta*) contains leucotylic, lyponephroarctin, and 16-O-acetyl-leucotylic acid. The latter compound is more potent and exhibits antiproliferative activity against HL-60

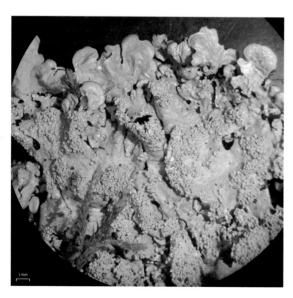

Myelochroa aurulenta
(Powdery Axil-Bristle Lichen)

human leukemia cell lines. Both are structurally related to the antitumor compound betulinic acid, found in birch bark (Tokiwano et al. 2009). There are four axil-bristle (*Myelochroa* species) in east-central North America.

NEPHROMA
Kidney Lichens

Geographic Range: colder and elevated zones of North America

Habitat: among moss in the arctic, elsewhere on mossy rocks and conifers, in humid forests

Practical Uses: food, dye

Medicinal Applications: weakness, tumor, liver and pancreatic conditions, *Candida*, colorectal cancer, sunscreen, antibacterial, antifungal

Notable Chemicals: emodin, fragilin, nephroarctin, and phenarctin

Arctic kidney lichen, or green light lichen (*Nephroma arcticum*), is one of only two *Nephroma* species containing green algae. The other is *N. expallidum*. Nephroma derives from the Greek *nephros*, for kidney.

Indigenous people of Alaska eat the stored, dried arctic kidney lichen by cooking it with crushed fish eggs. The Yup'ik call it *kusskoak*. An infusion is

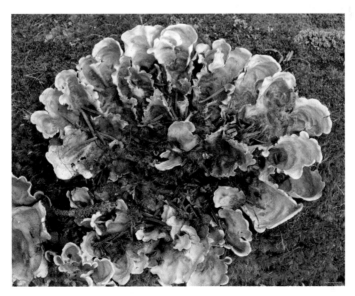

Nephroma arcticum (Arctic Kidney Lichen
or Green Light Lichen)

made with hot water and given to a person in a weakened condition (Oswalt 1957). The lichen is picked in summer and stored until needed. The lichen possess an antifreeze protein for which a patent has expired.

The arctic kidney lichen upper cortex forms an efficient solar radiation screen, providing high UVB tolerance (Váczi et al. 2018). It contains nephroarctin and phenarctin. This lichen exhibits activity against *Aspergillus fumigatus* (Furmanek et al. 2021) (see *Parmelia sulcata*, pages 158–61, for more information).

Mustard kidney lichen (*Nephroma laevigatum*) is abundant on Gabriola Island and other west coast islands. It contains two chlorinated anthraquinones not found in other *Nephroma* species. They are 7-choroemodin and 7,7'-dichlorohypericin (Cohen and Towers 2004). A recent paper by Lagarde et al. (2021) discusses these chlorinated anthraquinones, and new bianthrones. Other studies have identified 7-chloro-1-O-methylemodin, 1-O-methyl fragilin, 8-O-methyl fragilin, fragilin, emodin, 7-chloro-1-O-methylcitreorusein, and 2,2',7,7'-tetrachlorohypericin.

Emodin helps regulate cardiovascular function and atherosclerotic plaque. It has antioxidant, anti-inflammatory, antiproliferative, and lipid-modulating activity (Luo et al. 2021). Emodin shows antitumor effects in colon, liver, and pancreatic cancers (McDonald et al. 2022). The compound helps regulate the immune response in severe acute pancreatitis, in a mouse model. Emodin regulates the ratio of Th1, Th2, Th17, and interferon/interleukin-producing cells (Xiang et al. 2021).

Previous work by Lagarde et al. (2018) examined the antiproliferative and anti-biofilm potential of endolichenic fungi associated with this lichen. Four extracts were active against *Candida albicans*, but all were inactive against *Staphylococcus aureus* and *Pseudomonas aeruginosa* biofilm. However, extracts of two endolichenic fungi, *Nemania serpens* and *Nemania aenea* var. *aureolatum*, were active against human colorectal (HT-29 and HT116) and prostate (PC-3 and DU145) cancer cell lines. Induction of apoptosis was through activation of caspases 8 and 3, poly (ADP-ribose) polymerase cleavage, and DNA fragmentation (Legarde et al. 2018).

Mycosporines and mycosporine-like amino acids are UV protectants. The mycosporine hydroxyglutamicol was isolated from this lichen (Roullier et al. 2011).

Powdery kidney lichen (*Nephroma parile*) is widespread from northern Alaska, south to Oregon, and into the mountains south to Arizona. It is also found around the Great Lakes, east to Newfoundland, south to New England,

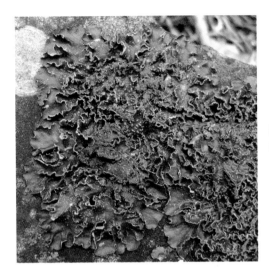

Nephroma parile
(Powdery Kidney Lichen)

and in the Appalachian Mountains. Few compounds have been identified, but it yields a blue dye, traditionally used in Scotland.

It should be noted that there is no correlation between the color of the lichen and the color obtained by boiling with wool. Gyrophoric, evernic and lecanoric acids, as well as erythrin, convert to a purple compound in the presence of oxygen and ammonia. The material yielding the richest dye is picked in August.

NIEBLA

Fog Lichen

The lichenist extracts nutriment from the very crust of the earth.

HENRY DAVID THOREAU

Armored fog lichen (*Niebla homalea* syn. *Desmazieria homalea*) is found on rocks in California and down the Baja peninsula. The Yuman of northern Mexico refer to this lichen as *Toji*. It contains various metabolites, including chlorine-rich nieblastictanes A–C, nieblaflavicanes A and B, other stictanes, and usnic, sekikaic, and divaricatic acids and divaricatinic acid methyl ester.

Usnic acid from this lichen exhibited moderately potent antiproliferative activity against A2780 (ovarian) and MCF-7 (breast) cancer cell lines (Zhang et al. 2020).

A fungal associate of the lichen, *Penicillium aurantiacobrunneum*, contains 4-epi-citreovirdin, auransterol, analogues of paxisterol, and

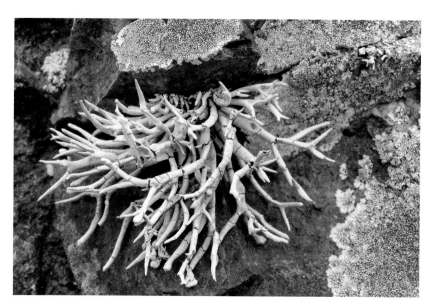

Niebla procera

two (15R˙,20S˙)-dihydroxyepisterols. 4-epi-Citreovirdin shows selective cyto-toxicity toward MCF-7 breast cancer and A2780 ovarian cancer cells (Tan et al. 2019). Auransterol and epi-citreovirdin (paxisterol derivatives) were incorporated with a fluorine atom, resulting in 7-monofluoroacetyl paxisterol. This compound may have increased pharmacological and pharmacokinetic benefits (Yamano and Rakotondraibe 2022).

Tumidulin was isolated from a *Niebla* species from Chile. Work by Yang et al. (2018) suggests tumidulin decreases the stemness potential of colorectal cancer cells. *Stemness* refers to the ability of cells to self-regenerate.

A study of this lichen by Diaz-Allen et al. (2021) identified five noncytotoxic new triterpenoids, and three known triterpenoids.

OCELLULARIA
Volcano Lichens

There are 12 volcano lichens (*Ocellularia* sp.) in North America, usually found on subtropical tree bark. They contain various ß-orcinol depsidones such as psoromic or hypoprotocetraric acid, or gyrophoric acid (depside).

Hollow volcano lichen (*Ocellularia cavata*) contains cinchonaric and concinchonaric acid. The species name derived from the Latin *cavō*, meaning "hollow out" or "excavate."

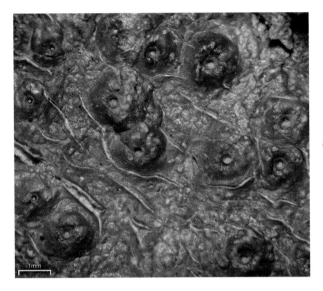

Ocellularia praestans

OCHROLECHIA

Saucer Lichens

Saucer lichens (*Ochrolechia* sp.) have been investigated for antibacterial and antioxidant activity (Kim et al. 2014).

Coral saucer lichen (*Ochrolechia yasudae*) is found on oak bark and granite in shaded Appalachian hardwood forests. Work by Joshi et al. (2010) found

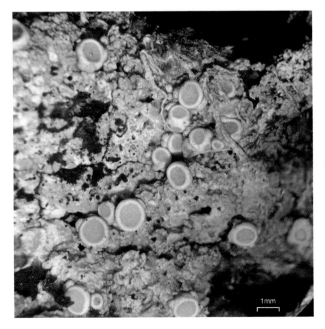

Ochrolechia mexicana

a lichenicolous fungus, *Dactylospora glaucomarioides*, growing on the thallus. More research is required. *Ochrolechia subisidiata* is a southwestern lichen species that contains variolaric acid, which shows potential to inhibit SARS-Cov-2 (Gupta et al. 2022).

OPEGRAPHA
Scribble Lichens

There are estimated to be, at last count, 42 *Opegrapha* species in North America. The genus name derives from the Greek *opê*, meaning "opening," and *grapha*, "to write," in reference to the scribbled appearance of the lichen on tree bark.

One member, *Opegrapha vulgata*, hosts cystobasidiomycete yeasts, a relatively rare occurrence (Lendemer et al. 2019).

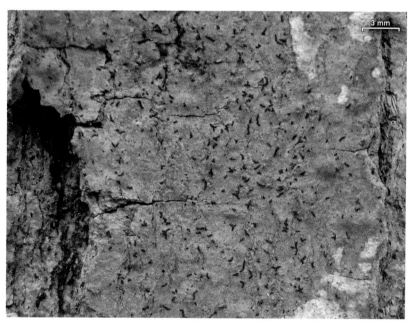

Opegrapha vulgata

OPHIOPARMA
Bloodspot Lichens

Alpine bloodspot lichen (*Ophioparma ventosa* syn. *Lecanora ventosa*) is used as a source of natural reddish-purple to magenta dye. It is found on noncalcareous rocks in arctic and alpine regions.

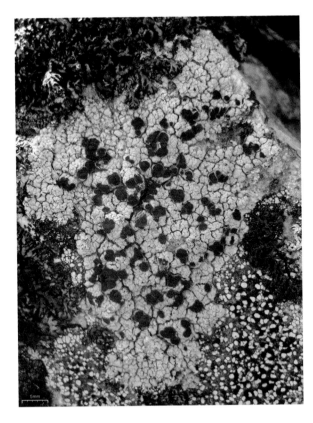

Ophioparma ventosa
(Alpine Bloodspot Lichen)

A secondary metabolite from this lichen has been identified as miriquidic acid (Le Pogam et al. 2016). Further research by Le Pogam et al. (2016a) isolated four quinonoid naphtopyranones from the lichen—ophioparmin, 4-methylhaemoventosins (2a and 2b), and 4-hydroxyhaemoventosin—as well as anhydrofusarubin lactone and haemoventosin. The latter compound is antioxidant, but also exhibits significant cytotoxicity against a panel of nine cancer cell lines.

OXNERIA

Hooded Sunburst Lichen

The lichen *Oxneria fallax* syn. *Xanthomendoza fallax* is known to the Yuman of northern Mexico as *ipa tebiyauup*, meaning "stick flower." The genus is named to honor the Ukrainian lichenologist Alfred Mycllayovych Oxner. The lichen contains parietin, fallacinal, emodin, teloschistin and parietinic acid. Parietinic acid exhibits potential against *Mycobacterium tuberculosis*, a pathogen becoming increasingly drug-resistant (Pant et al. 2021).

PANNARIA

Mouse Lichen   Shingle Lichen

There are 8 to 10 *Pannaria* species in North America at last count. Most of them contain (unsurprisingly) the compound pannarin. They are found on wood or soil, and rarely on rocks.

Mealy-rimmed shingle lichen (*Pannaria conoplea*) is found on tree bark in southern Nova Scotia and northern Ontario around Lake Superior, as well as at higher elevations in Colorado and along the southern borders of Arizona and New Mexico.

Work by Russo et al. (2006) found pannarin inhibits cell growth and induces apoptosis in human prostate carcinoma DU-145 cells. Activity on prostate cancer cells by sphaerophorin and epiphorellic acid-1 was noted, but the action was significantly weaker than with pannarin. When pannarin was tested against MRSA (methicillin-resistant *Staphylococcus aureus*) it was found to be synergistic with gentamicin, but antagonistic when combined with levofloxacin (Celenza et al. 2012).

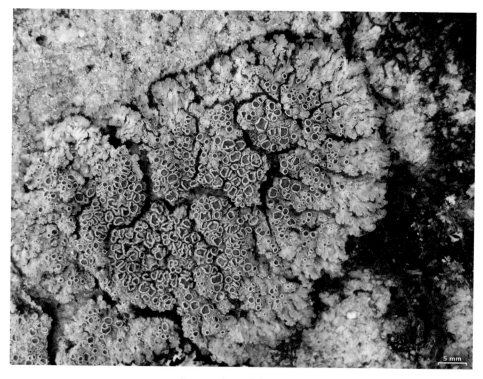

Pannaria rubiginosa

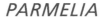

PARMELIA

Shield Lichens   Stone Flower Lichen   Waxpaper Lichen

Geographic Range: throughout North America

Habitat: tree bark, rocks, and soil

Medicinal Applications: antibacterial, antifungal, arthritis, burn treatment, cancer, colic, diabetes, epilepsy, teething, yellow fever

Notable Chemicals: atranorin, chloroatranorin; baeomycesic, diffractaic, gyrophoric, protocetraric, protolichesterinic, salazinic, pinastric, stictic, and usnic acids; ergosterol and tinctorinone

Common greenshield lichen (*Parmelia caperata* syn. *Flavoparmelia caperata* syn. *Pseudoparmelia caperata*) is present on tree bark, ranging from Manitoba to Nova Scotia, and south to Texas and Mexico. The Tarahumara (Rarámuri) of Chihuahua, Mexico collected and dried it into a powder to sprinkle on burns.

Reduction of paw edema inflammation and liver oxidative stress was noted by Salem et al. (2021). Levels of superoxide dismutase (SOD), glutathione peroxidase, and glutathione levels increased in this mouse study. Pinastric acid and ergosterol have been isolated from common greenshield lichen. The former is also found in *Vulpicida pinastri*, and possesses antiviral, antibacterial, and antitumor activity (Dias et al. 2007). Earlier work by Gupta et al. (2007) found ethanol extracts exhibit moderate activity against the *Mycobacterium tuberculosis* strains H37Rv and Ra.

Stone flower lichen (*Parmelia perlata* syn. *Parmotrema perlatum*) contains salazinic and stictic acids, atranorin, and chloroatranorin. Work by Bézivin et al. (2003) found that hexane fractions show the most activity against cancer cell lines. The methanol extract exhibited the highest free radical scavenging activity (Manojlovic et al. 2021). The polysaccharide fraction showed activity against the yellow fever virus, possibly through an attack on the viral envelope (Esimone et al. 2007).

Parmelia reticulata syn. *Parmotrema reticulatum* contains a number of antifungal constituents, including protolichesterinic acid, effective against *Rhizoctonia solani* and *Pythium debaryanum*, and atranorin, active against *Sclerotium rolfsii*. The antifungal activity of protolichesterinic was found comparable to the commercial fungicide hexaconazole (Goel et al. 2011). Other constituents, or secondary metabolites, in this lichen are isousnic acid, evernyl, ethyl hematommate, ethyl orsellinate, methyl hematommate, and baeomycesic and salazinic acids.

Rock shield or salted shield lichen (*Parmelia saxatilis*) accumulates the rare mineral beryllium from its host rocks. The James Webb Space Telescope has 18 hexagonal gold-plated beryllium mirrors, contributing to its ability to withstand severe temperature fluctuations.

The average human body contains 35 µg of beryllium, which displaces magnesium. Homeopathic *beryllium metallicum* was first proved by W. Lees Templeton in 1953 on seven healthy volunteers.

Rock shield lichen may have benefit in acute viral respiratory conditions, with symptoms of pneumonia or severe bronchitis (Stahl and Bagot 2020). It is relatively fast-growing as lichens go, increasing by an average of 3.4 millimeters annually.

The Nishinam (Nisenan) of Northern California call it *wa'-hat-tak* and collect it for a tea infusion to treat colic. Work by Kosanic et al. (2012) found it had a higher free radical scavenging activity than its cousin waxpaper lichen (*Parmelia sulcata*), which is a more active antimicrobial. Extracts from both of these lichens possess strong anticancer activity.

In terms of the components found in *Parmelia* species, salazinic acid shows stronger antioxidant activity than protocetraric acid, but both are active against FemX (human melanoma) and LS174 (human colon carcinoma) cell lines (Manojlovic et al. 2012). Protocetraric acid, found in *P. caperata* is, however, cytotoxic to human melanoma and colon carcinoma cell lines (Brandão et al. 2012).

Gyrophoric acid, derived from *Parmelia saxatilis*, is an angiotensin II type-1 receptor antagonist (Huo et al. 2019), suggesting cardiovascular benefit. The salazinic acid derived from this lichen inhibits *Mycobacterium aurum* (Ingólfsdóttir et al. 1998). Methanol extracts exhibit cytotoxic activity (Ingólfsdóttir et al. 1985). *Parmelia saxatilis* also contains diffractaic B, salazinin A, and usnic acid. It is used in Traditional Chinese Medicine and known as *shih hua*.

In fifteenth-century Europe, this lichen was known as *Muscus cranii humani* when found growing on human skulls. It was used to treat epilepsy and sold for its weight in gold (see also *Usnea*, page 240).

Hammered shield lichen (*Parmelia sulcata*) was used traditionally by the Metis of Alberta to comfort teething pain in children. It was simply rubbed on the gums to relieve restlessness and help them sleep (Marles et al. 2000).

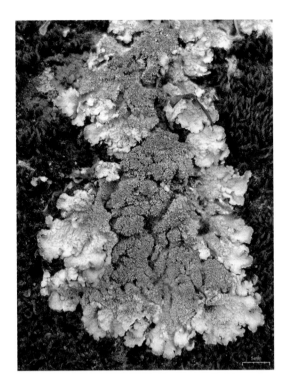

Parmelia saxatilis
(Rock Shield or
Salted Shield Lichen)

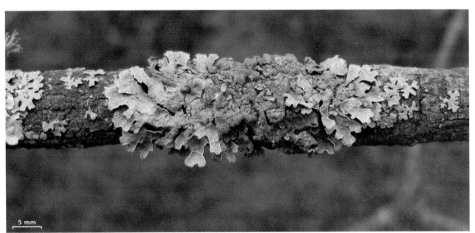

Parmelia sulcata (Waxpaper lichen)

The sulcate (parallel groove) markings on the surface are an example of the doctrine of signatures (which proposes that plants resembling a part of the body can be used to treat that part of the body), suggesting it may be useful for brain and cranial issues. Also known as waxpaper lichen, the Cree healer Russell Willier called it *waskwiya*. When found on diamond willow trees, hammered shield lichen is chewed and put on the gums for a half minute in babies with teething pain. The sap or syrup is used for sugar diabetes. Willier noted that it is an excellent fire starter. He passed on a few years ago.

Dr. David Young, Russell Willier, and I (2015) collaborated on the book *A Cree Healer and His Medicine Bundle*. The information shared was passed down orally to the oldest son for 10 generations, and Russell felt comfortable sharing this knowledge with others. The publication only came to fruition as I lived near Russell in northern Alberta for a number of years, and David Young et al. (1989) had previously written a book on Russell's life.

The Saanich of Vancouver Island know this lichen as *smexdales*. It is believed the tree it grows on gives it differing medicinal properties. The same name was used for lung lichen (*Lobaria pulmonaria*). Rufous hummingbirds use it to hide their small nests, and to disinfect them from mites, ticks, and other insects.

Hammered shield lichen may have been used traditionally for birth control (Turner and Hebda 2012). Methanol extracts of *Parmelia sulcata* were found to induce apoptosis in human lung (A549), prostate (PC3), and liver (Hep3B) and rat glioma (C6) cancer cell lines (Ari et al. 2014a). A year after that discovery, Ari et al. (2015) tested the lichen extract inhibition on MCF-7 and MDA-MB-231 cancer cell lines, with induced caspase-independent apoptosis.

This lichen shows activity against a vast range of bacteria and fungi (Candan et al. 2007; Rankovic et al. 2007). These include *Aeromonas hydrophila*, *Bacillus cereus*, *B. mycoides*, *B. subtilis*, *Enterobacter cloacae*, *Klebsiella pneumoniae*, *Listeria monocytogenes*, *Proteus vulgaris*, *Yersinia enterocolitica*, *Staphylococcus aureus*, *Streptococcus faecalis*, and 15 fungal species. This has added significance because *Enterobacter cloacae* is part of the normal human gut flora but has been implicated in hospital contagion scenarios that involved heparin paraphernalia. One interesting mouse experiment found bacteria-free mice retained their weight, while those with this gut bacteria were more obese.

Nanosilver-reinforced extracts of waxpaper lichen (*Parmelia sulcata*) are cytotoxic to MCF-7 breast cancer cells, but not to normal cells (NIH3T3). Such downregulation of inflammatory genes (TNF-alpha and IL-6) and cell cycle genes (PCNA and Cyclin-D1) promotes the intrinsic apoptotic pathway (Gandhi et al. 2021).

Waxpaper lichen shows antibacterial activity against *Bacillus subtilis*, *Pseudomonas aeruginosa*, *Escherichia coli*, and *Klebsiella pneumoniae* (Gandhi et al. 2022), and antifungal activity against *Aspergillus fumigatus* (Furmanek et al. 2021). This pathogenic fungus can create serious infection and death in immune-compromised individuals. Known as pulmonary aspergillosis, the illness is responsible for 600,000 deaths annually, with a 25–90% mortality rate. Azole-type drugs were at one time beneficial but their low-level use in agriculture has created drug resistance. Ironically, the fungus contains spirotryprostatin B, which is antimitotic and a novel cell cycle inhibitor (Cui et al. 1996).

Fascinating work by Johnson et al. (2011) found that extracts from waxpaper lichen, as well as from *Cladonia rangiferina* and *Lobaria pulmonaria*, degrade prion protein from transmissible spongiform encephalopathy (TSE)-infected hamsters, mice, and deer. Research suggests a serine protease is involved, and that freshly collected lichen or its water extracts reduce infected brain homogenates. Also known as chronic wasting disease (CWD), this misfolded prion protein disease affects mule and white-tail deer, moose, caribou, and elk. It is widespread in North America, due to elk ranching and its escape into wild animals. It has long been believed that CWD cannot be transmitted to humans, but recent work by Hannaoui et al. (2022) suggests potential transmission to humans is possible. Of course, there is now a concerted effort to create a vaccine. As they say, it is probably too late after the horse has left the barn, or in this case, after elk and deer disease has escaped the ranch.

PARMOTREMA

Ruffle Lichen   Scatter Rug Lichen

Geographic Range: mainly in southeastern United States, especially coastal plains
Habitat: bark and twigs, trees, mossy rocks
Medicinal Applications: antibacterial, anthelmintic, cancer, digestion
Notable Chemicals: atranorin, diffractaic, evernic, gyrophoric, isolecanoric, lecanoric, protocetraric, norstictic, salazinic, stictic, and usnic acids; lupeol, tinctorinone, zeorin

Medical Uses

Extracts from palm ruffle lichen (*Parmelia tinctorum* syn. *Parmotrema tinctorum* showed no activity against gram-negative bacteria, but inhibited methicillin-resistant *Staphylococcus aureus* (MRSA) (Shiromi et al. 2021).

Significant antioxidant activity and inhibitory potential against carbohydrate digestive enzyme and aldose reductase suggest use of palm ruffle lichen as a possible functional food or nutraceutical for diabetes (Raj et al. 2014).

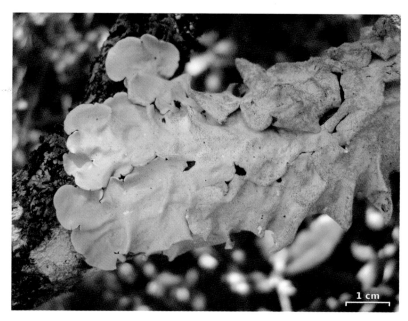

Parmotrema tinctorum (Palm Ruffle Lichen)

Amylase inhibition from extracts of this lichen was noted in work by Vinayaka et al. (2013) and Raj et al. (2014). Early work by Kumar and Müller (1999) found the palm ruffle lichen constituents gyrophoric, usnic, and diffractaic acids are potent antiproliferative agents and inhibit cancer cell growth. Palm ruffle lichen (*Parmotrema tinctorum*) also contains the phenol compounds 2-ethylhexyl orsellinate and tinctorinone. Work by Bui et al. (2022) found that tinctorinone showed strong inhibition of alpha-glucosidase, suggesting possible benefit in blood sugar dysregulation.

This lichen has been studied for reducing viability of cancer cells by Suresh and Nadumane (2021). At the cellular level, induction of apoptosis and inhibition of angiogenesis were confirmed. The bioactive fraction was found nontoxic to normal human peripheral lymphocytes. Two compounds, 5-methyl-1,3-benzenediol and its derivative methyl-2,4-dihydroxy-6-methylbenzoate, were identified in the bioactive fraction.

Phenolic derivatives isolated from this lichen by Kumar et al. (2020) show strong free radical scavenging (comparable to Trolox), and moderate inhibition of advanced glycation end products associated with blood sugar dysregulation. A study by Ahmed et al. (2019) investigated the potential of the lichen for treating arthritis, a traditional use. The lichen shows immune-modulating activity (Santos et al. 2004). Arthritis was induced in rats using Freund's complete adjuvant, and then treated with an extract of this lichen. Inhibition of edema and arthritic score were noted.

Methyl gamma-orsellinate, atranorin, and usnic acid were identified in this lichen, as well as a novel isophthalic ester derivative. Other work identified lecanoric and isolecanoric acid, evernic acid, ethyl orsellinate, and 3,5-dihydroxytoluene. The latter may be residual from the extraction. Lecanoric acid and its derivative orsellinates have been studied for cytotoxicity against Hep2 (larynx), MCF-7 (breast), and 786-0 (kidney) carcinoma, as well as B16-F10 murine melanoma cell lines (Bogo et al. 2010). The compound *n*-butyl orsellinate was the most active against all cell lines tested, and more active against melanoma cells than the chemotherapy drug cisplatin. Ethyl orsellinate was more active against Hep2 (larynx) cells than the other three compounds.

Palm ruffle lichen extracts also show activity against *Onchocerca ochengi*, a parasitic worm that affects cattle (Kang et al. 2022).

Lecythophora sp. FL1375 is an endolichenic fungus isolated from this lichen. Wijeratne et al. (2016) identified oxaspirol B from the fungus, which showed moderate p97 ATPase inhibition. Further work suggests this compound is a reversible, non-ATP-competitive, and specific inhibitor of p97. This is significant because p97 plays an essential role in homeostasis, and its mutations are associated with numerous neurodegenerative conditions, plus overexpression of wild-type p97 is associated with various cancers. This p97 is also essential for the replication of various viruses, including poliovirus, herpes simplex virus, cytomegalovirus (HCMV), and influenza (Huryn et al. 2020).

The human cytomegalovirus (HCMV) is a beta herpes virus and a leading cause of congenital infections. It inflicts a great risk on immune-compromised individuals, can result in mononucleosis, and is associated with development of various cancers and chronic inflammatory cardiovascular disease. The virus has coevolved with mammals for millions of years and perturbs macrophage identity. In newborn children it may cause hearing loss and is disproportionally associated with higher levels of mortality in African Americans and Native Americans.

Unwhiskered ruffle lichen (*Parmotrema austrosinense* syn. *Parmelia austrosinensis*) is found on bark and twigs in diverse areas, in the subtropical states of Texas, Mississippi, Louisiana, and neighboring states, as well as in pockets of New Mexico and California. It contains cristiferides A and B, lecanoric acid, orsellinic acid, 5-chloro-orsellinic acid, methyl haematommate, and methyl ß-orsellinate. Work by Pham et al. (2022) found that cristiferide B and methyl haematommate exert potent alpha-glucosidase inhibition. Cristifones A and B also inhibit this enzyme, which prevents the breakdown and absorption of glucose into the bloodstream (Do et al. 2023). Parmoferone A, a new depsidone from this lichen, is a potent noncompetitive inhibitor of alpha-glucosidase (Duong et al. 2023).

Atranorin found in this lichen increased growth of the probiotic *Lactobacillus casei* (Gaikwad et al. 2014). An endolichenic fungus isolated from this lichen was analyzed, and found to contain (3*R*)-5-hydroxymellein, which has UVA absorption activity. The antioxidant level was high when compared to ascorbic acid and butylated hydroxyanisole (BHA). No toxicity to normal cell lines was noted, and it recovered damage caused by UVB irradiation and inhibited melanin synthesis. This suggests development of a skin UV-protectant product (Zhao et al. 2016).

Fertile cracked ruffle lichen (*Parmotrema cetratum* syn. *Rimelia cetrata* syn. *Parmelia cetrata*) is found on oak and maple trees in the southeastern United States. It contains the unusual components threitol and volemitol, as well as galactose (2%) (Da Silva et al. 1993). Threitol is a four-carbon sugar ($C_4H_{10}O_4$) also found in the honey mushroom (*Armillaria mellea*). Its structure is a diastereomer of erythritol, an alcohol sugar widely used in sugar-free products. The Alaskan beetle *Upis ceramboides* uses threitol as an antifreeze protectant. Volemitol is a seven-carbon sugar alcohol found widely in moss, mushrooms, and elsewhere. It is a natural sweetener, identified originally by Émile Bourquelot from the mushroom *Lactarius volemus* in 1889.

This lichen also contains salazinic and hypostictic acid, which show antiproliferative activity against K562 (leukemia), HT29 (colon), and B16-F10 (melanoma) cancer cell lines. In vivo, mice fed this lichen showed no sign of systemic toxicity, and the metabolites inhibited tumor growth in relation to weight and 88% of tumor volume (Alexandrino et al. 2019).

Fertile cracked ruffle lichen exhibits antimicrobial activity against *Vibrio fischeri*, and anthelmintic activity against the nematode *Caenorhabditis elegans* (Nugraha et al. 2020). This *Vibrio* species is generally found in salt water and is bioluminescent. It is not a serious pathogen like its cousin *V. cholerae*. Research has shown it deregulates the expression of peroxidase in tissue. The nematode is used in laboratory work related to the nervous system, metabolism, and aging. Three Nobel Prizes, in 2002, 2006, and 2008, were rewarded for work involving this organism. It is often studied for nicotine dependency due to its reactions that parallel those of mammals.

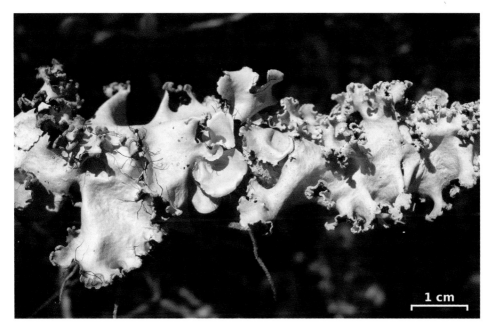

Parmotrema dilatatum (Cracked Ruffle Lichen)

Salted ruffle lichen (*Parmotrema crinitum* syn. *Pamelia proboscidea*) may be found on mossy rocks or on the bark of eastern cedar or other deciduous trees. Its range is from the Great Lakes to Nova Scotia and the throughout the southeastern United States, south to the tip of Florida. It is the only common isidiate *Parmotrema* containing stictic acid, but also atranorin, 9-alpha-hydroxymenegazziaic acid, and cryptoconstictic acid (3-O-methylsalazinic acid).

Cracked ruffle lichen (*Parmotrema dilatatum*) is restricted in North America to Florida and slightly north.

Dilatatone and sernanderin, found in the cracked ruffle lichen, also show weak inhibition of alpha-glucosidase (Phan et al. 2021). This lichen also contains protocetraric acid, usnic acid, and echinocarpic acid. Parmosidones F and G and three parmetherines, A–C, were also isolated from the lichen. The parmosidones inhibit alpha glucosidase and are more potent than acarbose, a drug prescribed for lowering blood sugar (Devi et al. 2020). Secondary metabolites from this lichen exhibited immune-modulating potential (Santos et al. 2004).

Cracked ruffle lichen (*Parmotrema dilatatum*) and *Parmelia tinctorium* (see pp. 161–2) were evaluated for their chemistry and activity against *Mycobacterium tuberculosis*. Diffractaic acid was the most active compound, followed by norstictic acid and then usnic acid. Hypostictic acid and protocetraric acid showed moderate activity (Honda et al. 2010).

Extracts of the ruffle lichen *Parmotrema hababianum* exhibit antioxidant and antihyperglycemic activity in streptozotocin-induced diabetic rats (Ganesan et al. 2016).

Powdered ruffle lichen (*Parmotrema hypotropum*) is found on tree trunks and branches in eastern and southeastern states and west to the Great Lakes and Texas. It contains atranorin and norstictic acid. Work by Lendemer et al. (2019) identified this lichen as one of the few hosting cystobasidiomycete yeasts. Its close cousin *Parmotrema subsumptum* syn. *Canomaculina subsumpta* hosts the same yeasts.

Perforated ruffle lichen (*Parmotrema perforatum*) is found in the southeastern United States. I can find no ethnolichenology information from North America. It is a food and medicine known as *chharila* in India and listed in that country's Materia Medica under this binomial and *Parmotrema chinense*. It has a wide range of use in medicine, including dyspepsia, spermatorrhea, amenorrhea, kidney stones, enlarged spleen, bronchitis, hemorrhoids, sore throat, and generalized pain. Smoke from this lichen is inhaled to relieve headache, or the lichen is powdered and used as snuff (Rogers 2011).

Black-edged leaf or powdered ruffle lichen (*Parmotrema perlatum* syn. *Lobaria perlata* syn. *Parmelia perlata*) is common around the world. It contains atranorin, stictic acid, and traces of norstictic acid.

In India, this is known as black stone flower, and when it is heated in oil, it releases an umami, earthy, smoky flavor. Also known as Kalpasi and Dagad Phool, the lichen is found in many curry powders in biryanis and Nalli Nihari dishes. It not only improves flavor, but aids digestion, giving relief from acidity and bloating. It is has become rare, due to over-exploitation.

This lichen has been used traditionally for gastrointestinal, respiratory, and vascular diseases. In North America, it is found on the east and west coasts, usually associated with oak.

Work by Hussain et al. (2021) investigated the antimuscarinic and calcium antagonistic mechanisms of this lichen. It exhibits antispasmodic, bronchodilator, and vasodilator activity. This suggests possible benefit in asthma and hypertension. Its amylase inhibition, determined in work by Valadbeigi and Shaddel (2016), prevents carbohydrate digestion by stopping hydrolyzation of starch and glycogen into maltose.

Polysaccharides isolated from this lichen show potent antiviral activity against yellow fever virus (the positive-sense RNA virus; Hosoya et al. 1991). The terpenes found here, parmelanostene and permelabdone, show activity against *Staphylococcus aureus* and *Escherichia coli* bacterial strains (Abdulla

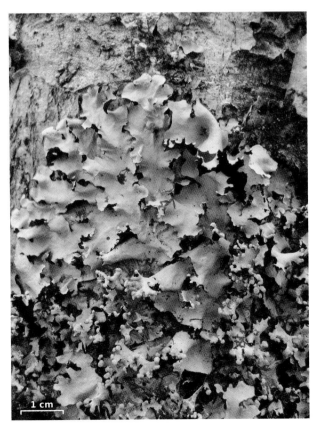

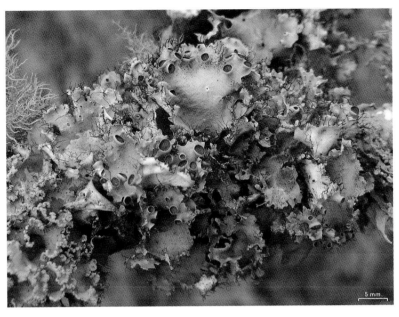

Parmotrema perforatum (Perforated Ruffle Lichen)

Parmotrema perlatum
(Black-Edged Leaf or
Powdered Ruffle Lichen)

et al. 2007). As a side note: Before traveling to Peru in 1982, I chose to receive a yellow fever vaccination. For four days and nights I suffered hot and cold sweats and suffered significant permanent hearing loss in my left ear.

An essential oil derived from *Parmotrema perlatum* shows activity against various species of *Staphylococcus*, *Streptococcus*, *Escherichia*, *Pseudomonas*, and *Candida* (Maqbul et al. 2019). This may be an extremely useful form in treatment for and/or prevention of various infections. Essential oils can be nebulized into the atmosphere, diluted in carrier oils for skin conditions, or encapsulated in enteric-coated capsules for oral benefit. In France, more than 10,000 medical doctors prescribe essential oil therapies, and entire wings of hospitals offer aromatherapy treatment for all manner of acute and chronic health conditions.

Powder crown ruffle lichen (*Parmotrema praesorediosum* syn. *Parmelia santae-crucis*) is found in Florida and neighboring Gulf states. This lichen contains diphenyl ethers, atranorin, praesorethers E–G, and protopraesorediosic acid.

Work by Huynh et al. (2022) tested the discovered compounds against HeLa (cervical), NCI-H460 (non-small-cell lung), and MCF-7 (breast) human cancer cell lines. Praesorethers E and F exhibited weak cytotoxicity against all three lines.

Praesordin, virensic acid, protocetraric acid, furfuric acid and 8'-O-methylprotocetraric acid were isolated from this lichen (Huynh et al. 2022a). These four compounds possess stronger anti-glucosidase activity than the standard drug acarbose. Extracts from this lichen show beta-glucosidase inhibition (Lee and Kim 2000).

Extracts of *Parmotrema praesorediosum* were tested for antimicrobial activity and were found active against *Bacillus cereus*, *Corynebacterium diptheriae*, *Shigella flexnerii*, *Staphylococcus aureus*, *Vibrio cholerae*, and *Candida albicans* (Balaji and Hariharan 2007).

Actinomadura parmotremmatis, isolated from this lichen, contains five derivatives of MK-9 (menaquinones) also known as vitamin K2 (Somphong et al. 2022). Research suggests small amounts of vitamin K2 daily help improve bone density and reduce cardiovascular risk by improving arterial flexibility in renal transplant patients (Mansour et al. 2017). This benefit is due, in part, to MK9 and other kallikrein-like enzymes that are hypotensive and counteract the renin–angiotensin system of regulating blood pressure. In one study, only MK9 was found to be regulated by thyroid hormone (Das et al. 2002).

Long-whiskered ruffle lichen (*Parmotrema rampoddense*) and palm ruffle lichen (*Parmotrema tinctorum*) are found on palm trees and occasionally on rocks in the extreme southeastern United States. Alectorialic acid, alectoronic

acid, atranorin, atraric acid, orcinol, and O-orsellinaldehyde have been identified in long-whiskered ruffle lichen. Atranorin derived from long-whiskered
ruffle lichen showed cytotoxicity against both MCF-7 and MDA MB-231
breast cancer cell lines (Harikrishnan et al. 2021).

Long-whiskered ruffle lichen contains nine endolichenic fungi (Tan
et al. 2020). Three of them, *Fusarium proliferatum*, *Nemania primolutea*, and
Daldinia eschsholtzii, possess antibacterial activity. *Fusarium proliferatum* was
most active against *Enterococcus faecalis* and *Staphylococcus aureus*.

Further purification of long-whiskered ruffle lichen revealed
bis(2-ethylhexyl)-terephthalate, fusarubin, and acetyl tributyl citrate in the
extract. The latter of these exhibited moderate activity against *Klebsiella
pneumoniae* and *Pseudomonas aeruginosa*.

Traditional Uses

Netted ruffle lichen (*Parmotrema reticulatum* syn. *Rimelia reticulata*) is
common in Quebec and the surrounding territory. It is listed as critically
endangered in Nova Scotia and threatened in Ontario.

Netted or cracked ruffle lichen grows on bark in well-lit woods from
Nebraska to Texas, south into northern Mexico, and over to Florida and up the
eastern states to Maine.

The Tepehuán of southern Chihuahua use a tea of this lichen to relieve
discomfort from kidney disorders, or to treat sexually transmitted infections.
The tea is prepared in the late afternoon and then set aside for a night before
use (Pennington 1969).

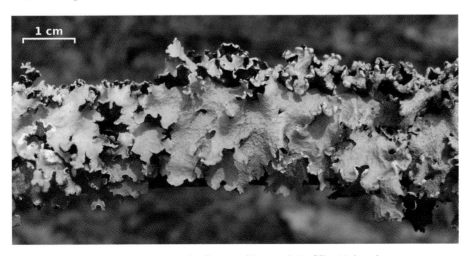

Parmotrema reticulatum (Netted Ruffle Lichen)

Additional Medical Uses

A methanol extract of this lichen was tested against breast (MCF-7) and lung (A549) cancer cell lines, and normal lung fibroblast (WI-38) tissue. Cytotoxicity was found against the breast cancer cells, but not the other two. The extract halted the MCF-7 breast cancer cells in the S and G2/M phases and induced apoptosis (Ghate et al. 2013).

It contains purpurin, which has antigenotoxic, anticancer, neuromodulatory, antimicrobial, and antioxidant effects (Singh et al. 2021). Reserpine is also found in the lichen. This compound can be derived from the herbal medicine *Rauwolfia serpentina* and was previously used to treat hypertension. Many years ago, I was given more than a hundred different plant tinctures by the widow of a deceased herbalist from central Alberta. Among the great finds was a liter of this tincture, and another of *Nux vomica*.

Six compounds of interest were isolated from netted ruffle lichen: reticulatin, zeorin, leucotylin, lupeol, betulinic acid, and dihydroreynosin. Reticulatin inhibits alpha-glucosidase at a much lower rate than acarbose, used for blood sugar control (Duong et al. 2022).

Extracts show anti-inflammatory effects and antibacterial activity against *Bacillus subtilis*, *Staphylococcus aureus*, *Escherichia coli*, and *Pseudomonas aeruginosa* (Jain et al. 2016).

Powder-edged ruffle lichen (*Parmotrema stuppeum* syn. *Parmelia maxima*) is isolated to the eastern United States and coastal California; it is nearly always found on the bark of deciduous trees.

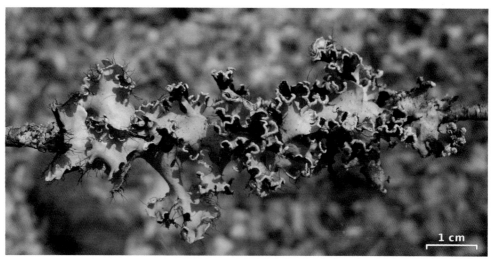

Parmotrema stuppeum (Powder-Edged Ruffle Lichen)

Work by Jayaprakasha and Rao (2000) identified four phenolic compounds in powder-edged ruffle lichen: methyl orsenillate, orsenillic acid, atranorin, and lecanoric acid. Moderate antioxidant activity was noted.

PECTENIA

Felt Lichens

Blue felt lichen (*Pectenia plumbea* syn. *Deglelia plumbea*) was recently chosen as the official lichen of Nova Scotia. The lichen has specific oceanic climate requirements with high humidity. It cohabitates with *Nostoc* cyanobionts, and other cyanolichen species, especially *Dendriscocaulon umhausense*, that reproduce asexually.

PELTIGERA

Dog Lichen   Liverwort   Pelt Lichen

Geographic Range: global
Habitat: rocks, logs, soil, moss
Medicinal Applications: reducing inflammation; skin burns and sores, mouth sores, insect stings
Notable Chemicals: aphthosin, gyrophoric acid, methionine, methyl evernate, and tenuiorin

There are presently 28 identified species in North America. *Peltigera* originates from the Greek and then Latin, meaning "shield shape" in reference to the appearance of apothecia. This lichen contains aphthosin, tenuiorin, methyl gyrophorate, gyrophoric acid, triterpenes, methyl evernate and dolichorrizin.

The Latin *aphthosa* refers to the resemblance of cephalodia to the disorder thrush, for which it was boiled in milk in Europe. Alternatively, it may have originally derived from the Greek *aphthai* meaning "pustule" or "eruption."

Traditional Uses

Various Indigenous peoples of North America used *Peltigera*, not identified to species, for medicine.

The *Tlingit* of Alaska dried and powdered this lichen to treat skin burns and scalds. They call it *ka wuh ghon* meaning "it burned up" (Emmons 1991).

The *Ditidaht* of coastal British Columbia call it *titidicc?a*, meaning "rocks growing on rocks." They chewed and ate the lichen for tuberculosis and used it as a poultice for leg sores (Turner et al. 1983).

The *Nlaka'pamux* from the province of British Columbia call it gall-colored frog moss, or frogs (on the) rocks. It was used fresh on bee stings (Turner et al. 1990).

Flaky freckle pelt lichen (*Peltigera britannica*) was used in a manner similar to *P. aphthosa* uses by the coastal *Ditidaht*. These lichens look similar, but the flaky one has a lobed cephalodia that easily detaches. It is largely confined to the coast from northern British Columbia to southern Oregon. Its constituents are similar to those of the common freckle pelt lichen.

In fact, flaky may be two different lichens, according to renowned lichenologist Trevor Goward. The Ways of Enlichenment website is highly recommended. I especially love Trevor Goward's *Twelve Readings on the Lichen Thallus*, which is brilliant and insightful.

The deciduous pelt lichen (*Peltigera britannica*) has *Coccomyxa* algae as its dominant symbiote. The panther pelt lichen resides with the cyanobacterium *Nostoc*.

Recent work by Almer et al. looked at thallus sectors that contain both green algal and cyanobacterial photobionts. They investigated the different gene expressions at different temperatures. Both fungus and cyanobacteria exhibited thermal stress at 15°C, and the green algae at 25°C.

The Dena'ina of Alaska call *Peltigera species* lichens *k'udyika'a*. Decoctions were prepared for tuberculosis and prolonged bleeding (Kari 1987). Residents of Haida Gwaii call lichens *hik'inxa kwii'awaay* (forest cloud) or *xil kwii. awaa* (cloud leaves). It was used in combination for several medicinal mixtures (Turner 2004).

The Oweekeno (Wuikinuxv), south of Bella Coola, used *xxwpiga* thallus, pounded with spruce pitch, to dress wounds (Compton 1993).

Membranous dog lichen (*Peltigera membranacea* syn. *P. canina* var. *membranacea*) was used as a love charm by the Kwakiutl (Kwakwaka'wakw) of northern British Columbia (Boas 1921). They call it *tl'extl'ekw'es,* meaning "seaweed of the ground." Both the Hesquiat and Nitinaht used this lichen for medicine (Turner and Efrat 1982).

Peltigera membranacea is found on mossy soil on both coasts, as well as in western Alberta and south into Idaho and Montana. This thin lichen has slender rope-like rhizines.

Many-fruited pelt lichen (*Peltigera polydactylon*) tea was prepared by the

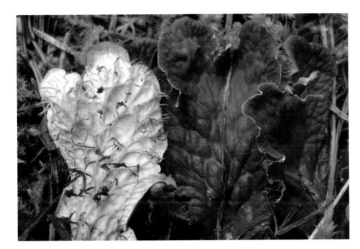

*Peltigera
membranacea*
(Membranous Dog
Lichen)

Haudenosaunee (people of the long house, Iroquois) in Ontario to induce vomiting, or as an anti-love medicine. The tea either makes a loved one return, or un-bewitches you (Herrick 1995).

In India, a paste of this lichen, known as *Jhau*, is applied to skin wounds to stop bleeding and acts as an antiseptic.

Dog pelt or ground liverwort (*Peltigera canina*) was traditionally used in Europe to protect against dog bites, hence the species name. Or perhaps the ruffled edges looked like dog teeth or ears, according to the doctrine of signatures.

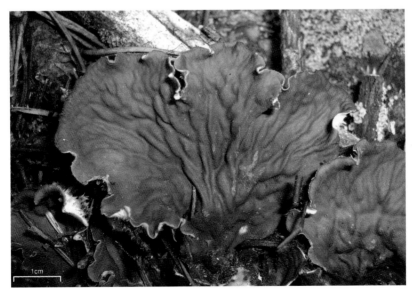

Peltigera canina
(Dog Pelt or Ground Liverwort)

The coastal Ditidaht (Nitinaht) used a gray *Peltigera* growing on rocks to induce urination (Turner et al. 1983). The Ditidaht name for this lichen translates as "flat against the rock" and "resembles whale baleen." This is probably either *Peltigera canina* or *Peltigera aphthosa*.

Medical Uses

Common freckle pelt, fairy pelt or lemon lichen (*Peltigera aphthosa*) is plentiful throughout North America, except in the extreme south.

Peltigera aphthosa contains ergosterol peroxide, which exhibits anti-inflammatory, antiviral, and antitrypanocidal activity. It contains the secondary metabolites aphtosin, tenuiorin, methyl, gyrophorate, gyrophoric acid, triterpenoids, and phlebic acids A–D.

Work by Zhou et al. (2019) found *Peltigera* significantly suppressed influenza A virus inflammation and apoptosis by blocking RIG-1 (retinoic acid-inducible gene 1) signaling. This molecule is an essential part of the innate immune system, recognizing cells infected with various viruses, including coronaviruses. Reducing inflammation may reduce unpleasant symptoms but may also reduce the elevated temperature (fever) that promotes viral destruction.

Ergosterol peroxide, found in *Peltigera aphthosa*, is toxic to *Trypanosoma cruzi*, which causes Chagas disease; the toxicity is due to a free-radical reaction leading to cell death (Meza-Menchaca et al. 2019).

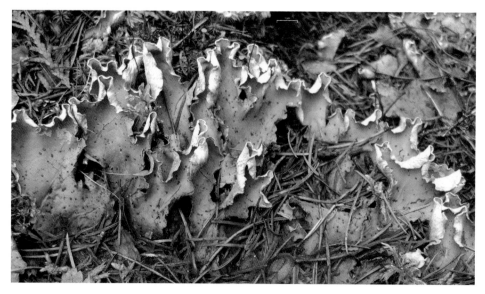

Peltigera aphthosa (Common Freckle Pelt,
Fairy Pelt, or Lemon Lichen)

In the mountains of New Mexico is found a *Peltigera* species the Navajo call Earth moss, or nihaaá.d. It was chewed in a manner like *Xanthoparmelia* species to treat canker sores, swollen gums, and decayed teeth (Wyman and Harris 1941).

Tree pelt lichen (*Peltigera collina*) contains tenuiorin, gyrophoric acid, methyl gyrophorate, and various triterpenes.

Concentric pelt lichen (*Peltigera elisabethae*) is found on soil and rocks from Alaska to southeastern United States. Its components sacrosomycin A–C and three analogues were tested against human cancer cell lines. One compound induced cell cycle arrest at the G2/M phase and promoted cell death. It also induced upregulation of the P53-P21 pathway. The compounds did not induce cell death in normal cell lines. The spirobisnaphthalene compounds, also present, deserve further study (Li et al. 2019).

Peltigera elisabethae, *P. leucophlebia*, *P. aphthosa*, and *P. britannica* contain tenuiorin, which shows moderate activity against human breast, pancreas, and colon cancer cell lines (Ingólfsdóttir et al. 2002).

Flat-fruited pelt lichen (*Peltigera horizontalis*) and scaly dog lichen/born-again pelt lichen (*Peltigera praetextata*) are found from Alaska south, and into eastern North America. Work by Nardemir et al. (2015) looked at the antimutagenic activity of these two lichens and examined whether their use is safe. Methanol extracts were tested for their genotoxic, antigenotoxic, and antioxidant properties. Flat-fruited pelt lichen (*Peltigera horizontalis*) has also been studied by Stajanovic et al. (2020) for constituents and biological activities.

The major constituents of the thallus of flat-fruited pelt lichen are gyrophoric acid and methyl gyrophorate, while the dominant component of the apothecia is tenuiorin. Gyrophoric acid produced the greatest decrease in micronuclei frequency, while an extract of the apothecia exhibited stronger antioxidant activity. Extracts of both of these lichens exhibited mild inhibitory effect on pooled human serum cholinesterase. This is significant because elevated levels of this enzyme are associated with hyperexcitation of the nervous system.

Ruffled freckle pelt lichen (*Peltigera leucophlebia*) grows on moist or dry moss, soil, logs, or rocks. It is widespread across Canada and follows the Rocky Mountains down to Arizona. Tenuiorin and methyl orsellinate are its active components, showing in vitro inhibition against 15-lipoxygenase. Activity against 5-lipoxygenase from porcine leucocytes was moderately active. Both tenuiorin and methyl orsellinate were tested for antiproliferative activity against human breast (T-47D), pancreatic (PANC-10), and colon (WIDR) cancer cell lines. Methyl orsellinate showed no activity, but tenuiorin showed moderate/weak inhibition of the pancreatic and colon cancer cell lines (Ingólfsdóttir et al. 2010). Earlier work by Ingólfsdóttir et al. (2000) found moderate inhibition of HL-60 human leukemia cell lines.

The phytobiont of this lichen, *Coccomyxa* sp., produces, in a culture medium, 16-fold more biotin (vitamin B7) than free-living *Chlorella*.

Tenuiorin, derived from this lichen and from *Umbilicaria* species, inhibits 50% of tau protein, which is associated with Alzheimer's disease (AD) and other neurodegenerative pathologies known as tauopathies (Salgado et al. 2020).

> Beta amyloid plaques and tau tangles are two issues associated with AD. The word amyloid is misplaced as it means 'starch.' These clumped, sticky protein molecules are outside neurons, but begin their life inside. Tau is a protein that forms inside the neurons, helping create microtubules that are flexible, but help maintain their shape. This led to scientists debating which is more important, leading to the intellectual challenge between tau and beta amyloid (BA) believers. The *Tau*ists versus *BA*ptists" (Rogers 2019, 148–49).

Phlebia fungal extracts, isolated from carpet pelt lichen (*Peltigera neopolydactyla*), show potential for being developed into an anti-inflammatory agent. Carpet pelt lichen is found on moss and tree bases in conifer forests throughout Canada. Alcohol extracts show activity against *Bacillus subtilis* and *Trichophyton mentagrophytes*, and cytotoxicity against murine leukemia and slow-growing BS-C-1 (African green monkey, ATCC CCL 26) cell lines (Perry et al. 1999).

Work by Lim et al. (2022) found *Phlebia* extracts reduced the production of pro-inflammatory cytokines (TNF-alpha, interleukin 6, and IL-1-beta), chemokine, nitric oxide, and prostaglandin E2 in macrophages. The inhibitory effect acts mainly via suppressing JNK-mediated AP-1 (activated protein 1) transcription factor, rather than the more well-known NFkB pathway.

Many-fruited pelt lichen (*Peltigera polydactylon* syn. *Peltigera dolichorhiza*) is found in scattered areas of the northern Pacific Coast, New Mexico, the Great Lakes and northeastern states and provinces, Appalachia, eastern British Columbia, and north-central Alberta. It grows on moss and mossy rocks in forests, with dark green thalli and bright red-brown apothecia. It contains tenuiorin, methyl gyrophorate, gyrophoric acid, and various triterpenes. Alcohol extracts exhibit cytotoxicity against murine leukemia cell lines (Perry et al. 1999).

Scaly dog lichen, also known as born-again pelt lichen (*Peltigera praetextata*), is widely distributed. No lichen secondary metabolites have been identified but the lichen definitely exerts antifungal action. Work by Shahi et al. (2003) found that acetone extracts test positive against various human dermatophytic fungi, *Epidermatophyton floccosum*, *Microsporum audounii*, *M. canisv*, *M. nanum*, *M. gypeum*, *Trichophyton mentagrophytes*, *T. rubrum*, *T. tonsurance*, and *T. violaceum*. Fungicides such as imazalil (enilconazole) are widely used in veterinary and agricultural practice, with serious toxic effects. In California such use is listed as a possible cause of cancer under Proposition 65. One of its main uses is in the citrus industry, and as a coating for barley seed. It is also a topical antifungal for animals. Lichens contain powerful antifungal compounds that require more intensive research.

Work by Valadbeigi and Shaddel (2016) found inhibition of amylase, which in turn slows down digestion and assimilation of sugars.

Field dog lichen (*Peltigera rufescens*) is found throughout Canada and down into parts of the United States, usually on sandy, calcareous soil, near roadsides

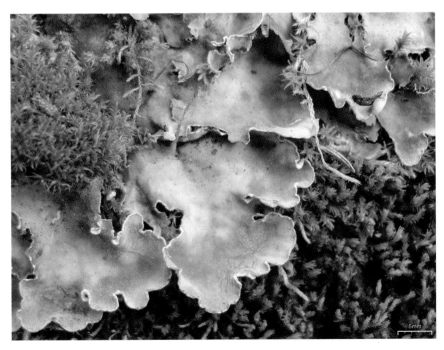

Peltigera rufescens (Field Dog Lichen)

or open fields, with full sun. A study by Tanas et al. (2010) involved a methanol extract of this lichen and testing against acute and chronic inflammation animal models. Research suggests the anti-inflammatory activity may involve reduced effect on neutrophil-derived free radicals and ameliorating the antioxidant defense systems. Its antioxidant activity is higher, considering the low levels of phenolics (Odabasoglu et al. 2005).

A study by Türkez et al. (2012) found an extract from field dog lichen is not toxic to normal cells but may have important application to protect lymphocytes from genetic damage in humans.

Fan lichen (*Peltigera venosa*) is widespread, found on bare mineral soil along the banks of creeks or roads, usually in areas of wet weather. Like all pelt lichens with green algae, it has cephalodia, which can detach and grow independently (Brodo et al. 2001). To my knowledge, it was not used by Indigenous healers of North America. It was mentioned, however, in the *Pharmacopeia Universalis* of 1846 (Vartia 1973).

Herbalism

The noble liverwort does not appear,
Without a speck, like the unclouded air,
A plant of noble use and endless fame,
The liver's great preserver, hence its name.

ABRAHAM COWLEY

Nicholas Culpeper, the famed English herbalist, wrote (1654):

Common Liverwort . . . is under the dominion of Jupiter, and under the sign Cancer. It is a singularly good herb for all the diseases of the liver, both to cool and cleanse it, and helps the inflammations in any part, and the yellow jaundice likewise. Being bruised and boiled in small beer and drank, it cools the heat of the liver and kidneys.

Powdered common liverwort lichen was mixed with black pepper and warm milk into Dr. Mead's *Pulvus Antilyssus*, a cure for rabies. Early settlers to North America mixed the dry powder with white wine and gave it to young boys suffering hernia. German settlers used this lichen to strengthen a weak liver, or to "cool" one that was inflamed. Sauer, in 1773, called it *Leberkraut*. In his book translation by Weaver (2001), he notes that "The distilled water of liverwort possesses similar virtues, but in particular it will cool an inflamed liver and withstand jaundice when a few tablespoons are taken several times a day."

This lichen can be decocted, cooled and strained, and the tea gargled with, for swelling of the tonsils and uvula. The vagus nerve raises the uvula, the dangling tissue at the back of our throat. When your doctor opens your mouth, they are looking for it to rise, and if the vagus nerve is weak, the rise is little or none. However, very few medical doctors use this important indication to strengthen digestion and brain function.

Dr. Kharrazian (2013) recommends a few exercises to help strengthen our vagus nerve. Gargle with four large glasses of healthy water. Sing loudly or use tongue depressors to stimulate the gag reflex. "Gag reflexes are like doing push-ups for the vagus, while gargling and singing loudly are like doing sprints" (Rogers 2019).

The liverwort lichen contains high amounts of the amino acid methionine (Subrahmanian and Ramakrishnan 1964). Recent work by Wu et al. (2023) and other scientists suggest that methionine-restricted diets may be a feasible strategy in chronic or age-related disease. Many studies over the past five years suggest benefit of a methionine-restriction in issues involving angiogenesis (cancer growth), neurodegenerative disease, and intestinal barrier function.

Work by Ingólfsdóttir et al. (1985) found extracts of dog pelt lichen cytotoxic, and active against *Bacillus subtilis* and *Pseudomonas aeruginosa* (Ingólfsdóttir et al. 2000). The polysaccharides in the extracts are immune modulating, influencing both the innate and adaptive systems (Omarsdottir et al. 2005).

Zucchini grown on DDT-contaminated soil shows more positive growth and development when crushed lichen powder is added to the soil (Akpinar et al. 2021).

Dog pelt lichen, or ground liverwort (*Peltigera canina*), has long been used in homeopathy. It is beneficial whenever there is throat congestion and hoarseness. The throat tickles and feels irritated, with a scraping, rough sensation. This lichen induces free and easy expectoration that relieves the feeling of something caught in the epiglottis. The dose of 2C, usually one or two sugar pellets under the tongue, is taken as needed.

PERTUSARIA
Wart Lichens

Wart lichen (*Pertusaria albescens* syn. *Lepra albescens* syn. *Marfloraea albescens*) contains (–)-dihydropertusaric acid.

Bitter wart lichen (*Pertusaria amara* syn. *Lepra amara*) is found along the U.S. Pacific Coast, as well as around the Great Lakes, usually on the bark of hardwoods, but occasionally on conifers or rocks. It is extremely bitter and contains arabitol, mannitol, emulsin, and picrolichenic acid. It was traditionally used for high fever, prepared in a decoction as a substitute for South American quinine. Bitter foods and herbs help alleviate dizziness and heated conditions such as fever through their descending property. Bitter taste receptors (T2Rs) are the target of more than 50% of drugs presently on the market. The expression of T2Rs and their signaling mediate the digestive, genitourinary, brain, respiratory systems and influence our innate immune cellular activity (Lu et al. 2017).

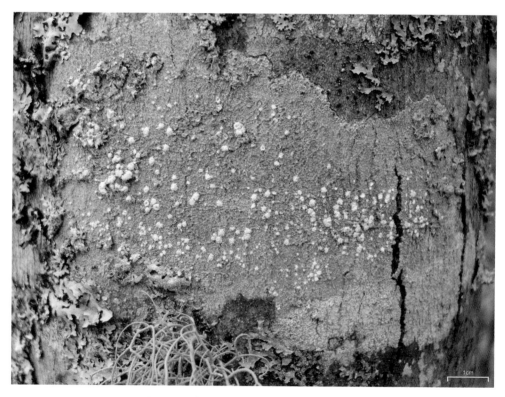

Pertusaria amara syn. *Lepra amara*
(Bitter Wart Lichen)

The bitter wart lichen extract is active against gram-positive bacteria and dermatophyte fungi (Taylor and Fourie 2019).

The related wart lichen *Pertusaria cicatricosa* from Columbia and other tropical forests contains 2-chlorlicexanthone.

Other *Pertusaria* species contain cryptothamnolic, thiophaninic, succinoprotocetraric, and decarboxyhypothamnolic acids. *Pertusaria moreliensis* contains haemathamnolic acid.

PHYLLOSPORA

Lace-Scale Lichens

There are 18 or more lace-scale lichens (*Phyllospora* spp.) in North America. They are generally found on tree bark, but occasionally on rocks in subtropical regions. They contain a variety of compounds, including zeorin, argopsin, atranorin, and pannarin.

Phyllospora beuttneri contains dechloropannaria. The lichen *Phyllospora furfuracea* syn. *Lecidia furfuracea* contains furfuraceic acid.

The lichen *Phyllopsora corallina* var. *ochroxantha* syn. *P. ochroxantha* syn. *Wolseleyidea ochroxantha* contains phyllopsorin.

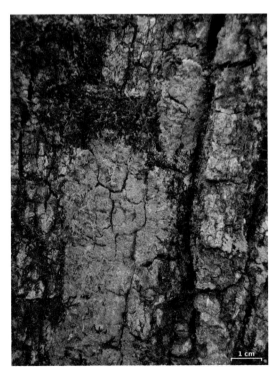

Phyllopsora corallina

PHYSCIA
Rosette Lichens

There are 36 rosette lichens in North America, mostly small light gray foliose lichens on various substrates. *Physcia* is derived from the Greek meaning "study of nature" or "natural things," and was also used as the title of an eight-volume set of lectures by Aristotle.

Hoary rosette lichen (*Physcia aipolia*) is widespread with white pruinose (frosted-looking) coating, explaining the common name. It grows on tree barks. Atranorin is its main secondary metabolite, with significant antimicrobial activity against *Bacillus mycoides*, *B. subtilis*, *Staphylococcus aureus*, *Enterobacter cloacae*, *Escherichia coli*, *Klebsiella pneumoniae*, and various fungi including *Aspergillus flavus*, *A. fumigatus*, *Botrytis cinerea*, *Candida albicans*, *Fusarium oxysporum*, *Mucor mucedo*, *Paecilomyces variotii*, *Penicillium purpurescens*, *P. verrucosum*, and *Trichoderma harzianum* (Rankovic et al. 2008).

Blue-gray rosette lichen (*Physcia caesia*) and star rosette lichen (*Physcia stellaris*) are widespread in North America. Blue gray rosette lichen is found on rocks, especially locations where birds perched, while star rosette lichen is rarely found on rocks, but on the bark of alder, poplar, and other hardwood trees.

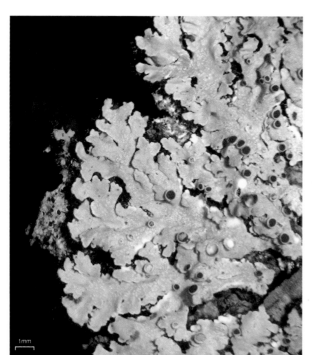

Physcia aipolia
(Hoary Rosette Lichen)

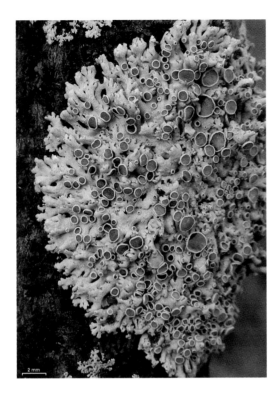

Physcia stellaris
(Star Rosette Lichen)

Physcia species lichens were traditionally combined with pine resin by Indigenous artists to produce a yellow-staining paint. *Physcia stellaris* is known to the Yuman of northern Mexico as *ipa teblyauup*, meaning "stick flower," or as *lama*.

Blue-gray rosette lichen, also known as powderback lichen, contains atranoric acid, haematommic acid, and zeorin. Star rosette lichen contains atranorin. Haematommic acid protects human umbilical vein endothelial cells from oxidative stress (Whang et al. 2005).

PLATISMATIA
Rag Lichens

Geographic Range: widespread but mainly coastal

Habitat: trees

Practical Use: brain tanning

Medicinal Applications: anti-biofilm, cancer

Notable Chemicals: atraric and caperatic acids; atranorinin and
    chloroatranorin

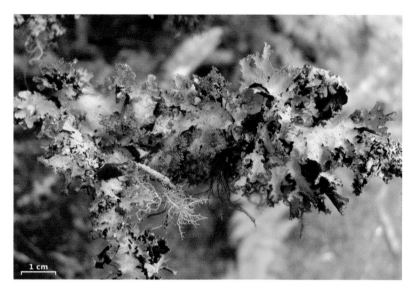

Platismatia glauca
(Ragbag or Varied Rag Lichen)

Ragbag, or varied rag lichen (*Platismatia glauca* syn. *Cetraria glauca*), is found on lodgepole pine, cedar, fir, Douglas fir, and white spruce. *Glauca* means "sea green." All the species have a green color due to the *Trebouxia* algae symbiont.

Elders of Haida Gwaii call the lichen "red cedar goat wool" or "light clouds."

Early work by Bézivin et al. (2003) identified in vitro anticancer activity. Extracts of this lichen induce cytotoxic effects on HCT-116 and SW-480 colon cancer cell lines (Seklic et al. 2018). Later work found the HCT-116 cancer cells were more responsive to the lichen extracts (Seklic and Jovanovic 2022).

This lichen contains caperatic and atraric acid, atranorin, and chloroatranorin. The lichen shows anti-biofilm activity against *Proteus mirabilis*, a deadly hospital-acquired bacterial infection (Mitrovic et al. 2014). A dear friend of mine died from complications of this pathogen, contracted in the hospital via an infected urinary-tract catheter. Mortality rates for geriatrics are over 50%, with no effective antibiotics. The bacteria hide inside urinary crystals, making them difficult to attack.

The lichen extract and isolated caperatic acid show inhibition of butyrylcholinesterase more strongly than acetylcholinesterase, but still suggestive of neurological benefit. The extract and caperatic acid exhibit cytotoxic and pro-apoptotic activity against T98G and U-138 MG glioblastoma multiforme cell lines (Studzinska-Sroka et al. 2022). This suggests possible benefit in brain and neurodegenerative conditions. The pro-inflammatory activation of leukocytes was inhibited by extracts of this lichen (Ingelfinger et al. 2020).

Antibacterial activity was strongest, in vitro, against *Staphylococcus saprophyticus*, *Staphylococcus aureus*, *Shigella flexneri*, *Streptococcus pneumoniae*, *Proteus vulgaris*, *Salmonella typhimurium*, *Bacillus cereus*, and *Escherichia coli*, respectively. The lichen also showed activity against *Candida albicans* (Abdallah 2019).

This lichen possesses antifungal activity against *Aspergillus flavus* (Furmanek et al. 2021). This is a soil-borne saprotrophic fungi aflatoxin commonly found in peanut butter and grains. It is responsible for aspergillosis, which is problematic for people with allergic reactions and patients with cystic fibrosis, asthma, and tuberculosis. The domesticated koji mold, used to make Japanese soy sauce and tamari, has a genome 99.5% identical to *Aspergillus flavus*.

Ragbag lichen, as well as *Cladonia convulata*, *C. rangiformis*, *Parmelia caperata*, and *Ramalina cuspidate*, demonstrates interesting activity on various human cancer cell lines (Bézlvin et al. 2003).

The lichen is widely used as a spice called *Kalpaasi* in Tamilian cuisine. In the Middle East it is known as *shibah*. It has not yet found its way into most North American markets.

Crinkled rag lichen (*Platismatia lacunosa* syn. *Cetraria lacunosa*) may have been used by the Wailaki of Northern California for brain tanning. (*Wailaki* was the name given to the tribe by the Wintun, meaning "north language," due to Athabaskan language spoken by this group.) Murphey (1959) referred to this lichen as *Usnea lacunosa*, which does not exist, so either the genus name is incorrect or the species is incorrect. Other authors believe the reference is to pitted beard lichen (*Usnea cavernosa*) (Chestnut, 1902). Traditionally, this gray-green lichen was wrapped around an animal brain, in brick form, and later rubbed into the ungulate hide. Brain-tanned and smoked hides are highly valued, compared to commercial leather.

PLEOPSIDIUM

Cobblestone Lichens

Gold cobblestone lichen (*Pleopsidium flavum* syn. *P. oxytonum*) grows on rocks in hot, dry regions from the southwest up to the Canadian prairies. It is highly prized by the Northern Paiute of Nevada for bright dyes. Their name for it

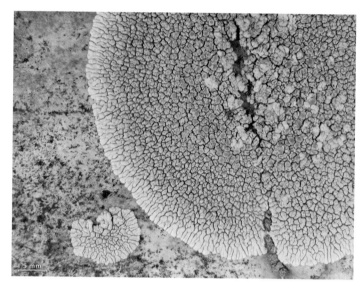

Pleopsidium flavum
(Gold Cobblestone
Lichen)

translates as "lizard semen," in reference to the motion lizards perform during courtship on the lichenized rocks.

PLEUROSTICTA

Saucer Lichens

Only two *Pleurosticta* species exist worldwide. The genus was first named by Franz Petrak in 1931.

Saucer lichen (*Pleurosticta acetabulum*) grows widely in Europe on tree bark, and in parts of Florida and California. It contains atranorin, salazinic, norstictic, protocetraric, and evernic acids. It also contains cytochalasin E, which exhibits antiproliferative activity against human HT-29 (colorectal) cancer cell lines (Delebassée et al. 2017).

This lichen, after being dried, chilled to $-196°C$ and deprived of oxygen, recovered and began to produce a high yield of hydrogen (see pages 10–11 in the Introduction regarding hydrogen as a green energy).

PORPIDIA

Boulder Lichens

North America has at least 28 boulder lichens (*Porpidia* sp.). As the name suggests, they grow on siliceous boulders and contain a wide variety of compounds. These include confluentic acid, 2'-O-methylsuperphyllinic acid,

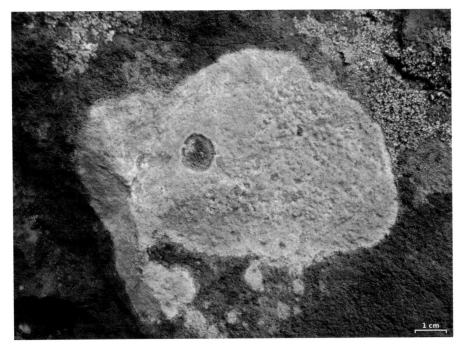

Porpidia ochrolemma

2'-O-methyperlatolic acid, 4-O-demethylsuperconfluentic acid, norstitic acid, and stictic acid.

Confluentic acid shows selective inhibition of monoamine oxidase B (MAO-B) with IC50 value of 0.22 microM (Endo et al. 1994). MAO-B inhibitors prevent an enzyme degrading dopamine, helping nerve cells have better access to this important neurotransmitter. Early stages of Parkinson's disease can benefit, as well as with carbidopa-levodopa therapy. Fava beans are also an important source of L-dopa.

The wrinkled boulder lichen (*Porpidia glaucophaea* syn. *P. rugosa* syn. *Huilia glaucophaea*) contains glaucophaeic acid, insignin, and superconfluentic acid.

The related *Porpidia carlottiana* lives on exposed rocks along the coast from Alaska south to Oregon. It contains glaucophaeic and 2'-O-methylsuperphyllinic acid.

PROTOPARMELIA

Chocolate rim lichen (*Protoparmelia badia*) is very common on arctic and alpine granite rocks. It contains lobaric acid also found in *Stereocaulon* species (see page 221).

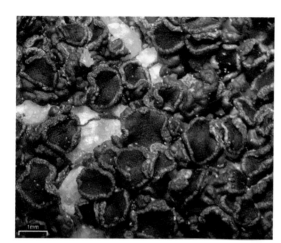

Protoparmelia badia
(Chocolate Rim Lichen)

PSEUDEPHEBE
Rock Wool Lichens

Fine rock wool (*Pseudephebe pubescens* syn. *Alectoria pubescens*) looks like black steel wool, appearing on granite rocks in alpine and arctic regions. The Indigenous Haisla of British Columbia used it to make a black wood paint.

This lichen was analyzed by Torres-Benitez et al. (2022) and 18 compounds

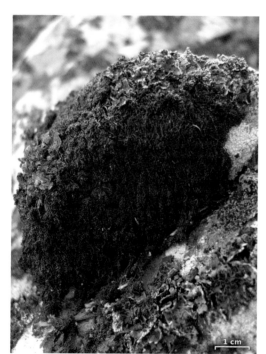

Pseudephebe pubescens
(Fine Rock Wool)

were identified. Ethanol extracts show high inhibition potential on the cholinesterase enzymes, including acetylcholinesterase and butyrylcholinesterase. This suggests potential application in neurodegenerative conditions.

PSEUDEVERNIA

Antler Lichens

From the height of this entirely naked summit from where I can barely distinguish a few lichens growing at its foot, I think how one is seized with such a strong feeling of solitude.

JOHANN WOLFGANG VON GOETHE (*ON GRANITE,* 1784)

Common antler lichen (*Pseudevernia consocians*) is usually found on conifer trees. It is mainly found in eastern North America, from New Brunswick south to Appalachia, but also in moist forests of northern Mexico. In the Nahua and mestizo communities from Tlaxcala, this lichen is used for heart conditions (Montoya et al. 2022). Only three species are found in North America, and this eastern lichen is the only one with isidia that can break off and re-establish.

Western antler lichen (*Pseudevernia intensa*) is found on conifers in open woodlands at higher elevation in Colorado, Arizona, and New Mexico.

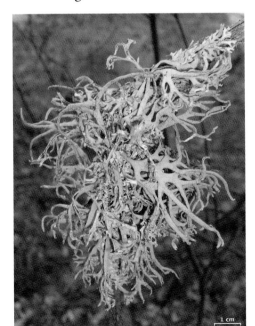

Pseudevernia intensa
(Western Antler Lichen)

The fungi *Geopyxis* aff. *majalis* and *Geopyxis* sp. AZ0066, isolated from this lichen, contain six new ent-kaurane diterpenoids, geopyxins A–F. Compounds obtained through methylation by Wijeratne et al. (2012) showed cytotoxicity against all five cancer cell lines tested.

PSEUDOCYPHELLARIA

Specklebelly Lichens

Geographic Range: mainly coastal North America and Appalachia

Habitat: trees, including old growth forests

Medicinal Applications: indigestion, potential anticancer components

Notable Chemicals: physciosporin; stictic acid, tenuiorin

Specklebelly lichens (*Pseudocyphellaria* sp.) number only seven species in North America. They are generally found in old growth, humid forests. In fact, specklebelly lichen (*Pseudocyphellaria rainierensis*) is extremely rare in old growth forests of the Pacific Northwest and is listed as vulnerable by the Committee on the Status of Endangered Wildlife in Canada. This lichen is the only west coast *Pseudocyphellaria* with green algae and isidia.

Green specklebelly lichen (*Pseudocyphellaria aurata* syn. *Crocodia aurata*) is found mainly in the southeastern United States, northern Florida, and across to East Texas. It is found on trees at low elevations. It contains calycin. It also contains fern-9(11)-ene-3ß,12ß-diol. In Madagascar, this lichen is prepared into tea to treat indigestion.

Yellow specklebelly lichen (*Pseudocyphellaria crocata*) was used as a yellow dye in Europe, due to the pigment calycin, but is too rare to use today. In North America it may be found in coastal forests from Alaska to Northern California, in parts of Appalachia, around the Great Lakes, and east to Nova Scotia and New England. This is not definite information, as Essinger does not believe the lichen is found in North America.

This lichen contains tenuiorin, methyl gyrophorate, gryrophoric acid, hopane-7ß,22-diol, physciosporin, norstictic acid, stictic acid, cryptostictic acid, constictic acid, pulvinic acid, pulvinamide, pulvinic dilactone, methyl lecanorate, orsellinic acid, calycinic acid, and calycin.

Physciosporin shows activity against human lung cancer motility (Yang et al. 2015; Yang et al. 2017). The expression of the metastasis suppressor

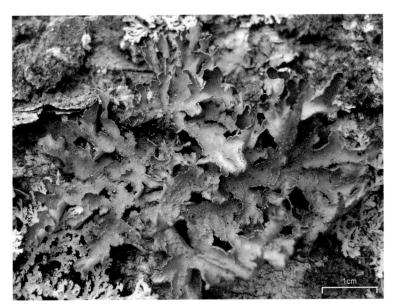

Pseudocyphellaria epiflavoides (*P. crocata* group)
(Yellow Specklebelly Lichen)

gene KAl1 was increased while the metastasis enhancer gene KlTENIN was dramatically decreased by physciophorin. Moreover, Cdc42 and Rac1 activities were decreased by this component. Physciosporin suppresses cell proliferation and motility and induces apoptosis in various colon and colorectal cancer cells, including Caco2, CT26, DLD1, HCT116, and SW620 (Tas et al. 2019).

Another study by Yang et al. (2019) found that physciosporin decreased the stemness potential of colorectal cancer cells. The most important stem marker, aldehyde dehydrogenase-1, was sharply downregulated at both the protein and mRNA levels. The authors suggest it suppresses stemness through the Sonic hedgehog and Notch signaling pathways. In general, physciosporin is a potent anticancer compound and markedly inhibits breast cancer cell viability.

Toxic doses of physciosporin trigger apoptosis by regulating the B-cell lymphoma-2 family proteins and activation of caspase pathway. At nontoxic levels, it potently decreased migration, proliferation, and tumorigenesis of cells in vitro.

Metabolic study reveals that the compound suppressed breast cancer growth in an implanted mouse model. The authors suggest it is promising against hormone-insensitive triple-negative breast cancer (MDA-MB-231) (Tas et al. 2021).

PSEUDOPARMELIA

Lemon-Lime Lichen

Lemon-lime lichen (*Pseudoparmelia uleana*) is subtropical and found in Georgia and Florida. It contains substances with antitubercular activity. Thus, various depsides, xanthones, orsellinic acids, and salazinic acid were evaluated for activity against *Mycobacterium tuberculosis* (Honda et al. 2010).

Another of its components, hypostictic acid, showed excellent antiproliferative activity against K562 (leukemia), B16-F10 (melanoma), and 786-0 (renal carcinoma) cell lines (Alexandrino et al. 2019).

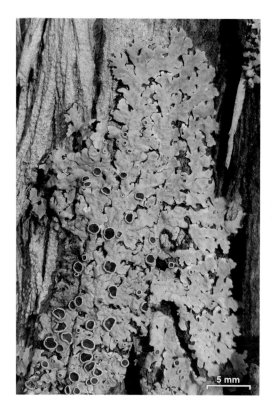

Pseudoparmelia uleana
(Lemon-Lime Lichen)

PSILOLECHIA

Sulfur Dust Lichen

Sulfur dust lichen (*Psilolechia lucida*) is found mainly around the Great Lakes and eastern North America, but also in the southern Northwest Territories. It is found on protected sides of overhanging cliffs, or in the crevices of old stone

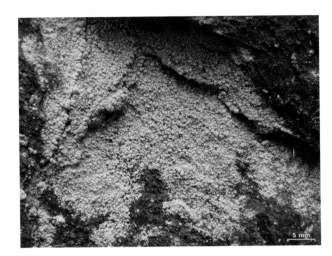

Psilolechia lucida
(Sulfur Dust Lichen)

walls, and rarely on wood. It contains the orange rhizocarpic acid. The lichen shows activity against various gram-positive bacteria (Taylor and Fourie 2019).

PSORA

Blushing Scale Lichen

Blushing scale lichen (*Psora decipiens* syn. *Biatora decipiens*) is found widespread in the arctic and most of the Midwest, south to Texas. It grows mostly on soil, but rarely on rock. As one of the biocrust lichens, it has been studied for the influence of global warming climate changes, when conditions are warmer and drier. When this lichen was exposed to the impact of ~2.3°C simulated warm treatment, the consequences for this important ground cover were impactful and negative (Raggio et al. 2023).

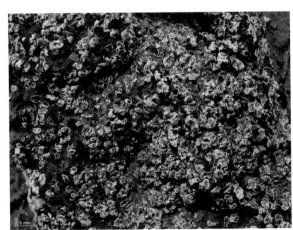

Psora decipiens
(Blushing Scale Lichen)

PSOROMA
Moss Shingle Lichens

Boreal moss shingle lichen (*Psoroma tenue* var. *boreale*) is an extremely rare species found in Banff National Park in Alberta, Canada. It contains pannarin and methyl porphyrilate. There are only six species in North America, among them the more widespread green moss shingle lichen (*Psoroma hypnorum* syn. *Pannaria hypnorum*).

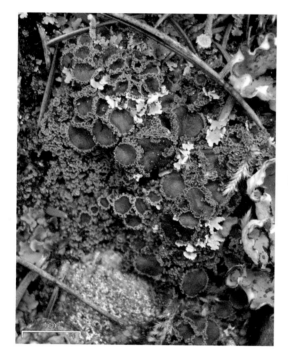

Psoroma hypnorum

PUNCTELIA
Speckled Shield   Speckleback Lichen

Geographic Range: North America

Habitat: trees, rocks

Medicinal Applications: antibacterial; potential for antibiotic-resistant infections, treatment of blurred vision, skin sores, uterine bleeding

Notable Chemicals: gyrophoric, lecanoric, lichesterinic, protolichesterinic, and usnic acids

Borrer's speckled-back lichen, or eastern speckled shield lichen (*Punctelia borreri* syn. *Parmelia borreri*), grows on hardwoods from California to Canada. The genus name is derived from the Latin *punctum*, meaning "small spot" or "dot." The species name honors William Borrer (1781–1862), the father of British lichenology.

This lichen is somewhat rare in Ohio and surrounding states. The Dakota (Sioux) name for it is *chan wiziye*, meaning "on the side of a tree." The lichen was used to produce a yellow dye (Gilmore 1977).

The lichen is also used in Traditional Chinese Medicine, where it is known as pink spotted plum, or spotted plum clothes. It is decocted and taken internally for blurred vision or uterine bleeding, and externally for chronic dermatitis, sores, and swellings.

The lichen contains gyrophoric, protolichesterinic, and lichesterinic acids. Work by Thadhani and Karunaratne (2017) and Valadbeigi and Shaddel (2016) confirms its amylase inhibitory activity, suggestive of benefit in blood sugar dysregulation.

Punctelia microsticta is tropical, found near Vera Cruz, Mexico, and elsewhere. This lichen's constituents include gamma-butyrolactone acid, (–)-dihydropertusaric acid, (–)-isomuronic acid, and gryphoric acid. The lichen exhibits activity against human melanoma M14 cells through induction of apoptosis (Maier et al. 1999).

Powdered speckled shield lichen, also known as forest speckleback lichen (*Punctelia jeckeri*), is found in open woods and occasionally on siliceous rocks from Manitoba to the southeastern United States, as well as Arizona and New Mexico, and along the Pacific Coast from Washington to California.

Rough speckled shield lichen (*Punctelia rudecta* syn. *Parmelia rudecta*) is common throughout eastern North America, on tree bark and shaded rocks. Its common presence is because it can tolerate urban pollution better than most lichens. It contains lecanoric acid.

Work by Bustinza et al. (1952) found extracts of this lichen inhibit *Alcaligenes faecalis* and *Escherichia coli* (see *Thamnolia vermicularis*, page 229, and *Xanthoparmelia conspersa*, page 259). The former bacteria is an opportunistic pathogen that is increasingly antibiotic-resistant. It is found in hospitals, usually associated with respirators, dialysis machines, and intravenous solutions. It has been found in urine, blood, wounds, stools, cerebrospinal fluid, and respiratory secretions. The bacteria is associated with endocarditis, bacteremia, meningitis, endophthalmitis, skin and soft tissue infections, urinary-tract infections, otitis media, peritonitis, and pneumonia. Its resistance to several antibiotics, including

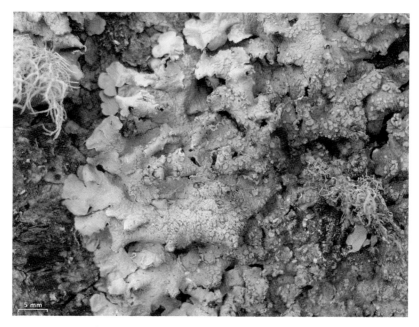

Punctelia jeckeri (Powdered Speckled Shield Lichen
or Forest Speckleback Lichen)

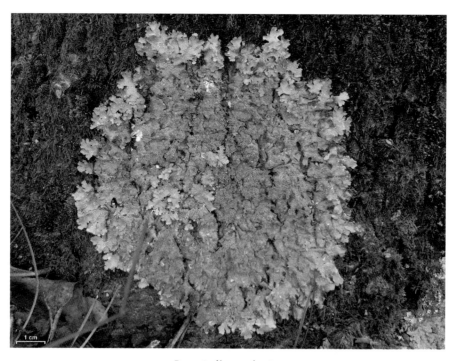

Punctelia rudecta
(Rough Speckled Shield Lichen)

anti-*Pseudomonas* penicillin, cephalosporins, carbapenems, aminoglycosides, and quinolones, is making treatment of infections more difficult. According to one report by Huang (2020), more than 60% of patients had received intravenous antibiotics within three months of diagnosis with this pathogen.

Rough speckled shield lichen contains lecanoric acid, orsellinic acid methyl ester, orcinol, and usnic acid. Activity against gram-positive and gram-negative bacteria, including MRSA and mycobacteria, was found for this lichen (Ivanova et al. 2010). Antiproliferative activity and cytotoxicity were also noted. Valadbeigi and Shaddel (2016) found that this species inhibits amylase, slowing down digestion and preventing release of sugars into the bloodstream.

While traveling on the Canary Islands more than 30 years ago, I found the related *Punctelia subrudecta* growing on rocks below the puffing, smoking volcano opening at the top of Tenerife. The snow at this elevation was colored a surreal pink! In North America it ranges from Manitoba to New England and down to Tennessee, as well as Colorado, New Mexico, and along the Pacific Coast.

PYRENULA
Rash or Pox Lichen

Bark rash lichen (*Pyrenula cruenta* syn. *Melanotheca cruenta* syn. *Trypethelium cruentum*) is a red lichen growing on broad-leaved trees in woodlands and hammocks in southeastern United States. The red anthraquinones coloring it include draculone and minor amounts of haematommone (Mathey et al. 2002).

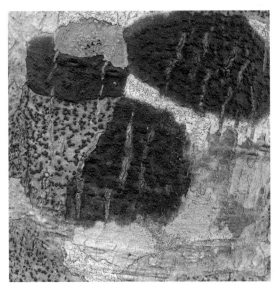

Pyrenula cruenta
(Bark Rash Lichen)

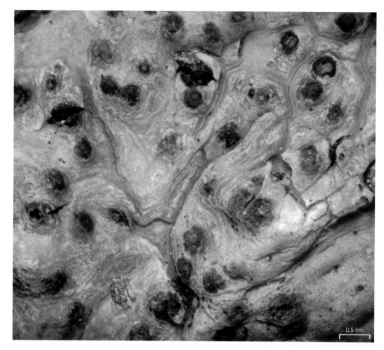

Pyrenula pseudobufonia
(Eastern Pox Lichen)

Eastern pox lichen (*Pyrenula pseudobufonia*) resides on beech, holly, and oak trees in eastern North America, from Nova Scotia to Florida and along the Gulf Coast. It contains lichexanthone, discussed below.

PYXINE

Button Rosette Lichens

Geographic Range: North America

Habitat: trees, tree bark, rocks

Medicinal Applications: antibacterial; potential treatment for
tuberculosis

Notable Chemicals: atranorin, lichexanthone

Buttoned rosette lichen (*Pyxine berteriana* syn. *Physcia meissneri*) is found on tree bark near Jacksonville and Key Largo, Florida.

Several interesting compounds have been isolated from this lichen genus, including fernane triterpenoids, with a carbonyl function at C-19, and lichexanthone (Maier et al. 2009). The two fernane triterpenoids are

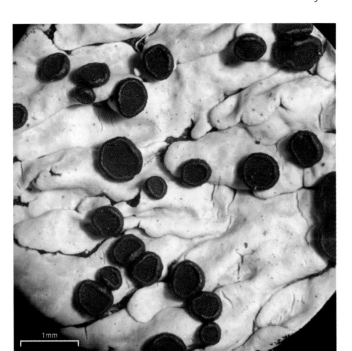

Pyxine berteriana
(Buttoned Rosette Lichen)

3ß-acetoxyfern-9(11)-ene-12ß-one and 3ß-acetoxyfern-9(11)-ene-19-one. It also contains fern-9(11)-ene3,19-dione, and testacein.

Lichexanthone is found in many species of *Pyxine*. Its presence causes yellow fluorescence under long-wave UV light. An ethanol extract reacts with iron(III) chloride to produce a purple color. The compound inhibits *Bacillus subtilis* and MRSA, and a dihydropyrane derivative showed activity against *Mycobacterium tuberculosis*, similar to pharmaceuticals. In vitro studies found that lichexanthone enhances the motility of sperm (Micheletti et al. 2013; Le Pogam and Boustie 2016b; Wang et al. 2012).

Another form of the buttoned rosette lichen (*Pyxine cocoes*) is similar to the one just described, but is sorediate, with a white medulla. It also grows on tree bark, and sometimes on rocks, in Florida, Alabama, and the eastern shore of Louisiana.

During the lockdown associated with COVID-19, it was found that the lichen population showed increases in pigments, the Fv/Fm ratio (a measure of variable fluorescence versus maximum fluorescence associated with photosynthesis), and levels of phytohormones. The reduction in transport vehicles was likely a causal effect of this change (Bajpai et al. 2023).

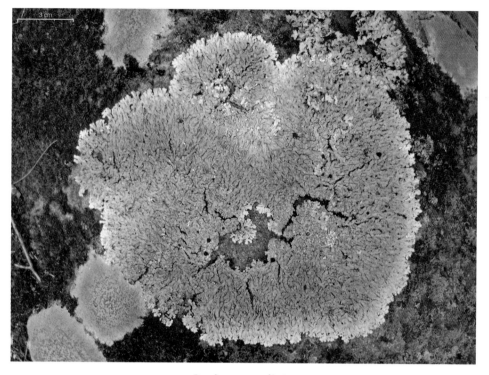

Pyxine sorediata
(Mustard Lichen)

The related mustard lichen (*Pyxine sorediata*) contains atranorin and diactylpyxinol. This is the largest of the *Pyxine* and is widespread in northeastern United States and maritime provinces of Canada on the bark of hardwoods and *Thuja occidentalis* (white cedar). The common name is derived from the mustard-yellow medulla.

RAMALINA

Strap or Cartilage Lichens

Burning Bush Lichen	Frayed Ramalina	Peruvian Ramalina
Chalky Ramalina	Lace or Fishnet Lichen	Sinewed Lichen
Dotted Ramalina	Obtuse Ramalina	Southern Strap Lichen
Fan Ramalina	Palmetto	Warty Ramalina

Huge lichens, rough as dragon's scales.

GEORGE SAND (1870)

Geographic Range: global

Habitat: trees, across widespread temperatures; rocks

Practical Uses: food, baby diapers, cosmetics

Medicinal Applications: antibacterial, antifungal

Notable Chemicals: atranorin, methyl evernate, divaricatic, evernic, norstictic, protocetraric, protolichesterinic, ramalic, sekikaic, salazinic, trivaric, and usnic acids

The *Ramalina* genus contains about 246 species around the world. A review by Moreira et al. (2015) looked at 118 species with published chemical or biological activity of extracts, or the isolated compounds. There are at last count about 50 species in North America. The genus name is derived from the Latin *ramalia* meaning "twigs."

In China, two species of *Ramalina* are prepared as a traditional cold dish served at marriage banquets. Couples who eat it will love each other more and never separate (Wang et al. 2001).

Sinewed Ramalina lichen (*Ramalina americana* formerly *R. fastigiata*) is found in eastern North America from the Great Lakes east to Nova Scotia and inland to Tennessee.

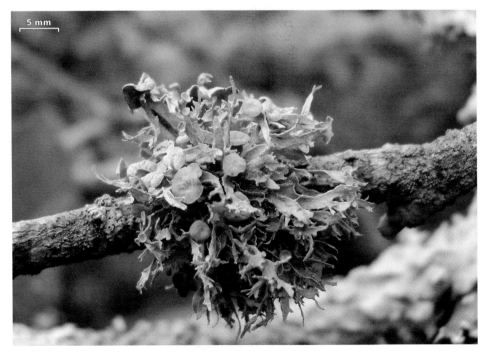

Ramalina americana (Sinewed Ramalina Lichen)

Medical Uses

The methyl evernate isolated from this lichen inhibited *Bacillus cereus, Staphylococcus aureus, Escherichia coli, Proteus mirabilis,* and numerous fungi species. The lichen also contains 4'-O-demethylsekikaic acid, dihydropicrolichenic acid, isonorobtusatic acid (noriscobtusatic acid), norisonotatic acid, ramalinaic acid, subdivaricatic acid, subsekikaic acid, trivaric acid, and 3'-methylevernic acid (isoobtusatic acid).

This lichen is cytotoxic, in vitro, to HeLa (cervical/epithelial), A549 (lung), and LS174 (colon) cancer cell lines (Ristic et al. 2016a).

Palmetto lichen (*Ramalina celastri*) is found in southern Texas on trees, sometimes rocks.

The palmetto lichen contains parietin, which exhibits activity against arenaviruses Tacaribe and Junin, and sekikaic acid, which is a potent inhibitor of respiratory syncytial virus (RSV) and RSV A2 (Fazio et al. 2007). In vitro work found extracts of the lichen inhibit HeLa (cervical) cancer cell lines (Camerio-Leão et al. 1997).

More interesting work involves the use of sulfated polysaccharides from this lichen for antischistosomal activity. Work by Araújo et al. (2011) encapsulated

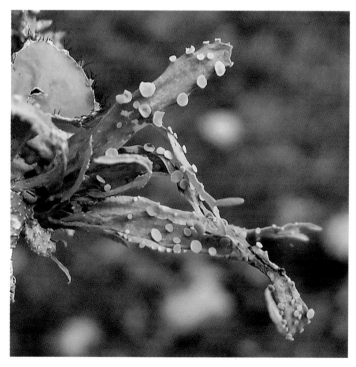

Ramalina celastri (Palmetto Lichen)

these sulfated polysaccharides into liposomes and then treated *Schistosoma mansoni*-infected mice. A decrease in the number of hepatic egg-granulomas and a change in the glycosylation profile of the egg-granuloma were noted.

Work by Verma et al. (2012) found that this lichen's extracts inhibit alpha-glucosidase, suggestive of benefit in reducing breakdown of oligosaccharides and disaccharides into glucose. This lichen's components sekikaic acid, sala-zinic acid, and the dibenzofuran derivative usnic acid exhibit promising antihyperglycemic effect.

A water-soluble alpha-D-glucan from this lichen exhibits cytotoxicity to HeLa cancer cells and sarcoma-180 cells. Work by Stuelp-Campelo et al. (2002) found the alpha-glucan exhibits immunomodulation as a biological response modifier.

The lichen species called dotted Ramalina or the dotted line lichen (*Ramalina farinacea*) is extremely variable. It grows on all types of trees in regions of mild, humid climate. But I have also found it in central Alberta, where temperatures go down to −40° C, so there are some exceptions. It is also found in the Atlantic provinces, in northern Ontario, and on the Pacific Coast from Alaska to Southern California.

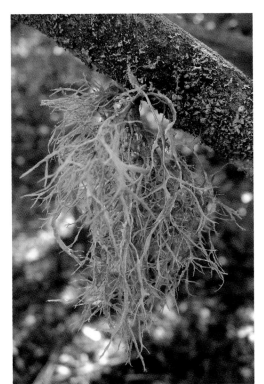

Ramalina farinacea
(Dotted Ramalina or
Dotted Line Lichen)

Its widespread habitat may be due to its ability to vary its coexisting phycobionts. Work by Casano et al. (2011) found two different algae taxa of *Trebouxia*, with one giving better physiological performance under high temperatures and irradiance, and another thriving in more moderate temperatures with less sunlight.

This lichen contains (+)-usnic, protocetraric, norstictic, obtusetic, ramalinolic, sekikaic, and protolichesterinic acids, as well as methyl evernate, arabitol, and mannitol. Work by Tay et al. (2004) found the (+)-usnic acid from this lichen active against *Bacillus subtilis*, *Listeria monocytogenes*, *Proteus vulgaris*, *Staphylococcus aureus*, *Streptococcus faecalis*, *Yersinia enterocolitica*, *Candida albicans*, and *C. glabrata*. Norstictic acid is active against all of the organisms just listed except *Y. enterocollitica*, as well as *Aeromonas hydrophia*. Protocetraric acid was active only against the *Candida* species.

Previous studies found that ethyl acetate fractions inhibit the infectivity of lentiviral and adenoviral vectors, as well as wild-type HIV-1. Work by Esimone et al. (2009) discovered the lichen fraction showed broad-spectrum activity against DNA viruses (adenovirus and herpes simplex) and the RNA viruses HIV-1 and respiratory syncytial virus (RSV). A follow-up study by Lai et al. (2013) also showed an extract active against RSV. That work led to the isolation of 13 phenolic compounds, including 5-hydroxysekikaic acid, and new orsellinic acid derivatives.

Sekikaic acid showed potent inhibition of the recombinant strain of RSV and RSV A2 strain. Lai et al. determined that sekikaic acid clearly interferes with viral replication at the viral post entry step and is over 1.3-fold more active than the control drug ribavirin at 4 hours post infection. Sekikaic acid did not display virucidal activity at concentrations below the TC50, but the extract did. It appears to work at the viral post entry stage of replication.

Sekikaic acid modulates pancreatic ß-cells in type 2 diabetic rats, by inhibiting digestive enzyme production. Both alpha-amylase and alpha-glucosidase were inhibited. Lowering of low-density lipoprotein (LDL), total cholesterol, and total glycerides was observed, as well as significant regeneration of pancreatic ß-cells compared to diabetic control (Tatipamula et al. 2021).

An extract of this lichen exhibits inhibition of *Streptococcus pneumoniae* and MRSA (methicillin-resistant *Staphylococcus aureus*). In vitro studies have found that obtusetic acid and methyl evernate inhibit A549 (lung), HeLa (cervical), LS174 (colorectal) and V79 (fibroblast) cancer cell lines (Ristic et al. 2016a). Protocetraric acid inhibits *Candida albicans* and *C. glabrada*. The latter fungus is increasingly resistant to drugs for treating urinary-tract infections.

Cartilage lichen (*Ramalina fraxinea*) contains atranorin, usnic, salazinic, sekikaic, obtusatic, and protocetraric acids. This lichen exhibits strong free radical scavenging ability and antimicrobial activity. Acetone extracts of cartilage lichen exhibit strong anticancer activity (Ristic et al. 2016).

Work by Yayla et al. (2023) found this lichen, among four *Ramalina* species tested, to be the highest in antioxidant activity. This species and *Ramalina fastigiata* (syn. *Ramalina americana*) and *Ramalina polymorpha* exhibit cytotoxic activity against human lung (A549) and breast (MDA-MB-231) cancer cell lines.

Prominent Species

Lace or fishnet lichen (*Ramalina menziesii*) lives on the west coast of North America, from British Columbia to California. The Pomo of that state used the lichen for baby diapers (Goodrich et al. 1980). (Pʰoʔma? or Pomo may have originally meant "those who live in a red earth hole.") This may be due to local deposits of red magnetite or hematite. Red ochre was commonly rubbed on bare skin by numerous Indigenous groups to minimize or prevent insect bites. The Yuman of northern Mexico refer to this lichen as *Toji*.

In 2016, California formerly named *Ramalina menziesii* their state lichen, the first official state lichen in the country.

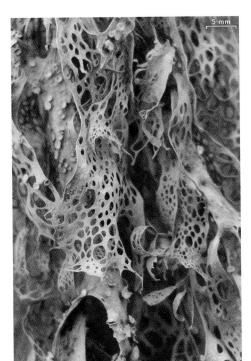

Ramalina menziesii
(Lace or Fishnet Lichen)

Work by Weiss-Penzias et al. (2019) found that this lichen, which is a source of food for deer and predatory pumas, contains high levels of mercury. With possible relevance, atmospheric fog in coastal California contains ocean-derived monomethylmercury, a problem affecting coastal food webs.

The obtuse Ramalina (*Ramalina obtusata*) contains obtusatic acid.

Warty Ramalina (*Ramalina paludosa*) is confined to the Atlantic coast south from North Carolina to southern Florida and across to Alabama. It is found on exposed trees and shrubs and is easily identified by its large, white papillae. It contains cryptochlorophaeic, subpaludosic, and paludosic acids.

Peruvian Ramalina (*Ramalina peruviana* syn. *Desmazieria peruviana*) was named by Eric Acharius for the location where it was first collected, and in North America is restricted to southern Florida and Texas. Recent work identified three new phenolic compounds for this lichen: peruvinides A–C (Huynh et al. 2022b).

Chalky Ramalina (*Ramalina pollinaria/Ramalina labiosorediata*) is found on the bark of older trees, and sometimes on rocks in shade. It is frequent in my part of Alberta, but also in British Columbia, and the northeastern and southwestern United States. It contains usnic, sekikaic, evernic, ramalic and obtusatic acids. The lichen extract inhibits the enzyme alpha-amylase, which in turn reduces the breakdown of carbohydrates, thus reducing blood-sugar spikes (Valadbeigi and Shaddel 2016).

An extract of this lichen shows activity against 11 bacteria and three fungi (Güllüce et al. 2006). The lichen and isolated usnic acid exhibit activity against *Escherichia coli*, *Enterococcus faecalis*, *Proteus mirabilis*, *Staphylococcus aureus*, *Bacillus subtilis*, and *B. megaterium* (Cansaran et al. 2007).

Both dotted line and chalky Ramalina were long ago used in cosmetics and perfumes in Europe.

Frayed Ramalina (*Ramalina roesleri* syn. *Fistulariella roesleri*) is confined mainly to disparate areas of Canada, and isolated parts of Wisconsin and California, on branches and twigs. It was recently designated the unofficial lichen of Prince Edward Island. It contains sekikaic acid complex and homsekikaic acid, usnic acid, atranorin, protolichesterinic acid, benzoic acid, and other minor compounds.

The maximum radical scavenging activity of an extract of this lichen was exhibited by sekikaic acid, followed by homosekikaic acid (Sisodia et al. 2013). Both of these acids exhibit antifungal activity. Moderate antibacterial activity was found against *Streptococcus mutans*, *Staphylococcus aureus*, and *Streptomyces viridochromogenes.* The latter bacterium led to isolation of the antibiotic strep-tazolin in 1981. It is not suitable for human use.

The components of the extract can be considered in terms of these observations: Work by Goel et al. (2021) found binding efficacy of uric acid with penicillin binding protein-PBP2a, which is responsible for conferring resistance to *Staphylococcus aureus* (SA). Scanning electron microscopic pictures show the cell wall disruption of methicillin-resistant SA by usnic acid. Binding potential with PBP2a suggests impressive inhibitory activity toward MRSA.

Fan Ramalina or burning bush lichen (*Ramalina sinensis*) is found on trees and shrubs in Wisconsin and southwestern states. It contains usnic acid, betulin, and betulinic acid. Work by Raj et al. (2014) found that this lichen inhibits the enzyme alpha-amylase, thus reducing the breakdown of starch to sugar, and slowing down digestion of carbohydrates. Both methanol and ethanol extracts of this lichen show significant activity against *Bacillus subtilis* (Sargsyan et al. 2021).

Both silver and iron oxide nanoparticles show inhibition of various bacteria, including *Staphylococcus aureus* and *Pseudomonas aeruginosa* (Abdolmaleki and Sohrabi 2016; Safarkar et al. 2020). This can be considered in the following context: The synthesis of nanomaterials using lichen extracts is a growing field of medicine that is ecofriendly, simple, and low cost. According to Hamida et al. (2021), lichens have great potential reducible activity to fabricate different nanomaterials, including metal and metal oxide products. These products show promising catalytic and antidiabetic, antioxidant, and antimicrobial activities.

Methanol extracts of this lichen when applied against HeLa (cervical) cancer cells were considered noncytotoxic.

The presence of betulin and betulinic acid in fan Ramalina is intriguing, as both compounds have been widely studied for their anticancer and antiviral activity. A common source for these components is birch bark.

Southern strap lichen (*Ramalina stenospora*) is confined to the subtropical regions of Georgia, Florida, and the Gulf Coast. It contains stenosporic acid, which exhibits activity against *Aeromonas hydrophila*, *Bacillus cereus*, *B. subtilis*, *Listeria monocytogenes*, *Proteus vulgaris*, *Staphylococcus aureus*, *Streptococcus faecalis*, *Yersinia enterocolitica*, *Candida albicans*, and *C. glabrata* (Candan et al. 2006).

Ramalina usnea derives its specific name from its usnea-like appearance, at least at first glance. It is found in southern regions of North America, associated with mainly hardwood trees. This lichen contains usnic, sekikaic, and homosekikaic acids, as well as 4-methyoxy-6-propyl-methyl benzoate. Work by Moreira et al. (2016) found methanol extracts of this lichen killed 100% of mosquito (*Aedes aegypti*) larvae.

RHIZOCARPON

Map Lichens

Geographic Range: North America

Habitat: usually on non-calcareous rocks

Practical Uses: dye for wool

Medicinal Applications: antibacterial, potentially anticancer

Notable Chemicals: psoromic, norstictic and rhizocarpic acid, beta-orcinol depsidones

There are, at last count, more than 70 species of map lichens (*Rhizocarpon* spp.) in North America. *Rhizo* is from the Greek meaning "root" and *karpos*, also Greek, means "fruit."

Yellow map lichen (*Rhizocarpon geographicum* syn. *Buellia geographica*) presents in various shades of yellow, with black apothecia. It is the most common and widespread of the yellow map lichens, ranging from the high arctic to Alaska, and at higher elevations south to Arizona and California.

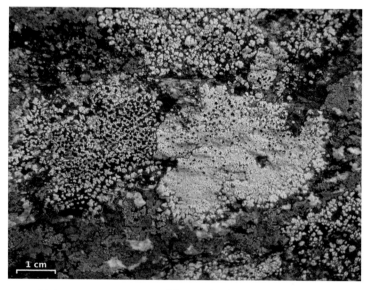

Rhizocarpon geographicum (Yellow Map Lichen)
and *R. lecanorinum*

Work by Miral et al. (2022a) examined the microbiota associated with this lichen. They isolated and identified 68 fungal isolates in 43 phylogenetic groups, 15 bacterial isolates in five taxonomic groups, and three microalgae belonging to two species. They could not identify 12 more fungal isolates from 10 different taxa, as they had never before been sequenced, described, or studied.

French scientists sampled the lichen after exposure to oil spills and found a set of bacterial strains resistant to a wide range of antibiotics and displaying tolerance to persistent organic pollutants (Miral et al. 2022).

The bacterium *Paenibacillus odorifer*, associated with this lichen, has two compounds containing *tert*-butylphenol groups. One compound exhibits significant cytotoxicity against B16 murine melanoma and HaCaT human keratinocyte cell lines (Nguyen et al. 2018).

Yellow map lichen yields a brown dye for wool. It contains the pigment rhizonic acid and tetronic acid derivatives, as well as psoromic, parellic, and rhizocarpic acids. The latter compound is weakly antibacterial against *Bacillus subtilis*, and possesses selective antitumor activity against the NS-1 (murine myeloma) cell line (James et al. 2023).

In 2014 this lichen and *Xanthoria elegans* (described later) survived for 18 months on walls inside the International Space Station. Upon their return to Earth, they began to grow! Some scientists speculate lichens may exist or could survive on Mars.

RHIZOPLACA
Rock Posy or Rockbright Lichens

Geographic Range: North America

Habitat: siliceous or calcareous rocks, or unattached on dry soil

Practical Uses: natural dyes for wool or silk

Medicinal Applications: antibacterial, cancer

Notable Chemicals: psoromic acid, usnic acid

Orange rock posy lichen (*Rhizoplaca chrysoleuca* syn. *Lecanora chrysoleuca*) is widespread on granite rock in western North America, from Alaska to New Mexico. Its content of secondary metabolites varies with location. Some lichens contain placodiolic or pseudoplacodiolic acid, others psoromic acid or combination, and others just usnic acid.

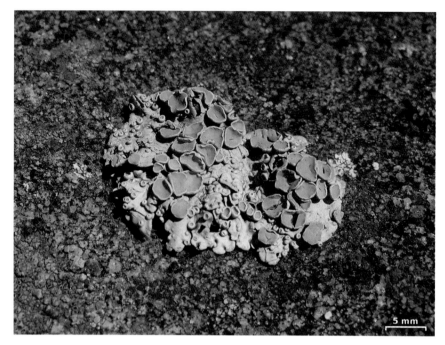

Rhizoplaca chrysoleuca
(Orange Rock Posy Lichen)

Hexane extracts of orange posy lichen exhibit high radical-scavenging capacity (Kumar et al. 2014).

Marginal rock posy lichen (*Rhizoplaca marginalis*) extracts exhibited significant activity against methicillin-resistant *Staphylococcus aureus* (MRSA) in a study of 34 North American lichens by Shrestha et al. (2014).

Green rock posy lichen (*Rhizoplaca melanophthalma*) is found on siliceous or calcareous rocks, ranging from the far northern arctic islands to Arizona. This lichen is active against *Bacillus subtilis* and *Staphylococcus aureus*. Psoromic acid, isolated from the lichen, was investigated for its potential in treating glioblastoma multiforme cancer. Cytotoxicity was noted on human U87MG-GBM cell lines in vitro (Emsen et al. 2016). Psoromic acid also showed activation of apoptosis against human prostate androgen-insensitive DU-145 and androgen-sensitive LNCaP cancer cells lines (Russo et al. 2012).

Recent work by Cometto et al. (2022) found a high diversity of basidiomycetous yeasts in the green rock posy lichen mycobiome. Between this lichen and *Tephromela atra*, they isolated and cultured 76 new strains of yeast.

Orange rock posy, green rock posy, and brown rock posy (*Rhizoplaca peltata*) lichens have been studied by Cansaran et al. (2006) in terms of their

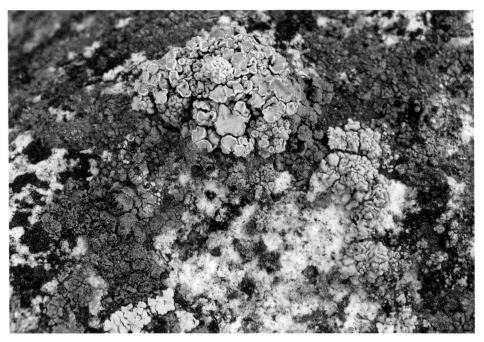

Rhizoplaca melanophthalma
(Green Rock Posy Lichen)

usnic acid content. In these three species, usnic acid varied from 0.19% to 4.0% dry weight. Antibacterial activity was determined against *Escherichia coli, Enterococcus faecalis, Proteus mirabilis, Staphylococcus aureus, Bacillus subtilis, B. megaterium (Priestia megaterium),* and *Pseudomonas aeruginosa.*

RIMELIA
Cracked Ruffle Lichens

Geographic Range: southeastern North America

Habitat: bark of deciduous trees, sometimes rocks

Practical Uses: food component, probiotic growth in yogurt and cheese, spice

Medicinal Applications: kidney conditions, sexually transmitted infections

Notable Chemicals: atranorin, beta-orcinol depsides and depsidones, diffractaic acid, fatty acids, lichexathone, orcinol, salazinic acid

Cracked ruffle lichen (*Rimelia cetrata* syn. *Parmotrema cetratum*) is found on deciduous trees in the eastern and southeastern United States, and west to east Texas.

Increasing awareness of the importance of a healthy gut microbiome has led to increased ingestion of functional foods and supplements. An example is the probiotic *Lactobacillus casei*, with uses as follow:

> *Lactobacillus casei* is found in cheese and yogurt products and prevents antibiotic-induced diarrhea and *C. difficile* infections. Human studies show improvement in depressive moods in only ten days, after consumption of yogurt containing *L. casei*. It increases microbiome Bifidobacterium levels, as well. The bacterium reduces anxiety and improves gut health in patients suffering chronic fatigue syndrome and produces GABA and acetylcholine in the transverse colon. The microbe helps relieve constipation and improves the quality of life in patients with Parkinson's disease (Rogers, 2019). An extract of cracked ruffle lichen, along with three others, was tested for its growth-promoting effects on this probiotic (Gaikwad et al. 2014).

Reticulated ruffle lichen (*Rimelia reticulata* syn. *Parmotrema reticulatum*) is found on bark in well-lit woods in the same Southern regions as its cousin. This lichen is known in the West Sahel of Africa as part of a four-lichen food mixture called *yari*. On that continent it grows on ebony trees (*Diospyros mespiliformis*). It contains protein, calcium, and iron (Glew et al. 2005). Almost all the essential amino acids, except lysine, were found at a high level.

Its use in North America for food is unknown. The Tepehuan of Mexico use this lichen to treat symptoms of kidney and sexually transmitted infections. It is an ingredient in the Kabu garam masala spice used in many Indian dishes.

RINODINA
Pepper-Spore Lichens

The pepper-spore lichens (*Rinodina* spp.) make up a large and diverse genus, numbering at least 80 species. Many have no noted chemistry, while others contain pannarin, zeorin, or atranorin. The lichen *Rinodina intermedia* contains deoxylichesterinic acid.

The pepper-spore lichen called common moonglow (*Rinodina oreina*

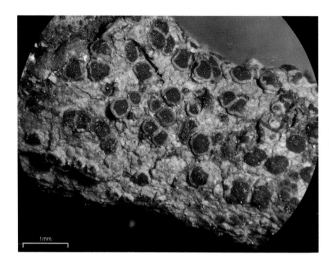

Rinodina polyspora
(Pepper-Spore Lichen)

syn. *Dimelaena oreina*) contains gyrophoric and fumaroprotocetraric acids.

The pepper-spore lichen *Rinodina stictica* contains, as the name suggests, stictic acid. Work by Pejin et al. (2017) found this acid gave moderate inhibition of HT-29 (colon) adenocarcinoma cell lines.

Tundra pepper-spore lichen (*Rinodina turfacea*) contains sphaerophorin, which possesses antioxidant activity (Yañez et al. 2023).

> *This herb is called Slime [Stune]; it grew on a stone*
> *It resists poison, it fights pain,*
> *It is called harsh [stiff], it fights against poison.*
>
> ANCIENT ANGLO-SAXON RECIPE
> TRANSLATED BY R. K. GORDON

ROCCELLA
Orchil Lichens

Geographic Range: Baja California into the Mexican states of Sonora and Sinoloa

Habitat: rock, bark in full sun

Practical Uses: dyes (especially litmus)

Medicinal Applications: asthma, antiviral, burns, potential inhibitor of *Mycobacterium tuberculosis*

Notable Chemicals: lecanoric acid, methyl orsellinate, portentol, roccellic acid

The *Roccella* genus is quite rare in North America, with only a few species identified. *Roccella* species lichens were, and still are harvested in the Mediterranean region, the Canary Islands, and South America for purple dyes called orchil.

Around the beginning of the fourteenth century, the Spanish physician Arnaldus de Villa Nova discovered the possible use of *litmus*. The term derives from the old Norse *litmos,* meaning "dye-moss." Litmus, a pigment that turns red from acid, and blue from alkaline, is manufactured from a European *Roccella* species. The development of litmus paper was invented during the sixteenth century in Holland.

"In modern times, the *litmus test* has been used in a philosophical sense as well. We may say something is a litmus test of success, or love, or commitment, meaning that it is a discriminating test that will produce a definitive answer" (Mohammed 2002).

Roccella dyes may replace or collaborate with others: Before 1500 BCE, two species of the shellfish/snail *Murex* were harvested to produce Tyrian or royal purple. In fact, the term *Phoenician* may be related to the Greek word

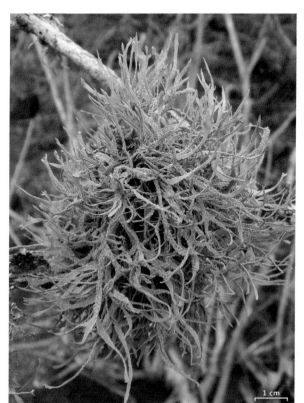

Roccella gracilis

for purple. The dye and clothing were reserved for royalty and the wealthy in Rome and Greece. Eugenia Bone (2011) notes, "'Tyrian purple' is still made by some manufacturers, from another species of snail, *Purpura lapillus*. The secretions of 10,000 snails make 1 gram of dye." The related *Purpura or Stramonita haemastoma* and *Murex or Bolinus brandaris* species produce a compound that oxidizes and changes from yellow, to green, then red or blue-black.

The lichen-derived dye is initially much brighter but fades from solar exposure, and the expensive snail-derived dye becomes richer with exposure to the sun, making a great combination.

Theophrastus, a Greek author, wrote in 320 BCE of a "seaweed" for a purple dye. This is believed to have been a coastal lichen, most likely *Roccella tinctoria*. The process involved lichens soaked in urine and various amounts of slaked lime to obtain shades of blue and purple.

Orchil lichen (*Roccella decipiens* syn. *R. babingtonii*) is found in Southern California, the coast of Texas, and south into Mexico. It was used traditionally for burns and asthma (Godinez and Ortega 1989), and contains lecanoric acid. A related species containing methyl orsellinate and montagnetol exhibits antiviral activity against Herpes simplex type-1 (Bhat et al. 2023).

Another orchil lichen, or Canary weed (*Roccella portentosa*), is found only in the southern Baja peninsula, usually on rocks or bark in full sun, and contains erythrin, lecanoric acid, roccellic acid, and portentol. Portentol has been identified as a potential potent antigen 85C (Ag85C) inhibitor of *Mycobacterium tuberculosis*. Due to the existence of drug-resistant tuberculosis (TB), the need for novel compounds is increasing. Portentol's inhibition of Ag85C represents an attack on the cell wall envelope, which is essential for virulence and survival (Pant et al. 2021).

SARCOGRAPHA
Warty Script Lichens

Warty script lichen (*Sarcographa tricosa*) is found on tree bark in Florida. The genus name may derive from the Greek *sarx*, meaning "flesh," and *graphis* for "write" or "record."

Spore-derived mycobionts were cultivated on malt yeast extract by Le et al. (2013). This led to the isolation of three eremophilane-type sesquiterpenes, 3-epi petasol, dihydropetasol, and sarcographol, along with six known eremophilanes and ergosterol peroxide.

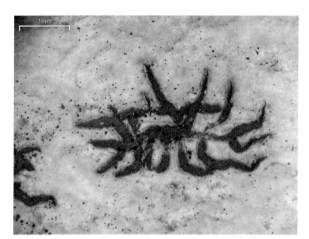

Sarcographa tricosa
(Warty Script Lichen)

SARCOGYNE

Grain-Spored Lichen

Grain-spored lichen (*Sarcogyne similis* syn. *S. reebiae*) is widespread in North America, growing on calcareous and noncalcareous (sandstone) rocks. It ranges from Nova Scotia south through the eastern states and westward to the Sonoran Desert.

Grain-spored lichen contains psoromic acid, found elsewhere in only a few *Psoroma* and *Alectoria* species. Psoromic acid inhibits the replication of herpes simplex virus type 1 and 2, as well as HSV-1 DNA polymerase, which is a key enzyme in the virus replication cycle (Hassan et al. 2019). Psoromic acid is active against HIV and possesses antitumor and antimalarial activity.

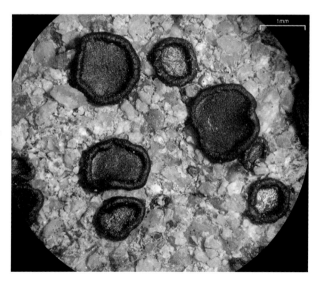

Sarcogyne similis
(Grain-Spored Lichen)

Rab geranylgeranyl transferase (RabGGTase) inhibitors have potential as selective compounds for the treatment of cancers and osteoporosis. Work by Deraeve et al. (2012) found that psoromic acid potently and selectively inhibits RabGGTase with an IC_{50} of 1.3 μM.

SCHIZOPELTE
Fog Finger Lichen

Fog finger lichen (*Schizopelte californica* syn. *Combea californica*) is restricted to coastal California from San Luis Obispo to central Baja. The former genus *Combea* was named in honor of Francesco Comba (1845), an Italian who worked in the Turin Zoological Museum. The lichen contains isoschizopeltic acid, various dibenzofurans, schizopeltic acid, erythrin, lecanoic acid, pannaric acid, and pannaric acid 2-methyl ester, as well as 3-O-methyl pannaric acid.

Erythrin has been found to be a potential antidiabetic compound, faring better than metformin, repaglinide, or sitagliptin (Rao and Hariprasad 2021).

SIPHULA
Waterfingers Lichen

Waterfingers lichen (*Siphula ceratites*) is a beautiful finger-like oceanside species on the arctic coast south to Haida Gwaii and extending east to northern Labrador. It contains the homoflavone siphulin, protosiphulin, and oxysiphulin. It is the only North American species.

Work by Joshi et al. (2020) identified siphulin as a potential inhibitor of SARS-CoV-2, with high affinity to main protease and angiotensin-converting enzyme 2. The research has not yet been peer-reviewed.

SOLORINA
Chocolate Chip or Owl Lichens

Orange chocolate chip lichen (*Solorina crocea*) is found throughout the arctic and in alpine regions of the Rocky Mountains. It is unmistakable with its bright orange medulla and red borne apothecia.

It grows on moist soil, due to seepage or retreating snow. It contains at least two laccases, and solorinic acid, norsolorinic acid, 4,4'-disolorinic acid, averantin, averythrin, methyl gyrophorate, gyrophoric acid, 6-O-methylaverantin,

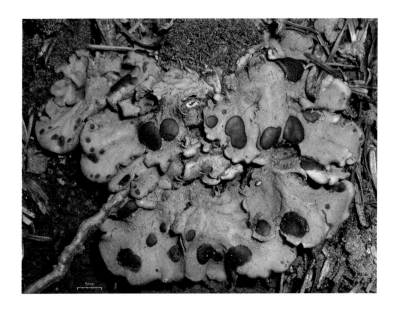

Solorina crocea
(Orange Chocolate
Chip Lichen)

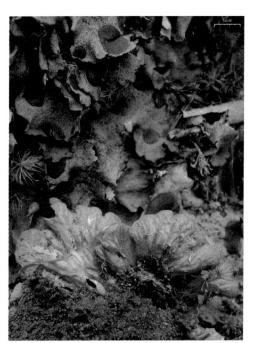

Solorina crocea
(background)

2-O-methylnorstenosporic acid, 2-O-methylglomelliferic acid, norsolorinic acid, and 2-O-methylnordivaricatic acid.

Work by Ingólfsdóttir et al. (2000) found the methanol extract of this lichen exhibits anticancer and cytotoxic activity. Averythrin and averantin exhibit activity against *Bacillus subtilis* (Liu et al. 2014).

SPHAEROPHORUS
Coral Lichens

Geographic Range: the arctic, alpine regions

Habitat: rocks, soil; humid coastal forests

Medicinal Applications: cancer; potentially treating hormone-sensitive cancers; neurodegenerative conditions

Notable Chemicals: hypothamnolic acid, pannarin, squamatic acid, sphaerophorin

Fragile coral lichen (*Sphaerophorus fragilis*) is found on rocks or soil in arctic and alpine regions. As the species name suggests, it grows in dense cushions with very fragile branches.

This species contains sphaerophorin and pannarin, which inhibits cell growth and induces apoptosis in human prostate carcinoma (DU-145) cells (Russo et al. 2006). Pannarin is moderately synergistic with gentamicin against MRSA, but antagonistic when combined with levofloxacin (Celenza et al. 2012). Sphaerophorin prevents DNA damage from UV light or nitric oxide and induces apoptosis in human melanoma cells (Russo et al. 2008). In more recent work, sphaerophorin was found to exhibit antioxidant and UVB protection. It is lipophilic, which suggests good diffusion across the skin barrier (Valencia-Islas et al. 2021).

Globe ball lichen (*Sphaerophorus globosus*) is found in the arctic and

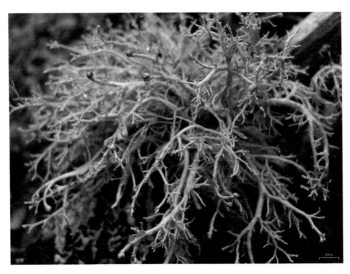

Sphaerophorus venerabilis

Antarctic on rocks, among moss. However, it also is found on mossy tree bark in humid coastal forests of both coasts. Both geographic varieties contain hypothamnolic acid, and sometimes squamatic acid. Extracts of both varieties prevented estrogen formation from estrogen precursors by inhibiting the enzymatic activities of aromatase (Ingólfsdóttir et al. 2000). Fragile coral lichen inhibition showed 95% inhibition, and coral lichen 74%.

The presence of pannarin and inhibition of aromatase suggest benefit in preventing or treating hormone-sensitive cancers, including breast, prostate, and uterine growths.

Recent work by Torres-Benitez et al. (2022) identified 14 compounds in coral lichen that show high inhibition potential on cholinesterase enzymes. This suggests possible benefit in neurodegenerative conditions, including Alzheimer's disease.

SQUAMARINA

Rim Lichens

Notable Chemicals: psoromic acid

White rim lichen (*Squamarina lentigera*) shows activity against *Enterobacter cloacae*, *Enterococcus faecalis*, and *Staphylococcus aureus* (Mendili et al. 2021). Cartilagenous rim lichen is rich in proanthocyanidin content, and a methanol extract of it exhibited high DPPH antioxidant capacity (Mendili et al. 2021a).

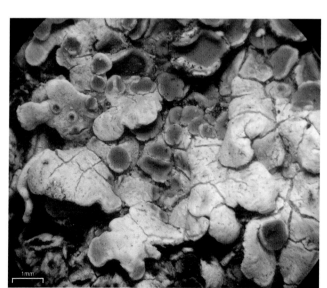

Squamarina lentigera
(White Rim Lichen)

Cartilagenous rim lichen (*Squamarina cartilaginea/S. crassa*) is somewhat rare in North America. It grows on calcareous rocks. Despite being somewhat rare, it was found in a river valley in Saskatchewan, Canada. It contains usnic, squamarone, psoromic, and 4-O-dimethylpsoromic acids.

STEREOCAULON

Alpine Lichens   Easter Lichen   Foam Lichens

Geographic Range: North America

Habitat: rocks, soil

Medicinal Applications: antibacterial, arthritis, cancer, diabetes, inflammation, respiratory conditions, skin conditions

Notable Chemicals: atranorin, lobaric acid, lobarstin, methyl 3'-methyllecanorate, norstictic, perlatolic, protolichesterinic, stictic, and usnic acid

> *To the lichenist is not the shield (or rather the apothecium) of a lichen disproportionally large compared to the universe.*
>
> HENRY DAVID THOREAU

Stereocaulon is derived from the Greek *stereos*, meaning "hard" or "firm," and *kaulos*, meaning "stem," referring to the texture of dry lichen.

Alpine foam or alpine coral lichen (*Stereocaulon alpinum*) was screened for in vitro activity against *Mycobacterium aurum*, a nonpathogenic organism with similarity of sensitivity to *M. tuberculosis*. Work by Ingólfsdóttir et al. (1998) found that lobaric acid and atranorin exhibit inhibition of this pathogen.

Protolichesterinic acid, isolated from this lichen, shows antiproliferative and cytotoxic effects against breast (T-47D and ZR-75-1) and leukemia (K-562) cancer cell lines (Ogmundsdóttir et al. 1998).

This lichen also shows activity against the gram-positive bacteria *Bacillus subtilis* and *Staphylococcus aureus* (Paudel et al. 2008).

Lobaric acid, isolated from this lichen, was tested for anti-inflammatory activity. Lobaric acid treatment of lipopolysaccharide (LPS)-stimulated macrophages decreased their nitric oxide (NO) production and expression of COX-2 and prostaglandin E2. It also significantly reduced production of tumor necrosis factor-alpha (TNF-a) and interleukin-6 by inhibiting activation of mitogen-activated protein kinases (MAPKs) and nuclear factor-kappa B (NF-$_k$B). This suggests inhibition of inflammation and an alternative approach to modulating inflammatory disease (Lee et al. 2019).

Work by Phi et al. (2022) identified bioactive terphenyls from this lichen. One compound, 2-hydroxy-3,6-dimethoxy-*p*-terphenyl, exhibits cytotoxicity against the HCT116 (colorectal) cancer cell line, and inhibits NO production in lipopolysaccharide (LPS)-induced macrophages.

Lobastin, isolated from this lichen, downregulates the TNF-alpha-mediated induction of vascular cell adhesion molecules, suggesting it could provide an important regulator of inflammation associated with atherosclerosis (Lee et al. 2016). Lee et al. concluded that lobastin may be an important regulator of inflammation in atherosclerotic lesions, and might be a novel treatment.

Other compounds found in this lichen include usimines A–C, which are usnic acid derivatives. These three as well as usnic acid show moderate inhibitory activity against therapeutically targeted tyrosine phosphatase 1B (PTP1B) (Seo et al. 2008). The same lab (Seo et al. 2009) identified lobaric acid and two pseudodepsidone-type compounds with similar inhibitory activity on protein tyrosine phosphatase 1B (PTP1B). Inhibition of PTP1B is crucial in type 2 diabetes, as it has a regulatory effect on insulin and leptin signaling transduction.

Lobaric acid and lobarstin have been extracted from this lichen. Work by Hong et al. (2018) found that both compounds inhibit proliferation of HeLa (human cervix adenocarcinoma) and HCT116 (human colon carcinoma) cell lines. Significant apoptosis followed cell cycle perturbation and arrest in G2/M cycle. Significant downregulation of the apoptosis regulator B-cell lymphoma 2, and upregulation of the cleaved form of the poly (ADP-ribose) polymerase, indicated a DNA repair and apoptosis regulator.

Lobaric acid is also found in grand foam lichen (*Stereocaulon grande*), pixie foam lichen (*S. pileatum*), snow foam lichen (*Stereocaulon rivulorum*), rock foam lichen (*Stereocaulon saxatile*), *Stereocaulon intermedium*, *Stereocaulon sterile*, bony foam lichen (*Stereocaulon tennesseense*), and other species.

The lichen *Stereocaulon evolutum* may or may not be found in North America, but the Consortium of Lichen Herbaria, Lichen Portal website does suggest a collection from Maine. This lichen contains atranorin, atranol, lobaric acid, ursolic acid, and methyl 3'-methyllecanorate. Work by Huyen et al. (2017) found the latter compound the most cytotoxic against seven cancer cell lines: HuH7 (hepatoma), CaCo-2 (colon), MDA-MB-231 (breast), HCT116 (colorectal), PC3 (prostate), NCI-H727 (lung), and HaCaT (epidermal/skin). To put this into perspective, consider that in 2020, some 1.4 million men were diagnosed with prostate cancer worldwide. One in eight American men will be diagnosed with prostate cancer in their lifetime. Nearly 2.3 million women worldwide were diagnosed with breast cancer in 2022, with nearly one in every eight diagnosed with breast cancer in their lifetime. Worldwide, over 685,000 deaths from breast cancer occurred in 2020.

Protein tyrosine phosphatase 1B plays a key role in type 2 diabetes and other diseases. An extract from this lichen showed strong inhibition. Fractionation by Huyen et al. (2021) identified lobaric acid and norlobaric acid as the most potent components.

Greenland foam lichen (*Stereocaulon groenlandicum*) is found in central Alaska. It contains a mixture of porphyrilic, miriquidic, anziatic, and perlatolic acids.

Easter lichen (*Stereocaulon paschale*) is found throughout most of Canada. This lichen and other flat lichens were used by the Barrens-Keewatin Inuit as a filler in caribou skins to make rafts to cross rivers and streams.

The Mistissini Cree of northern Quebec call Easter lichen *wapskirnok*. It is made into a beverage for arthritis and rheumatism associated with diabetes (Fraser 2006; Leduc et al. 2006). Traditional Chinese Medicine uses this lichen for various skin and respiratory conditions.

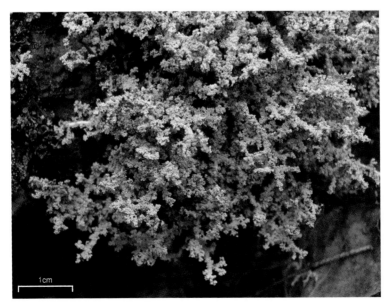

Stereocaulon paschale (Easter Lichen)

Ascomatic acid dibenzofuran derivatives isolated from the Easter lichen show antibacterial activity against the oral pathogens *Porphyromonas gingivalis* and *Streptococcus mutans* (Carpentier et al. 2017).

Lobaric acid and pseudodepsidones from the same lichen were found to inhibit the NF-kB activation and secretion of the pro-inflammatory cytokines IL-Ibeta and TNF-alpha in LPS-stimulated macrophages. They inhibit the NF-kB pathway via the activation of PPAR-gamma (Carpentier et al. 2018). Other secondary metabolites and compounds are atranorin, and dextro-mannose and dextro-galactose.

Ramulose foam lichen (*Stereocaulon ramulosum*) is found no further north than Mexico. It contains methyl haematommate. Ramulose means "many small branches."

Woolly foam lichen (*Stereocaulon sasakii*) is a beautiful, turquoise-colored species living on soil or mossy rocks from Alaska to Northern California. It has also been identified in Colorado and Wisconsin. This lichen contains lobaric acid and sakisacaulon (benzofuran). Lobaric acid inhibited the polymerization of tubulin (Morita et al. 2009), suggesting antimitotic activity.

Variegated foam lichen (*Stereocaulon vesuvianum*) attaches to newly exposed rocks. It contains stictic and norstictic acid.

STICTA

Moon Lichens   Crater Lichens

Moon or crater lichens (*Sticta* spp.) are not very common in North America (7 species), but reside on mossy rock or bark, in areas with high humidity.

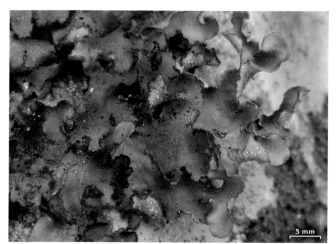

Sticta beauvoisii
(Fringed Moon Lichen)

Work by Widhelm et al. (2018) estimates the genus *Sticta* originated about 30 million years ago.

An unidentified *Sticta* species was found to contain stictamides A–C (Liang et al. 2011). Stictamide A was evaluated against a panel of disease-relevant proteases; it inhibited MMP12 and significantly reduced invasion in human glioma (U87MG) cell line. A docking study suggests stictamide A inhibits MMP12 by a non-zinc-binding mechanism. This is unusual, as zinc is usually involved. Macrophage elastase (MMP12) suggests its cellular source, an enzyme that degrades elastin.

Stictamide A has been tested in various cancers, including colorectal, non-small-cell lung, prostate, liver, and head and neck squamous cell carcinoma. Inhibition modifies the response to inflammation and limits the growth of tumor metastases.

TELOSCHISTES

Golden Lichens   Orange Lichens

Geographic Range: North America
Habitat: branches, shrubs, soil
Medicinal Applications: inhibiting leukemic cell proliferation, antitumor effect
Notable Chemicals: flavicansone, parietin

Golden-eye, or gold-eye, lichen (*Teloschistes chrysophthalmus*) contains parietin, which exhibits a virucidal effect against the Junin and Tacaribe arenaviruses (Fazio et al. 2007). The lichen is most common in the Mississippi River valley, on branches and shrubs. It is also found in Baja and northern Mexico. This beautiful orange lichen is designated as Manitoba's unofficial provincial representative. The genus name means "split ends."

Powdered orange bush or golden hair lichen (*Teloschistes flavicans*) is becoming rare on the east coast of North America but is still found on branches and the ground on the west coast and in the south.

Flavicansone, rhizonic acid, parietin, falacinol, falacinal, teloschistin (fallacinol), and vicanicin have been identified in *Teloschistes flavicans*. Flavicansone showed the highest rate of inhibition of all these compounds against leukemic (HL-60) cell proliferation (Sanjaya et al. 2020).

The anthraquinone parietin is found in several other lichens. The compound

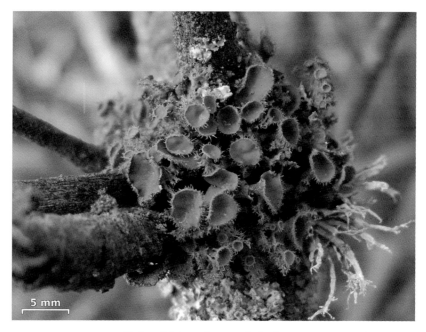

Teloschistes chrysophthalmus
(Golden-Eye or Gold-Eye Lichen)

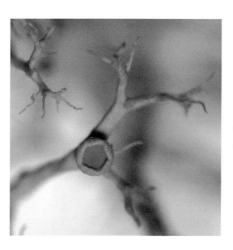

Teloschistes flavicans
(Powdered Orange Bush
or Golden Hair Lichen)

is being studied for its promising photosensitizing action in photodynamic therapy on leukemic cells. Work by Mugas et al. (2021) looked at its effect in mammary carcinoma LM2 cells both in vitro and in vivo. Combining parietin with blue light impaired cell growth and migration in vitro. It also induced a significant decrease in cell migration. In detail, when parietin was applied to the skin of mice subcutaneously implanted with LM2 cells and then illuminated with blue light, a significant tumor reduction was determined by day three.

More study is required, but it appears the natural anthraquinones administered topically to cutaneous malignancies may be beneficial against skin cancer.

Cogno et al. (2020) found that parietin derived from *Teloschistes flavicans* induced apoptosis in human colorectal (SW480) cancer cell lines.

This lichen increases its saturated fatty acid content in summer, and increases unsaturated fatty acids during winter, in order to maintain membrane fluidity (Reis et al. 2005).

Acetone extracts of this lichen and the compound vicanicin were compared to quercitin, examining antidiabetic activity (Maulidyah et al. 2020).

TEPHROMELA
Black-Eye Lichen

Black-eye lichen (*Tephromela atra*) is widespread in North America and is one of only five species in this genus identified to date. It is well named for its

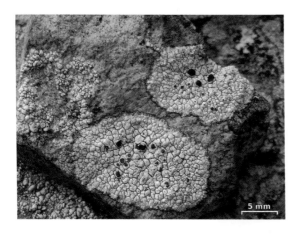

Tephromela atra
(Black-Eye Lichen)

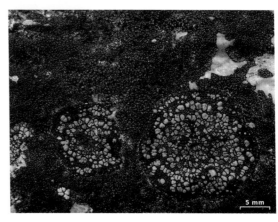

Tephromela armeniaca syn. *Calvitimela armeniaca*

appearance on siliceous rocks and sometimes on bark. It contains antranorin, *a*-collatolic, and at times alectoronic acid.

THAMNOLIA
Worm Lichens

Geographic Range: arctic and colder climates, northern Pacific Northwest and rugged parts of Eastern Canada

Habitat: arctic and alpine rocks, exposed gravel soil between mosses and heath, on windy slopes near sea level

Practical Use: skincare

Medicinal Applications: cancer; cough and hoarseness; immune modulation; weight reduction

Notable Chemicals: atranorin, baeomycesic, squamatic, and thamnolic acids; thamnolan

White worm lichen (*Thamnolia vermicularis*) occurs in two different chemotypes. One, var. *vermicularis*, contains thamnolic acid and is found in Yukon and coastal mountains. The other variation, *subuliformis,* is richer in squamatic and baeomycic acid and is found in the Rocky and Appalachian mountains.

White worm lichen is the unofficial territorial lichen of Nunavut. Birds like the golden plover use the lichen as part of nesting material.

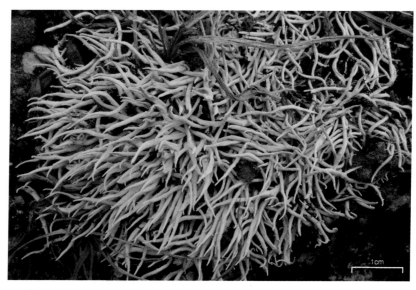

Thamnolia vermicularis (White Worm Lichen)

I lived and worked in Peru, from 1982 to 1984, and traveled to Ecuador and Bolivia on holidays. In the street markets of La Paz, this lichen is sold and used for cough and hoarseness.

Some taxonomists separate the variants into *Thamnolia vermicularis* and *Thamnolia subuliformis*. The latter lichen has a wider range of antibacterial activity and better inhibition of gram-positive bacteria (Wang et al. 2022).

A new polysaccharide from *Thamnolia subliformis*, named thamnolan, exhibits immune modulation in an in vitro phagocytosis assay and in the classic anticomplementary assay (Olafsdottir et al. 1999). Earlier work by Ingólfsdóttir et al. (1997a) identified baeomycesic acid in this species, or subspecies. The compound showed potent inhibition on 5-lipooxygenase in vitro.

Analysis of *Thamnolia vermicularis* by Xiang et al. (2013) isolated three beta-orcinol-type depsides, as well as the known hypothamnolic acid 3'-methylevenic acid, baeomyoesic acid, squamatic acid, methyl 3'-methyllecanorate, barbatinic acid, and atranorin. Other studies have found decarboxythamnolic acid.

Work by Bustinza (1952) identified activity against *Alcaligenes faecalis*, a pathogenic, drug-resistant pathogen (see *Punctelia rudecta*, page 195, and *Xanthoparmelia conspersa*, page 259).

Yamamoto et al. (1998) found methanol extracts of *Thamnolia vermicularis* inhibit Epstein–Barr virus activation-induced teleocidin B-4, a potent tumor promoter.

This lichen is edible, and when given to high-fat diet mice for three months, it significantly reduced visceral fat mass and body weight compared to the control. It increased the "good" high-density lipoprotein (HDL) and cholesterol levels, and lowered insulin resistance. This suggests a natural treatment for syndrome X, which involves obesity, cholesterol, and blood sugar issues (Choi et al. 2017).

Work by Haraldsdóttir et al. (2004) found slight antiproliferative activity from whole extracts against AGS (stomach), Capan-1, Capan-2 and PANC-1 (pancreas), HL-60 (leukemia), K-562 (myelogenous leukemia), and JURKAT (T cell leukemia), NCI-H1417 (lung), NIH:OVCAR-3 (ovarian), PC-3 (prostate), T47-D (breast) and WiDr (colorectal) cancer cell lines.

Thamnoliadepside A, isolated from this lichen, inhibits the growth of prostate cancer cells (Guo et al. 2011). The compounds thamnolic acid A, everninic acid, baeomycesic acid, beta-orcinol, beta-resorcylic acid, ethyl orsellinate, squamatic acid, and vermicularin were also isolated and identified.

Ethanol extracts of *Thamnolia vermicularis* were able to improve learning ability in APP/PSI transgenic mice by inhibiting both amyloid beta levels and tau protein hyperphosphorylation. The extracts markedly reduced the number of senile plaques in the hippocampus and cortex. This suggests a natural tincture for the treatment of Alzheimer's disease (Li et al. 2017).

Follow-up work by Yu et al. (2022) prepared a water extract of the lichen and its inhibition of amyloid fibrillation was followed. Three small molecules were identified, but not named or revealed. (This secrecy could be because there is a patent pending.)

This lichen has been used in Traditional Chinese Medicine for aging skin. Vermicularin and beta-sitosterol have both been identified from the lichens as important for preserving skin health. Vermicularin prevents the loss of collagen type I and inhibits the production of matrix metalloproteinases-1. Beta-sitosterol is common in nature and increases the expression of hyaluronic acid synthases in fibroblasts (Haiyuan et al. 2019).

THELOMMA

Nipple Lichens

Rock nipple lichen (*Thelomma mammosum* syn. *Cypheliopsis bolanderi*) is found on the Pacific Coast and coastal mountains from Vancouver Island to central California. It looks at first appearance somewhat like miniature barnacles on

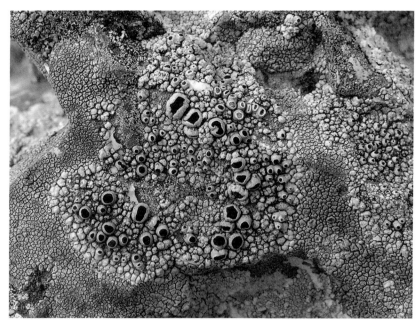

Thelomma mammosum (Rock Nipple Lichen)

rocks, with volcano or nipple-shaped verrucae. It contains norstictic, salazinic, 3-chlorodivaricatic, and 5-chlorodivaricatic acids.

TONINIA
Blister Lichen

There are at least 24 blister lichens in North America, most found on lime-based soil or rocks.

Blister lichen (*Toninia candida* syn. *Lecidea candida* syn. *Thalloidima candidum*) is found on calcareous rocks, mainly in alpine and arctic regions. The genus name honors the Italian botanist/lichenologist Carlo Tonini (1803–1877).

It contains norstictic acid, exhibiting higher antioxidant activity than *Usnea barbata* (Rankovic et al. 2012). Norstictic acid shows a strong cytotoxic effect and induces apoptosis on FemX (melanoma) and LS174 (colorectal) cancer cell lines (Rankovic et al. 2012).

TRYPETHELIUM

The *Trypethelium* genus comprises about 50 subtropical and tropical species.

The speckled blister lichen (*Trypethelium eluteriae*) is extremely rich in colored pigments. Research by Basnet et al. (2019) identified the yellow pigment as trypethelonamide A and the dark violet-red pigment as 5'-hydroxytrypethelone. Other pigments previously identified include (+)-8-hydroxy-7-methoxytrupethelone, (+)-trypethelone, and (–)-trypethelone. All five were tested for their cytotoxicity against various cancer cell lines, and all showed moderate and weak activity against the RKO (colon) cancer cell line.

Work by Srinivasan et al. (2020) identified various trypethelone derivatives, and screened them against *Mycobacterium tuberculosis* and non-tuberculosis mycobacteria. One compound inhibited *Mycobacterium tuberculosis* strain H37Rv with a minimal inhibitory concentration of 12.5 µg/mL.

TUCKERMANNOPSIS
Fringed Wrinkle Lichen

There are seven *Tuckermannopsis* species on the continent. The genus is named in honor of Edward Tuckerman (1817–1886), best known for his *Synopsis of North American Lichens* (1882).

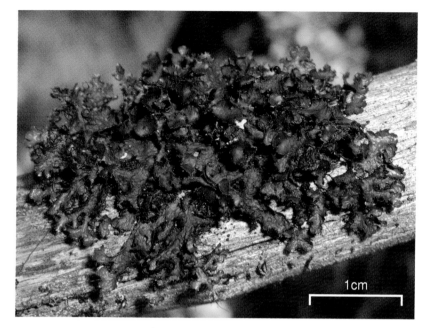

Tuckermannopsis americana
(Fringed Wrinkle Lichen)

Fringed wrinkle lichen (*Tuckermannopsis americana* syn. *Cetraria halei* syn. *C. ciliaris* var. *halei*) is commonly found on twigs and branches of conifers and birch trees. Its range extends from the Northwest Territories to Newfoundland and south along the eastern seaboard. I have found it growing on birch bark in central Alberta, near where I live.

Alectoronic acid has been found in this lichen. Work by Ureña-Vacas et al. (2022) found that *Tuckermannopsis americana* methanol extracts conveyed neuroprotection on neuroblastoma cells, in a hydrogen peroxide oxidative stress model. *Vulpicida pinastri* and *Dactylina arctica* showed even more promise to treat and prevent oxidative stress-related neurodegenerative diseases. Another effect of alectoronic acid derived from this lichen is inhibition of acetylcholinesterase and butyrylcholinesterase, suggestive of benefit in neurodegenerative diseases (Ureña-Vacas et al. 2022a).

The related *Tuckermannopsis ciliaris* (syn. *Cetraria ciliaris*) contains olivetoric and protolichesterinic acids. This lichen is distributed in temperate areas around the Great Lakes and Appalachian Mountains, with a disjunction in northern Alaska. It is more abundant than *Tuckermannopsis americana* in the southern regions of its range.

Work by Shrestha et al. (2015) found extracts of this lichen to be cytotoxic to Burkitt's lymphoma (Raji) cells. The extracts decreased proliferation, accumulated cells at the G0/G1 stage, and caused apoptosis. They upregulated p53 and the expression of TK1.

UMBILICARIA
Navel Lichens   Rock Tripe Lichens

Geographic Range: from high arctic down to Arizona
Habitat: on granite and other siliceous rocks
Medicinal Applications: antibacterial, cancer, cleaning wounds and skin, treating tuberculosis and prolonged bleeding, eliminating intestinal parasites, treating stomach conditions, treating mouth sores
Notable Chemicals: atranorin, evernic, gyrophoric, lecanoric, norstictic, salazinic, stictic, umbilicaric, and usnic acids; parietin

There are some 35 species of *Umbilicaria* lichens in North America. The genus name relates to its umbilicus or belly button shape, very fitting for one of the planet's first fetal life forms. It is also known as rock tripe, which suggests edibility.

The best known and most studied *Umbilicaria* species is the Japanese *iwatake* (*U. esculenta*). This is a prized and pricey commercial delicacy.

Members of the Franklin expedition of 1820–1821 survived the first winter by eating *tripes de roche*, which they harvested each day, until exhaustion and starvation brought an end to their suffering.

The Chipewyan call it *waac*.

Fur trader Daniel Harmon describes it as a crucial food source, but especially important to the Nipigon First Nations who were "frequently obliged, by necessity, to subsist on [it]." It was "a kind of moss, which they find adhering to the rocks, and which they denominate As-se-ne-Wa-quon-uck, that is eggs of the rock . . . this moss when boiled with pimicin, &c. dissolves into a glutinous substance, and is very palatable; but when cooked in water only, it is far otherwise, as it then has an unpleasant, bitter taste" (Harmon 1904, 280–81).

In North America, of the more than 35 *Umbilicaria* species, nine contain gyrophoric acid, which shows cytotoxic and antiproliferative properties against several cancer cell lines and is a broad-spectrum antimicrobial agent (Singh et al. (2022).

Umbilicaria species have been used in North America to treat tuberculosis. The Inuit of northern Quebec brewed a tea for this (Stevens et al. 1984; Sharnoff 1997), as did the Dena'ina of Alaska. Known as rock ear, or *qalnigi jegha*, the lichen was decocted to treat tuberculosis and for prolonged bleeding (Kari 1987).

Rock tripe is known to the Inuit as *quajautit*, a word associated with slipperiness underfoot. The lichen absorbs blood when cleaning a wound and applied to ripening skin boils. On Baffin Island, the lichen helps absorb oil from skins of baby seals. The boiled water was drunk by the spoonful, but the lichen was generally not eaten. The decoction may be used for soothing canker sores and bleeding gums (Rogers 2011).

A number of *Umbilicaria* species are synonymous with *Gyrophora*. I will not bore you with any synonyms unless disparate, or different, from the same species. Information on some species is found in a paper by Posner and Feige (1992).

Frosted rock tripe lichen (*Umbilicaria americana*) grows on steep, granite rock faces in protected shady sites. It is one of the thickest rock tripes, with a texture similar to firm cardboard. It looks somewhat like *Umbilicaria vellea*, which is smaller and rarer in the alpine and arctic regions.

Methanol extracts of both this lichen and *Cladonia rangiformis* were found protective against various mutagens in work by Gulluce et al. (2011). Strong antioxidative and antigenotoxic mechanisms were noted for the extracts in damage caused by aflatoxin B on human lymphocytes (Aslan et al. 2012). Aflatoxin, mentioned in an earlier chapter and noted for its presence in peanut butter, is is also found at low levels in corn products. This is significant because over time aflatoxin can lead to cirrhosis and is a leading cause of liver cancer. In fact, some sources estimate it kills more people each year than malaria.

Starred rock tripe lichen (*Umbilicaria angulata*) contains gyrophoric and umbilicaric acids.

Arctic rock tripe lichen (*Umbilicaria arctica*) contains gyrophoric and norstictic acids.

The endolichenic fungus *Ulospora bilgramii* inhabits several *Umbilicaria* species. Xie et al. (2020) identified nine heptaketides, ulsporin A–G, one diphenyl compound, ulophenol, and palmarumycin (spirobisnaphthalene). Ulosporin G inhibits the growth of A549 and of MCF-7 (breast) and KB (epithelial) human cancer cell lines, and induced A549 (lung) cancer cell apoptosis.

Folded rock tripe lichen (*Umbilicaria caroliniana* syn. *Lasallia caroliniana*) is found on exposed rocks at high elevations in the Appalachian Mountains, but also in northern Yukon and Alaska. It contains gyrophoric and lecanoric acids, as well as unknown substances.

Questionable rock tripe lichen (*Umbilicaria cinereorufescens*) is found on siliceous rocks from northern Alaska and Nunavet, and in elevated regions of Arizona. It contains gyrophoric acid.

Crusty navel lichen (*Umbilicaria crustulosa* syn. *Omphalodiscus crustulosus*) contains gyrophoric acid, crustinic acid, and unknown substances. It grows on rocks in the high arctic.

Fringed rock tripe lichen (*Umbilicaria cylindrica*) contains depsidone, salazinic acid, norstictic acid, methyl-beta-orcinol carboxylate, ethyl haematommate, atronorin, and usnic acid (Manojlovic et al. 2012). Ethanol extracts exhibit cytotoxicity against slow-growing BS-C-1 cells (African green monkey kidney, ATCC CCL 26) (Perry et al. 1999).

Netted rock tripe lichen (*Umbilicaria decussata*) is found in the high arctic, but also in the Rockies and south to Arizona and New Mexico, at elevated altitude. It contains gyrophoric acid.

Work by Vaez et al. (2021) studied 42 lichens for potential anticoagulation. This lichen showed the longest clotting time in both activated partial thromboplastin time and prothrombin time assays. Atranol, orsellinic acid, D-mannitol, lecanoric acid, and evernic acid were found to be possible anticoagulants. The authors suggest potential use for issues related to cardiovascular disease.

Peppered rock tripe lichen (*Umbilicaria deusta* syn. *Gyrophora flocculosa*) is widespread, from Alaska down to Washington state, and across to Newfoundland and northeastern states on exposed rocks. It contains gyrophoric and umbilicaric acid.

Hairy navel lichen (*Umbilicaria hirsuta*) is rather rare, but found in the Rocky Mountains, northern Alaska, southern Ontario, and northern Appalachians. It is the only sorediate species in North America. It is rich in gyrophoric acid, which has been purified for cancer studies. Work by Goga et al. (2019) found antiproliferative activity by gyrophoric acid against HeLa (human cervix carcinoma) and other cell lines. Gyrophoric acid induced ROS and apoptosis related to cancer cell death.

This lichen is rich in parietin, umbilicaric acid, atranorin, and usnic acid. The latter two compounds induced massive loss in the mitochondrial membrane potential, caspase-3 activation, and phosphatidylserine externalization in

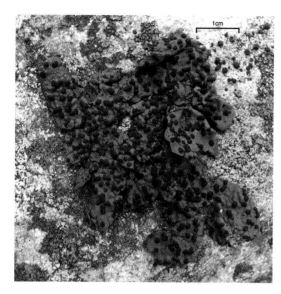

Umbilicaria hyperborea
(Blistered Rock Tripe Lichen)

test cancer cell lines. They were more effective than parietin and gyrophoric acid in inducing apoptosis in HT29 (colon) and A2780 (ovarian) human cancer cell lines. The lichen extract was very effective against ovarian, leukemia (HL-60), and Jurkat (lymphocyte leukemia) cell lines (Backorová et al. 2012).

Blistered rock tripe lichen (*Umbilicaria hyperborea*) is found on rocks in the far north (*hyperborea* means far north) but also in elevated regions south into California and the Rockies, as well as eastern Canada. It contains gyrophoric and umbilicaric acids.

Smooth rock tripe lichen (*Umbilicaria mammulata* syn. *Gyrophora dillenii*) is known as *asine-wakunik* to the Attikamekw of Quebec, and was boiled and placed on a woman's belly during a difficult childbirth (Raymond 1945). The Nihitahawak Cree of eastern Saskatchewan use the very similar name *asiniwakon*. Among this group, this lichen has been made into a soup that did not upset the stomach and added to fish broth as a thickener (Leighton 1985).

Smooth rock tripe lichen contains glycophoric, constictic, and lecanoric acids. Acetone extracts show activity against the virulent *Pseudomonas aeruginosa* (Shrestha et al. 2014). This is among the drug-resistant strains that are becoming more common, especially acquired in hospitals, associated with wounds from surgery or burns, and found as contaminants in catheters and ventilators. In the United States in 2017, about 32,600 cases of drug-resistant infection were recorded, with 2,700 deaths.

Plated rock tripe lichen (*Umbilicaria muehlenbergii* syn. *Actinogyra muehlenbergii*) is known to the northern Chipewyan as *thetsi*. The species name honors Henry Muhlenberg (1753–1815), a botanist and Lutheran minister in Pennsylvania. The famous Edward Tuckerman (mentioned earlier) preserved his herbarium.

Plated rock tripe lichen, called "rock dirt," is burned slightly in a frying pan, then mashed and boiled into a syrup that is cooled and consumed. Alternatively, it can be chewed for the same purpose (Marles 1984; Marles et al. 2000). It was also burned to ash and boiled into a syrup taken orally to remove intestinal parasites by northern Indigenous peoples.

The Cree of Manitoba call it *asinîwâkon*, the same name given to smooth rock tripe by the neighboring Cree in Saskatchewan. A decoction is given to someone to clean out their stomach (Marles et al. 2000) or to soothe an upset stomach. Wood ash helps neutralize the bitterness and acidity.

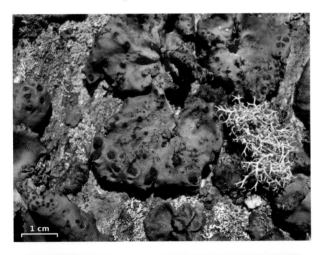

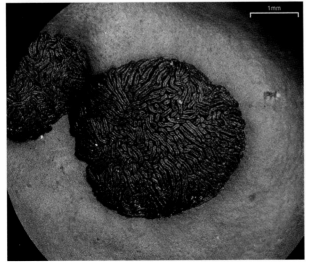

Umbilicaria muehlenbergii (Plated Rock Tripe Lichen)

The Dehcho (Dene) of the Northwest Territories refer to the plated rock lichen as *kwechi*. A soup using this lichen is eaten as a tonic and to help respiratory conditions (Rebesca et al. 1994; Uprety et al. 2012).

Plated rock tripe lichen contains a number of cytotoxic and antibiotic compounds, including glycophoric, constictic, and lecanoric acids. In vitro anticancer studies by Mohammadi (2021; Mohammadi et al. 2022) showed positive activity. A crude extract showed activity against gram-positive *Staphylococcus aureus* (Letwin 2017). An acetone extract exhibited cytotoxic activity against MCF-7 breast cancer cells at 2.3 times higher dose than cisplatin. Isolated fractions caused cell cycle arrest in 73.1% of cancer cells (Letwin et al. 2020).

Ascerbic rock tripe lichen (*Umbilicaria nylanderiana*) growth is widespread and contains gyrophoric and umbilicaric acids.

Emery rock tripe lichen (*Umbilicaria phaea*) is named for its rough, emery-like texture. This common western rock tripe is found on rocks in the Northwest Territories, but also thrives in dry, hot desert regions from British Columbia to California. Various viruses are hosted, including *Caulimovirus*, associated with the green algae photobionts (*Trebouxia*) (Merges et al. 2021).

Three *Umbilicaria* species were tested for antioxidant, antimicrobial, and anticancer activity (Kosanic et al. 2012). All three lichens, including fringed rock tripe lichen (*Umbilicaria cylindrica*) and crusty navel lichen (*Umbilicaria crustulosa*), showed strong anticancer activity against FemX (human melanoma) and LS174 (human colon carcinoma) cell lines (Kosanic et al. 2012). Petaled rock tripe lichen (*Umbilicaria polyphylla*) showed the greatest free radical scavenging activity, similar to the standard antioxidants.

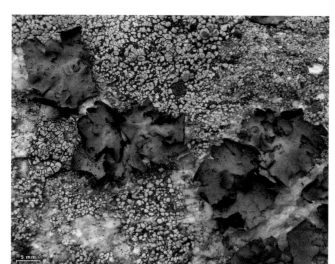

Umbilicaria polyphylla (Petaled Rock Tripe Lichen)

This lichen contains gyrophoric, umbilicaric, and lecanoric acids, and possesses antimicrobial activity.

Ballpoint rock tripe lichen (*Umbilicaria polyrrhiza*) contains gyrophoric, umbilicaric, and lecanoric acid.

Netted rock tripe lichen (*Umbilicaria proboscidea*) is found on exposed rocks in alpine regions of British Columbia, and across the arctic from Alaska to Baffin Island and northern Quebec. This lichen contains glucosides with mono- and diprenylated xanthones (Rezanka et al. 2003), as well as gyrophoric, umbilicaric, and norstictic acids.

Punctured rock tripe lichen (*Umbilicaria torrefacta* syn. *Gyrophora erosa*) is the only North American rock tripe that regularly produces ß-orcinol depsidones (i.e., stictic acid). It also contains gyrophoric, umbilicaric, and ovoic acid.

Navel lichen (*Umbilicaria vellea*) is found in high alpine and arctic regions. It is found in only one place in Iceland and is on Iceland's endangered list. It contains gyrophoric and umbilicaric acid.

Blushing rock tripe lichen (*Umbilicaria virginus* syn. *Gyrophora rugifera* syn. *Omphalodiseus virginis*) lives on rocks in the high arctic, including Alaska, and south along western North America to the Mexican border and beyond at elevated locations. The lichen contains gyrophoric and norstictic acids.

USNEA
Beard Lichens

Geographic Range: North America

Habitat: trees, shrubs, rocks

Practical Uses: bedding; diapers and toilet paper; dye; salves and ointments; tanning leather; wiping slime off fish

Medicinal Applications: antibacterial, antifungal

Notable Chemicals: atranorin, diffractaic, evernic, lecanoric, lobaric, norstictic, physodic, protocetraric, and salazinic, stictic, and usnic acids; xanthones, zeorin

Warnings: pregnant women may not take in their first trimester; skin irritant

My heart is wounded: the sun sets and two ducks fly off.
For you, I spread and then cooked the lichens [niu-lo,
medicinal Usnea].
KOUO YU (FOURTEENTH-CENTURY CHINESE POET)

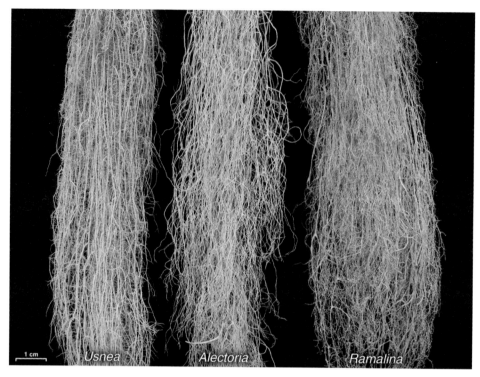

Comparison of *Usnea, Alectoria,* and *Ramalina*

Usnea is perhaps the most well-known lichen by the average layperson. It is widespread with 90 or more species identified in North America. The name may derive from the unani *ushna* or Arabic *ušna,* meaning "moss."

Historical Uses

A bit of an aside is best addressed here. *Usnea* or *Muscus ex craneo humano,* lichens or moss growing on human skulls, was popular medicine for epilepsy from the mid sixteenth century until the end of the eighteenth century in Europe. The concept was first recorded in work by Paracelsus, published in 1536. Numerous herbalists added to the idea of human skull "moss," using terms such as *Usnea Cranii Humani, U. humana, U. officinarum nostratium, U. microcosmi,* and *usnée humaine. Usnea* was an important ingredient in the Weapon Salve, which was believed to heal remotely over distances. Christopher J. Duffin (2022) has contributed a well-researched article on this strange period of magic and medicine. The term *Usnea,* in this case, does not pertain to the lichen species, but refers to the so-called "periwig of the dead cranium."

Alternative Medicine

The energy of *Usnea* lichens is bitter and cold, making it suitable for clearing hot, inflamed, damp conditions of the lungs and bladder. Herbalists, such as myself, have long promoted the use of *Usnea* lichen tinctures to treat *Streptococcus, Staphylococcus*, and *Mycobacterium tuberculosis* infections, orally and externally.

Usnic acid and its derivatives are the most plentiful compounds in this genus of lichens but are very poorly soluble in water. Ethanol extractions are richer, and oil extraction gives the highest degree of usnic acid efficacy. That is, usnic acid is more plentiful in low-polarity extracts such as methanol (Snyder Polarity) 6.6, ethanol 5.2, and ethyl acetate 4.3, as opposed to the high polarity of water, 9.0.

I make my *Usnea* tincture by stuffing a glass jar with the freshly picked and cleaned lichen and covering with 96% ethanol. The idea of a dual extraction to maximize the content of immune-modulating polysaccharides is in my opinion a nonstarter. In fact, if you have access to a Soxhlet extractor, the high heat of ethanol will extract, most efficiently, the active compounds.

Gram-positive bacteria are most sensitive to *Usnea* extracts, whereas gram-negative bacteria such as *Escherichia coli* are more resistant. Antiviral activity is limited (Sepahvand et al. 2021). This explains why the traditional use in parts of Europe involved oil-based salves and ointments for fungal infections, including athlete's foot, tinea, and ringworm. Modern-day uses include deodorant, mouthwash, toothpaste, and sunscreen products.

Usnea complanata, grown in submerged fermentation, developed psoromic acid, which in turn inhibited HMGR (cholesterol formation) and angiotensin-converting enzyme, suggesting this acid may also provide cardiovascular protection (Behera et al. 2012).

Usnic acid exhibits antiprotozoal, antiproliferative, anti-inflammatory, and analgesic activity (Ingólfsdóttir 2002).

Usnea species contain numerous compounds, including monosubstituted phenyl rings, depsides, anthraquinones, dibenzofurans, steroids, terpenes, fatty acids, and polysaccharides, with biological activity including antitumor, antibacterial, anti-inflammation, antioxidation, and antithrombosis activity (Laxinamujila et al. 2013).

They can easily be distinguished from other lichens by the presence of a central, stretchy, elastic central cord, most notable when wet. The outer green-gray cortex contains the active antibacterial and antifungal compounds, while the interior contains more of the immune-enhancing (water-soluble) polysaccharides.

Modern-day herbalists make widespread use of *Usnea* preparations. The late, great Dr. William Mitchell, Jr., combined it with parsley as an effective diuretic. It also combines well with Oregon grape root, dandelion root, and uva ursi for damp heat strangury, and with skullcap and elecampane root for respiratory phlegm heat. For *Giardia*, or amoebic dysentery, it combines well with elecampane and Oregon grape root.

Usnea species were widely used by Indigenous healers of North America. Brenda Holder (Indigenous Knowledge Keeper) is a former student and good friend. She shares the following:

> My grandmother gently picked some Usnea from the side of a tree and laid it in her open palm and told me "This medicine speaks to our bodies to teach us to be well. It starts in the neck, once we swallow the medicine, then it tells the body it is there to help heal." I often thought in later years that in her own wise way, she understood that there are lymph nodes all around the neck like gate keepers. She didn't know what the lymphatic system was, but she certainly knew it well in her amazing ways of knowing the land.

Traditional Uses

The Siksikaitsitapi (Blackfoot) call it *e-simatch-sis*, and use the lichen to stop nosebleeds, and bleeding wounds. Cree healers in Wabasca, Alberta, use a cooled and strained decoction of this lichen to wash skin sores and infected eyes (Marles et al. 2000). The call it *miyapakwn*.

Usnea species are susceptible to polycyclic aromatic compounds (PACs) and polycyclic aromatic hydrocarbons. They also concentrate mercury and selenium, noted in studies conducted on the Bigstone Cree Nation (Golzadeh et al. 2020; 2021). This may be related to the nearby Athabasca Oil Sands.

The neighboring Nihithawak or Saãwithiniwak (Cree) in Saskatchewan have a similar name, *mithāpäkwan*. They insert the fresh lichen to stop a nosebleed (Leighton 1985), similar to the use of the medicinal herb yarrow.

The Dakota call *Usnea* species *chan wiziye*, roughly translating as "on the north side of the tree" or "spirit of the north wind."

The Northern Chipewyan know it as *k'I tsaju*. The Dena'ina call it spruce hair, *ch'vala amdazi*.

People of Nitinaht, on Vancouver Island, call it *P'u7up*, and incorporated it traditionally into diapers and sanitary napkins and to dress skin wounds.

The Haida used old man's beard lichen for bedding. The Salish used *Usnea* species to produce a dark green dye. The Haisla mixed different yellow and black lichens with salmon eggs to color spoons, bowls, and totem poles (Turner 1998).

All *Usnea* species contain usnic acid.

Warty beard lichen (*Usnea ceratina*) is known to the Pomo of California as *kôchih*. It was used for diapers and toilet paper. It contains diffractaic acid.

The neighboring Wylackie used pitted beard lichen (*Usnea cavernosa*) to tan leather. Animal brains were wrapped in the lichen to hold it together and rubbed vigorously into the hide.

The Diné (Navajo) of the four corners area of Utah, Arizona, Colorado and New Mexico refer to this lichen as *cin bidayai* or "wood mustache" and use infusions to treat frostbite (Wyman and Harris 1951). It contains salazinic acid.

Various west coast tribes used *Alectoria* or *Usnea* lichens to wipe the slime off fish (Turner 1998). The Quinault of Washington, for example, used a lichen they call *ts' o' o' tc* to wipe and clean salmon. Washing fish toughens the skin and was avoided (Gunther 1988).

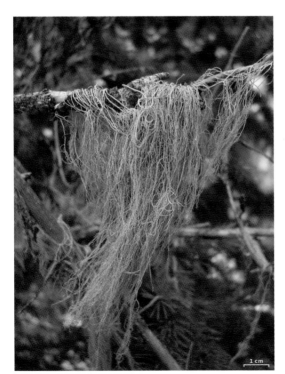

Usnea cavernosa
(Pitted Beard Lichen)

Kahlee Keane (2003), also known as Root Woman, wrote in her book *The Standing People* that *Usnea* would make a good heartworm medicine for wolves, and perhaps for domestic dogs.

Medical Uses

Usnic acid misuse in dietary supplements for weight loss has led to 20 incident reports to the Food and Drug Administration of liver toxicity (Kwong and Wang 2020). This misuse of a valuable medicine probably followed research on rats that found water-soluble *Usnea* significantly increased hepatic lipase activity (Zhu et al. 2017).

Work by Piska et al. (2018) notes that certain hepatoxic drugs generate reactive metabolites that damage the liver. *Usnea* enantiomers form two reactive metabolites that form adducts with glutathione, partially explaining the toxicity of usnic acid. This suggests a lichen/drug interaction that needs further examination in humans.

Dolichousnea longissima syn. *Usnea longissima* is the most well researched. Commonly known as Methuselah's beard lichen, it is extremely sensitive to pollution. Traditional Chinese Medicine writings from the sixth century suggest this lichen (known as "pine gauze" or "Lao-Tzu's beard") for its healing benefit. Today, both *Dolichousnea longissima* and *Dolichousnea diffracta* are known as *Sung-lo*.

The *Usnea* species on our continent deserve more study. One species from India, *Usnea pictoides*, contains 17,087 ppm calcium, 1,474 ppm potassium, and 1,937 ppm iron, as well as high levels of copper, zinc, chromium, and lithium (4.73 ppm).

Usnea species are effective against a broad spectrum of bacterial and fungal organisms. They are very effective for trichomoniasis, giardia, and candida infections, and particularly effective as a cooled water decoction prepared as a vaginal douche for cervical dysplasia. *Usnea* is also often part of herbal formulas treating cystitis, an infection of the urinary bladder, Weissbuch (2014) notes.

"Indeed, under the Scanning Tunneling Microscope, usnic acid is seen dissolving these biofilms and killing the pathogenic bacteria therein, validating an empirical usage dating back over 3,000 years" (Francolini et al. 2004).

Usnea species contain polysaccharides, which are water soluble. The polysaccharide CSL-0.1, isolated from this species, was tested for intestinal immunity and antioxidant activity (Wang et al. 2021). It increased spleen and thymus indices and conferred immune modulation on reversing the Th1/Th2-related cytokine imbalance in immunosuppressed mice. It also enhanced levels of secretory immunoglobulin A. Antioxidant levels in the liver and intestine increased 20 to 50%.

Work by Wang et al. (2018) examined the pharmacokinetics of usnic acid, compared to an ethanol extract of *Dolichousnea longissima*. The bioavailability after oral administration was 69.2% for usnic acid only, and 146.9% for the ethanol extract of the lichen. This suggests the full-spectrum ethanol extract is more bioavailable, confirmed by examining blood plasma. The same study found diffractaic acid reached 103.7% bioavailability, while barbatic acid and evernic acid levels were minimal.

Usnic acid derivatives are cytotoxic on human hepatoma HepG2 cell lines, inducing apoptosis comparable to methotrexate (Yu et al. 2016a). Usnic acid disrupts the cell membrane against methicillin-resistant *Staphylococcus aureus* (MRSA) (Gupta et al. 2012). It also disrupts biofilm formation (an extracellular l polymeric matrix) by disrupting the quorum sensing circuit of *Pseudomonas aeruginosa* (Müh et al. 2006).

There is evidence that the antibacterial activity of usnic acid is due to inhibition of RNA transcription (Campanella et al. 2002). Other scientists think usnic acid disrupts cellular metabolism, either by preventing the formation of ATP or by uncoupling oxidative phosphorylation (Lawrey 1986).

Bacteria walls are composed of peptidoglycans, and penicillin prevents their linkage and ability to hold together. Resistance to antibiotics occurs when a few surviving organisms find a way to integrate antibiotics into their cell wall, while dying, and then continue to replicate. Usnic acid can bypass cell walls and shut down ATP production at the mitochondrial level, and thus kill bacteria.

The tuberculin mycobacteria, for example, form heavily waxed coats and stiff cell walls that allow them to survive and divide inside macrophage cells. This can prevent the host's lysosomes from taking in the hydrogen ions needed to create an acidic environment, thus neutralizing their effect.

Noted herbalists and colleagues Christopher Hobbs and Chanchal Cabrera mention the use of usnic acid in tuberculosis lymphadenitis.

Alexander Fleming, the Scottish physician who noticed penicillin mold, noted the dangers of overusing the wonder drug in a June 26, 1945, speech, reported in *New York Times*.

> The greatest possibility of evil in self-medication is the use of too-small doses, so that, instead of clearing up the infection, the microbes are educated

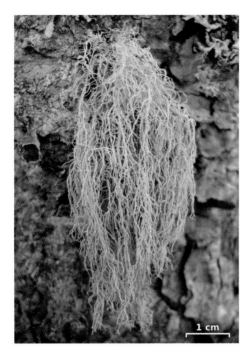

Usnea lapponica
syn. *U. perplexans*

to resist penicillin, and a host of penicillin-fast organisms is bred out which can be passed on to other individuals and perhaps from there to others until they reach someone who gets a septicemia or pneumonia which penicillin cannot save.

An in vitro study found intracellular adriamycin accumulation to be remarkably increased by usnic acid, including apoptosis and intracellular ROS level. This suggests usnea acid use for multidrug resistance found with human chronic myelogenous leukemia (Wang et al. 2021), and the need to explore lichen medicine as adjuvant synergists with numerous drug-resistant bacteria and cancer. Very little clinical research or application has been done on this to date.

Usnic acid inhibits the alpha-glucosidase enzyme, suggesting benefit in blood sugar control in diabetics (Maulidiyah et al. 2022).

Usnic acid is an effective inhibitor of PD-L1. The programmed cell death 1 (PD-1) ligand 1 (PD-L1) is abnormally expressed in cervical cancer cells. The blockade reduces apoptosis and exhaustion of T cells and inhibits the development of malignant tumors. Sun et al. noted enhanced cytotoxicity of cocultured T cells toward tumor cells and decreased expression of PD-L1 in HeLa (cervical) cells. Usnic acid inhibits cancer cell proliferation, angiogenesis, migration, and invasion (Sun et al. 2021).

Usnic acid and benzylidene analogues are potential mechanistic (formerly mammalian) targets of rapamycin (mTOR) inhibitors, suggestive of benefit in treating breast malignancies (Ebrahim et al. 2017). Rapamycin inhibitors regulate cell proliferation, autophagy, and apoptosis, and binds with the drug rapamycin. The mTOR pathway is implicated in cancer, diabetes, osteoporosis, and other health concerns.

Usnic acid possesses a vasodilating effect on blood vessels, and relaxes the muscles of the intestine, bronchi, and uterus.

> *Toxoplasma gondii* is a parasitic organism transmitted by outdoor cats eating an infected prey (rats or mice) and then spread in their feces. It is now found in raw meat including pork. In humans, acute infection with *T. gondii* can produce symptoms similar to Schizophrenia Spectrum Disorder (Rogers 2019).

Usnic acid and usnic acid liposome have an inhibitory effect on the viability of this pathogen (Si et al. 2016).

Both usnic acid and atranorin exert selective cytostatic and anti-invasive effects on human prostate and melanoma cancer cells (Galanty et al. 2017). Both lichen compounds inhibit DU-145 and PC-3 prostate cancer cells and HTB-140 melanoma cells, but usnic acid was found more efficient than atranorin. Polymeric micelles of usnic acid inhibit SH-SY5Y (human neuroblastoma) cell migration (Vasarri et al. 2022).

Prominent Species

The beard lichen (*Usnea aciculifera*) is rare in North America but has possibly been found in Texas. Early work by Tuong et al. (2014) on its components aciculiferin and diffractaic acids identified them as having good and strong cytotoxicity, respectively, to three cancer cell lines: HeLa (human epithelial carcinoma), NCI-H460 (human lung) and MCF-7 (human breast). This lichen also contains four unusual heterodimeric tetrahydroxanthones named usneaxanthones A–D. Of these, usneaxanthone D shows potent cytotoxicity against HT-29 (human colorectal) cancer cell lines (Tuong et al. 2019). Usneaxanthones E–H in these lichens were evaluated for cytotoxicity against four cancer cell lines. All four compounds exhibited good cytotoxicity against HCT116 (colorectal), MCF-7 (breast), and A549 (lung) cancer cell lines. They were especially potent against colorectal cancer cells (Tuong et al. 2020).

Western bushy beard lichen (*Usnea arizonica* syn. *Usnea intermedia*) is common on trees in restricted areas of the American Southwest. Extracts of this lichen exert the strongest proliferative effects observed in H1299 (lung) and MDA-MB-231 (breast) cancer cell lines. They induced apoptosis via phosphatidylserine translocation, and increased caspase 3/7 activity, loss of mitochondrial membrane potential, and the formation of pyknotic nuclei (Ozturk et al. 2019).

In North America hollow beard lichen (*Usnea baileyi* syn. *Usnea antillarum*, syn. *Usnea implicita*) is confined to northern Florida, growing on exposed trees and shrubs. It is named for its hollow axis. In India, it is combined with *Valeriana jatamansi* and other aromatic herbs to flavor and cure tobacco. Extracts of this lichen exhibit activity against *Staphylococcus aureus*, but not against *Escherichia coli* (Santiago et al. 2021). This lichen contains the compounds eumitrin A_1, A_2, and B, usnic acid, norstictic acid, salazinic acid, connorstictic acid, and traces of galbinic and hyposalazinic acid. Relatedly, three new xanthone dimers were identified in work by Nguyen et al. (2022). Eumitrins F–H were evaluated, and all showed moderate antimicrobial and weak tyrosinase inhibition. Eumitrin H showed significant inhibition of alpha-glucosidase, preventing blood sugar uptake. The next year, Nguygen et al. (2023) identified three new xanthone dimers, eumitrins I–K. All showed weak inhibition against alpha-glucosidase and tyrosinase, as well as weak antibacterial activity.

Pitted beard lichen (*Usnea cavernosa*) is widespread, hanging mainly from spruce trees. It contains the endolichenic fungal strain *Corynespora* sp. BA-10763. Work by Paranagama et al. (2007) identified herbarin, corynesporol, and 1-hydroxydehydroherbarin in the fungus. Aerial oxidation of corynesporol yielded herbarin. Acetylation of herbarin yielded dehydroherbarin. This compound inhibited migration of both human metastatic breast (MDA-MB-231) and prostate (PC-3M) cancer cell lines. This lichen also contains usnic acid and/or salazinic acid.

From the pitted beard lichen, Wang et al. (2010) identified six new polyketides in the endolichenic fungus *Corynespora* species. Four conioxepinols A–D, coniofurol A, and conioxanthone A were discovered and named. Conioxepinols 2–4 (oxepinochromenones) showed the most cytotoxicity against a small panel of human tumor cell lines.

Warty beard lichen (*Usnea ceratina*) is found around the Great Lakes and in parts of the eastern states. It contains ceratinalone, bailesidone, stictic acid, 8'-O-methylstictic acid, 8'-O-ethylstictic acid, isousnic acid, orsellinic acid, diffractaic acid, methyl orsellinate, and usneaceratins A and B. Of these, the compounds ceratinalone and 8'-O-methylstictic acid show moderate cytotoxicity against HeLa (cervical/epithelial), NCI-H460 (human lung), HepG2 (liver hepatocellular) and MCF-7 (human breast) cancer cell lines (Bui et al. 2022). Usneaceratin B possesses better inhibition of alpha-glucosidase than does acarbose (Bui et al. 2022a).

Inflated beard lichen (*Usnea cornuta*) is restricted in North America to parts of Arizona and New Mexico, as well as tiny populations in Appalachia. It is found on trees, usually conifers in open, elevated forests. Usnic acid derived from this lichen showed cytotoxicity against multiple human cancer cell lines in work by Kumari et al. (2023). When the cells were co-treated with an autophagy inhibitor, the potential increased by 12–16%, and caspase 3/7 activity by 40%.

The lichen *Usnea dasaea* contains galbinic acid, also known as alpha-acetylsalazinic acid.

Fishbone beard lichen (*Usnea filipendula* syn. *Usnea dasopoga*) is widespread on conifer trees across Canada, from Yukon to Nova Scotia. Research by Ari et al. (2014) found methanol extracts of this lichen induce apoptosis-like cell death in human lung (A549), prostate (PC3), liver (Hep38), and rat glioma (C6) cell lines. A significant increase in genetic damage was noted, indicating DNA damage to the cancer cells. This lichen contains salazinic, usnaric, barbatic, and *d*-usinic acids and emulsin. The latter is also found in almonds. Usnic acid and salazinic acid from this lichen show activity against *Serratia marcescens*.

The lichen *Usnea florida* is more widespread than the species name would suggest. It is certainly present in Mexico, but also possibly further south. When I lived in Peru, I bought a beautiful crimson-orange *serape* (blanket) made of wool and dyed with this lichen and other orange rock lichens. It is known as *qaqa sunkha*.

Work by Luedtke et al. (2002) examined nearly 100 extracts of plants and lichens, looking for activity on dopamine receptors. Alas, no such potential influence on the brain was found for this lichen.

However, inhibition of non-small-cell lung cancer metastasis was found for an extract of *Usnea florida* by Yang et al. (2016). The lichen extract was tested on human blood cells and no mutagenic effect was found on lymphocytes. The extract did exhibit antioxidant properties (Türkez et al. 2012a).

The lichen *Usnea florida* contains usnic, thamnolic, evernic, physodic, and 3-hydroxyphysodic acids, as well as 5,7-dihydroxy-6-methylphtalide. Work by Cansaran et al. (2006a) isolated usnic acid and tested it against seven bacteria, with positive results against *Bacillus subtilis* and *B. megaterium*. Work by Yilmaz et al. (2017) examined the activity of thamnolic acid, derived from this lichen, on 13 gram-positive and gram-negative bacteria and 9 fungi.

A California specimen of *Usnea fulvoreagens* contains the rare depsidone neotricone, as well as conneotricone (Burt et al. 2022).

Bristly or shaggy beard lichen (*Usnea hirta* syn. *Usnea variolosa*) is widespread and is found on hard weathered wood, conifers, and at times even on rocks.

Work by Renzaka and Sigler (2007) found that the compound hirtus-neanoside, isolated from *Usnea hirta*, showed inhibitory activity against gram-positive bacteria. Other secondary metabolites are 3% (+)-usnic acid, alectoric, hirtic, thamnolic, diffractaic, hertillic, and usnaric acids, anthraquinones, hirtus-neanoside, and fatty acids.

Methuselah's beard lichen (*Usnea longissima* syn. *Dolichousenea longissima*) was recently designated the unofficial lichen of New Brunswick. Useanol and two other phenolic constituents from *Usnea longissima* show significant anti-inflammatory activity, comparable to the controls curcumin and indomethacin (Yu et al. 2016). Longissiminone A, also isolated from this lichen, possesses potent anti-inflammatory activity in vitro (Choudhary et al. 2005), and in another study showed moderate in vivo anti-inflammatory activity and moderate antiplatelet aggregation (Azizuddin et al. 2017).

Other compounds in this lichen include orcinol, ethyl everninate, arabitol,

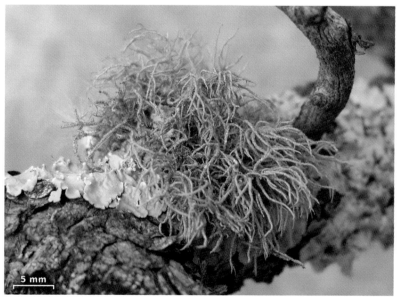

Usnea hirta (Bristly or Shaggy Beard Lichen)

apigenin 7-O-beta-D-glucuronide, friedelin, barbatic acid, neuropogolic acid, usnic acid, glutinol, hematommate, beta-amyrin, beta-sitosterol, barbatinic acid, zeorin, ethyl orsellinate, orsellinic acid, barbatic acid, evernic acid, diffractaic acid, oleanolic acid, usnic acid, 8-hydroxydiffractiac acid, and methyl-orsellinic acid.

From a crude extract of this lichen (1.2 g), various amounts of acids were found: orsellinic acid (74 mg), 4-O-methylorsellinic acid (55.5 mg), evernic acid (353.5 mg), usnic acid (44.9 mg), diffractaic acid (19.4 mg), and barbatic acid (102 mg), all with over 92% purity (Sun et al. 2016).

Water extracts of this species inhibit the growth of U87MG human glioblastoma cells (Emsen et al. 2019). Work by Mammadov et al. (2019) found ethyl acetate extracts prevented gastric and esophageal cancer induction in rats. The authors suggest the extract is not toxic and is selective to cancer tissue. Water extracts show protection against indomethacin-induced gastric ulcers in rats, probably due to antioxidant activity (Halici et al. 2005).

Various compounds in this lichen, especially (+)-usnic acid, show inhibition of Epstein–Barr virus activation (Yamamoto et al. 1995). Epstein–Barr virus infects almost all humans during their lifetime, and after an acute episode remains latent and dormant. It infects B lymphocytes but is prevented from reactivating through healthy immunity. The infected cells act as a safe harbor for the dormant virus, making them less sensitive to apoptosis, which is part of the virus strategy for long-term survival. But the virus can reactivate and is associated with a variety of cancers, including Burkitt's lymphoma, Hodgkin's lymphoma, gastric cancer, and nasopharyngeal carcinoma (Wyzewski et al. 2022). The virus is implicated in autoimmunity disorders, including chronic fatigue syndrome and possibly multiple sclerosis (Soldan and Lieberman 2023). The virus is rarely tested for, but inhibiting reactivation is an important step.

Methuselah's beard lichen lichen contains glutinol (Choudhary et al. 2005), which has been found to inhibit the proliferation of human ovarian cancer cells via P13K/AKT signaling pathway (Chen and Li 2021). Barbatic acid, also present, manifested doxorubicin-equivalent activity against A549 lung cancer cells (Reddy et al. 2019).

This lichen also contains usenamine A, which shows prominent antiproliferative activity and resulted in G2/M phase arrest in MDA-MB-231 breast cancer cells. It also induced autophagy and endoplasmic reticulum stress. Usenamine A inhibits ubiquitin-like modifier-activating enzyme 5, which impedes tumor growth (Fang et al. 2021).

The endolichenic fungus *Aspergillus quandricinctus* isolated from this lichen has been studied for its medicinal potential. Work by Prateeksha et al. (2020) found metabolites of the fungus disturbed the biofilm formation of *Pseudomonas aeruginosa* (PAO1), a pathogenic multi-drug-resistant strain that uses a quorum sensing network. Inhibiting quorum sensing in managing human infections could be an alternative or adjuvant approach to conventional antibiotics.

Recent work by Bharti et al. (2022) found lichen extracts inhibited quorum sensing in *Chromobacterium violaceum*, and effectively reduced biofilm formation in *Bacillus cereus*, *Escherichia coli*, *Pseudomonas aeruginosa*, *Staphylococcus aureus*, and *Candida albicans*.

Red beard lichen (*Usnea rubicunda*) is mainly confined to forests of the southeastern United States. Work by Salgado et al. (2017) identified 38 compounds in this species. Bézivin et al. (2003) found extracts of this lichen were active against murine and human cancer cell lines.

Usnea steineri lichen contains diffractaic and (+)-usnic acid. Extracts of the lichen show strong activity against resistant strains of *Staphylococcus epidermidis* and *Enterococcus faecalis*. A combination of penicillin and tetracycline did not exhibit a synergistic antimicrobial effect (Tozatti et al. 2016). Usnic acid and penicillin were antagonistic against *S. haemolyticus*, meaning the antimicrobial activity did not improve but was considerably reduced.

Earlier work by Lucarini et al. (2012) found this lichen and (+)-usnic acid strongly inhibitory of *Mycobacterium tuberculosis*, *M. avium*, and *M. kansasii*. There are about 440,000 cases of tuberculosis (TB) reported annually, with 150,000 deaths. About 5% are multi-drug-resistant strains. More than 8% of global TB cases are associated with alcohol abuse. Alcohol impairs the immune function of the alveolar macrophage, and chronic use increases oxidative stress in lower respiratory tract (Wigger et al. 2022). Avian TB (*M. avium*) is an increasingly opportunistic pathogen, with increasing levels of drug resistance (Mattoo 2021). *Mycobacterium kansasii* is also highly virulent, but a nontuberculous mycobacterium affecting increased numbers with lung disease worldwide. Clarithromycin-resistant strains are becoming prevalent (Huang et al. 2020).

Bush beard lichen (*Usnea strigosa*) is found from Nova Scotia to Florida and west to Texas. It prefers deciduous trees and shrubs, including oak. This lichen is used in Mexico as a diuretic, and to treat fevers, colds, indigestion, mouth ulcers, skin burns, and lung conditions (Guzman 2008). It contains norstictic acid, which significantly suppressed MDA-MB-231/GFP tumor growth on breast cancer xenograft mice. Norstictic acid also significantly inhibits cell proliferation, migration, and invasion, with minimal toxicity to nontumor mammary epithelial cells (Ebrahim et al. 2016).

This species of *Usnea*, and two others, inflated beard lichen (*Usnea cornuta*) and *Usnea subgracilis*, host cystobasidiomycete yeasts, a relatively rare occurrence. In a study of 339 lichen species by Lendemer et al. (2019), only nine showed the presence of this yeast.

The beard lichen *Usnea subcavata* (syn. *Usnea perplectata*) contains atranorin, and usnic, diffractaic, lecanoric, protocetraric, salazinic, hypostictic, and norstictic acids. In vitro tests found diffractaic acid the most active against *Mycobacterium tuberculosis* cells. Both usnic and norstictic acid were fourfold less potent (Honda et al. 2010).

Boreal beard lichen (*Usnea subfloridana*) is widespread in North America. The lichen contains five known depsidones, galbinic acid, conprotocetraric acid, constictic acid, salazinic acid, and lobaric acid, as well as usnic and norstictic acids. The Raramuri in Chihuahua, Mexico, use the lichen to heal heart discomfort and other affections (Moreno-Fuentes et al. 2004). In India, it is mixed with tobacco and butter, boiled, cooled, and applied as a lotion to painful and red eyes, as well as to swelling and bleeding from external injury. In New Hampshire, it was known as "brighten" and at one time was used to treat weak eyes, similar to the tradition in Ireland (Wise 1863). Conprotocetraric and lobaric acid inhibit COX2 enzymes, suggestive of anti-inflammatory activity, and perform better than the reference drug indomethacin. All five of these depsidones inhibit xanthine oxidase, indicating potential benefit in treating gout (Nguyen et al. 2021).

This lichen and usnic acid, extracted with acetone, exhibit activity against *Escherichia coli*, *Enterococcus faecalis*, *Proteus mirabilis*, *Staphylococcus aureus*, *Bacillis subtilis*, and *B. megaterium* (Cansaran et al. 2006a).

Work by Popovici et al. (2022; 2022a) examined the potential of *Usnea* dry acetone extracts in either canola oil or isopropanol to treat oral squamous cell carcinoma (CLS-354). *Usnea* in canola increased oxidative stress, diminished DNA synthesis, and induced cell cycle arrest in G0/G1. With *Usnea* in isopropanol, cellular oxidative stress, caspase 3/7 activity, nuclear condensation, lysosomal activity, and DNA synthesis were investigated and found suitable for application on oral mucosa. Antimicrobial potential against *Pseudomonas aeruginosa*, *Candida albicans*, and *C. parapsilosis* was also noted.

Usnea barbata is in the homeopathic materia medica but is not a North American species.

Methuselah's beard lichen or *Usnea* (*Usnea longissima* syn. *Dolichousnea longissima*) lichen essence is for people in the healing profession. There is a danger of empathizing or identifying too strongly with patients and beginning to take on their "illness." The essence helps one retain boundaries. It may help relieve the *tuberculinum miasm*, recognized in homeopathy. This exists on a cellular or predisposed genetic level or trait (Rogers 2016).

Caution: Pregnant women can take small amounts of *Usnea* after the first trimester. The fresh or dry lichen can irritate the skin of some individuals. Remember, do not pick *Usnea*, nor any lichen, for medicine within 200 meters of a highway.

VULPICIDA
Sunshine Lichens

Geographic Range: some species in high arctic and others only in southeastern United States

Habitat: bark, wood, rocks, soil

Practical Use: dying mountain goat wool

Medicinal Applications: antibacterial, cancer; colds, coughs, respiratory ailments,

Notable Chemicals: pulvinic, usnic, and vulpinic acids

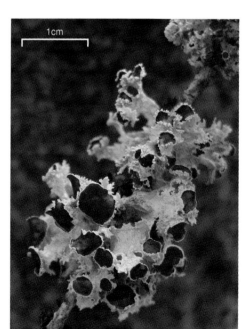

Vulpicida canadensis (Brown-Eyed Sunshine Lichen)

Brown-eyed sunshine lichen (*Vulpicida canadensis* syn. *Cetraria canadensis*) is found in conifer forests, mainly in western North America. Vulpicida is derived from *vulpes*, meaning "fox," and *cida* (who kills). A Swedish myth suggests it kills foxes, but not dogs and wolves. Who knows for sure!

The Ulkatcho of British Columbia know this as *dahgha*, "limb hair." It was prepared as tea for coughs and colds, or chewed fresh for respiratory complaints (Hebda et al. 1996).

This lichen contains usnic, pulvinic, and vulpinic acids. Vulpinic acid significantly induced apoptosis of PC-3 (prostate) cancer cell lines (Cansaran-Duman et al. 2021).

Extracts of brown-eyed sunshine lichen appear to be neuroprotective, based on work by Fernández-Moriano et al. (2015). When tested against astrocytes damaged by hydrogen peroxide, the lichen was able to reverse the oxidative damage and improve survival. Cytotoxicity was noted against human hepatocellular carcinoma (HepG2) and human breast adenocarcinoma (MCF-7) cell lines.

Extracts from wolf lichen and the fertile sister species brown-eyed wolf lichen (*Letharia columbiana*) were effective against *Escherichia coli*, *Staphylococcus aureus*, MRSA, and *Pseudomonas aeruginosa* (Shrestha et al. 2014). Brown-eyed sunshine lichen (*Vulpicida canadensis*) was also effective against the same bacterium. This is significant because about 70% of the world's bacteria have some antibiotic resistance. According to a study in *Lancet Planetary Health*, global antibiotic rates increased by 46% from 2000 to 2018. Another UK study found that the number of people given antibiotics between 2012 and 2017 had increased an average of 8.9% prescriptions in the previous three years.

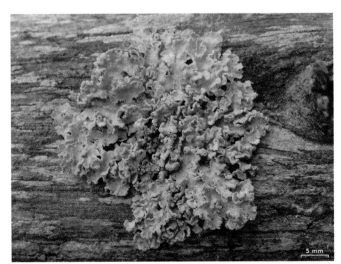

Vulpicida pinastri (Powdered Sunshine Lichen)

Powdered sunshine lichen (*Vulpicida pinastri* syn. *Cetraria pinastri*) is green with yellow tips and found on bark, wood, and rocks in both open and shaded regions. It was recently chosen as Ontario's unofficial provincial lichen. In boreal forests it is found at waist height, or a little higher, possibly due to using snowdrifts to protect against drying, cold winter wind chill.

Work by Ureña-Vacas et al. (2022) found methanol extracts of *Vulpicida pinastri*, at only 5 μg/mL, prevented cell death and morphological changes in neuroblastoma cell lines. Usnic, pinastric, and vulpinic acids have been identified in this lichen. This is significant because vulpinic and gyrophoric acids show photoprotection for human keratinocytes, suggestive of benefit in UVB cosmetic products (Varol et al. 2016). A combination of usnic acid, vulpinic acid, and pinastric acid increased photoprotective activity against UVA and UVB radiation (Legouin et al. 2017). Vulpinic acid is also found in limestone sunshine lichen (*Vulpicida tilesii* syn. *Cetraria tilesii* syn. *V. juniperina*), also known as Goldtwist. It is found from the high arctic, including Alaska, south along the alpine regions of the Rocky Mountain trench. As the name suggests, it is found only on soil with a high pH, like limestone.

XANTHOPARMELIA

Rock Frog Lichens   Rock Shield Lichens

Geographic Range: widespread in North America, mainly in the United States with a few exceptions

Habitat: siliceous rocks, soil

Practical Uses: dye

Medicinal Applications: cancer, antibacterial, impetigo

Notable Chemicals: salazinic, stictic, and norstictic acids

No words that I know of will say what mosses and lichens are. None are delicate enough, none rich enough . . . Yet as in one sense the humblest, in another they are the most honored of the earth children . . . Strong in lowliness, they neither blanch in heat nor pine in frost. To them, slow fingered, constant hearted, is entrusted the weaving of the dark eternal tapestries of the hills . . . Sharing the stillness of the unimpassioned rock, they share also its endurance . . . the silver lichen-spots rest, starlike on the stone; and the gathering orange stain upon the edge of yonder western peak reflects the sunsets of a thousand years.

JOHN RUSKIN (1819–1900), *MODERN PAINTERS*

There are more than 50 rock shield lichens in North America.

Meagre rock frog lichen (*Xanthoparmelia angustiphylla*) contains stictic and norstictic acids. It has wide distribution, ranging from Appalachia to the Great Lakes and in the southwest. It has also been found near Spokane, Washington, and in parts of Idaho. The Greek *xanthos* means "yellow."

The endolichenic fungus *Talaromyces* sp. found in this lichen contains several compounds isolated by Yuan et al. (2020). These include talarolactone A, which shows selective anti-migratory activity in a wound-healing assay without appreciable cytotoxic activity.

Talaromyces species are both terrestrial and marine. A review of the literature by Zhai et al. (2016) cited the identification of 221 secondary metabolites, including 43 alkaloids and peptides, 88 esters, 31 polyketides, 19 quinones, 15 steroids and terpenoids, and 25 other compounds.

Tumbleweed shield lichen (*Xanthoparmelia chlorochroa*) is found in Yukon and the Northwest Territories, but mainly in western deserts and high, dry plains, rolling around like tumbleweed. It contains salazinic acid and traces of norstictic acid.

Tumbleweed shield lichen is prized by the Navajo of Arizona and New Mexico for the red-brown dye it yields from boiling. They also used the dry

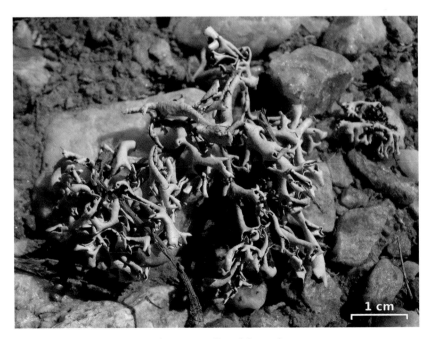

Xanthoparmelia chlorochroa
(Tumbleweed Shield Lichen)

powder to treat impetigo, due to the presence of norstictic and salazinic acids.

Much further north, in Saskatchewan, tumbleweed shield lichen was recently designated the unofficial lichen of the province. As the common name suggests, the lichen detaches from rocks and tumbles around dry regions. Presence of the lichen suggests good antelope country.

In Arizona it is known as rock flower, *owa'si,* or rock manure, *owa'huru'suki.* In New Mexico, it goes by *tschetlaat* (rock covering), earth moss, or rock moss. *Tschetlaat* was used as a dry powder applied to impetigo, a *Staphylococcus* infection (Elmore 1943).

The Crow of southern Montana recognize this lichen as *a wa ga chilua.*

"Judging from the symptoms, I think it was diphtheria . . . And that is how a lichen, *Xanthoparmelia chlorchroa,* a foliose lichen that grows on the rocks or rocky ground around here came to be used for sore throats, even to this day" (Snell 2006).

This lichen contains salazinic acid and traces of norstictic acid. Work by Shrestha et al. (2015) found extracts of this lichen induce apoptosis in Burkitt's lymphoma (Raji). They found accumulation of cells in the GO/G1 stage and an increase in p53 protein, a protective gateway that determines whether aberrant cells live or die (apoptosis).

However, this lichen should not be taken internally by humans until more studies have been conducted. In the 1930s, the consumption of the lichen by range-stressed sheep and cattle was believed to result in sickness and deaths.

During the spring of 2004, an estimated 400–500 free-ranging elk (*Cervus elaphus*) developed paresis, became recumbent and died, or were euthanized in Wyoming. Gross lesions were limited to degenerative myopathy, with pallor and streaking in skeletal muscles. Tumbleweed shield lichen was found in the rumen of several elk, and when three captive elk were fed this lichen, two exhibited signs of ataxia, which progressed to weakness and recumbency after a week, and a degenerative myopathy was observed (Cook et al. 2007).

Ironically, the lichen is an important food for pronghorn antelope and an indicator of good habitat for management.

Peppered rock shield lichen (*Xanthoparmelia conspersa* syn. *Parmelia conspersa* syn. *P. isidiata*) grows on siliceous rocks, especially granite, in both the eastern and western United States.

Peppered rock shield lichen is taken internally and applied externally by the Xhosa of Africa as a snake bite remedy. A decoction and powder of this lichen were also used in attempts to treat sexually transmitted infections,

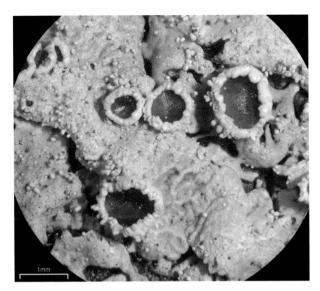

Xanthoparmelia conspersa (Peppered Rock Shield Lichen)

especially syphilis (Watt 1962). It contains cryptostictic acid, also found in *Ramalina siliquosa*. This lichen was utilized by the Haudenosaunee (Iroquois) for inflamed gums and sore throat. A cup of cold water with the lichen and the bark of the tree the lichen was collected from was combined with gold thread (*Coptis trifolia*) and black ash (*Fraxinus nigra*). One teaspoon was taken and held in the mouth until warm and then swallowed; repeat and finish the full cup (Herrick 1995).

This lichen was carried as a good luck charm in Arizona. Known as *jievut hiawsik*, or *jewed hiosig*, meaning "earth flower," the lichen was mixed with tobacco to smoke and to "make young men crazy." Hawksworth (2003), however, disagrees. It was also ground into powder and sprinkled on wounds and cuts, but not bound or it may cause blisters. It was also applied for several days to rattlesnake bites (Curtin 1949).

An extract of this lichen exhibits activity against pathogenic *Alcaligenes faecalis* (Bustinza 1952) (see *Punctelia rudecta*, page 195, and *Thamnolia vermicularis*, page 229). This lichen and the related *Xanthoparmelia chlorochroa* syn. *Parmelia chlorochroa* contain constictic acid.

Cumberland rock shield lichen (*Xanthoparmelia cumberlandia*) is a sexualized species. In an amusing paper by Pringle et al. (2003) a significant correlation was found between size and reproductive effort. This lichen allocates a disproportionate share of resources to reproduction. This suggests sexual fecundity is correlated to size—a trait that does cause anxiety and concern in some of the human male populations. It contains stictic, constictic, and norstictic acids.

Salted rock shield lichen (*Xanthoparmelia mexicana*) is basically found in the entire western side of the United States, with a little bump into the desert of southern British Columbia. It is found on arid or semi-arid land, often on exposed rock in oak or pine forests.

Extracts of *Xanthoparmelia mexicana* were found to inhibit gram-positive bacteria, including *Staphylococcus aureus* and *Enterococcus faecalis*, but not gram-negative species (Yeash et al. 2017; Letwin 2017).

The Yuman of northern Mexico used various species of *Xanthoparmelia* lichens for heart, urinary, and gastrointestinal issues (Baustista-González et al. 2022). Included are salted rock shield (*Xanthoparmelia mexicana*), tight rock shield (*Xanthoparmelia lineola*), New Mexican rock shield (*Xanthoparmelia novomexicana* syn. *Xanthoparmelia arseneana*), *Xanthoparmelia joranadia*, and Maricopa rock shield (*Xanthoparmelia maricopensis*) lichens. Various local names are used for these lichens, including *uja' tebiyauup*, or *flor de piedra*; *wui tabsh* or *wui mokual*, meaning "rock skin;" or *zacatito*, "little grass." Other names from this region of Mexico are *alfombrita* (little carpet), *hongo de piedra* (stone mushroom), *wuiy tapsh* (stone flower), *wuiy ugtapch chpach* (flower that comes out of the stone), *jam shkual* (born in the water), *wui tabsh*, *wui tab* or *iwuil taosh* (stone flower), and *wui shishai* (lying on the stone or stone rug). All are common on exposed rocks throughout the American Southwest.

Issues involving kidney, bladder, and scanty or painful urination were resolved with decoctions of these lichens. Conditions of the urinary tract are known as *sitam micha*, *sit jam ju'looy* (sit = go out; *u'looy* = bad), or *mal de orin* (bad urine). Blood may be present in worse cases. *Mal de orin*, in the Kiliwa dictionary, is *pamaay cheen*; *pamaay* means "to urinate." According to Baustista-González et al. (2022), kidney issues may be caused by eating acid-containing foods, such as immature fruit, or walking barefoot. Lime is sometimes added to the tea in cases of kidney stone formation.

Liver conditions and gallstone disintegration is another use for these lichens. *Lepée* (liver) conditions such as cirrhosis are helped.

Gallstones (*wui wui bjá* in Paipai) are disintegrated by lichen tea, which also treats stomach pain associated with eating spoiled food. The lichen tea also helped relieve overeating, or feeling embarrassed or disgusted while consuming a meal.

The treatment of hypertension and heart issues associated with anger, depression, or intense feelings are helped. The Yuman believe negative feelings

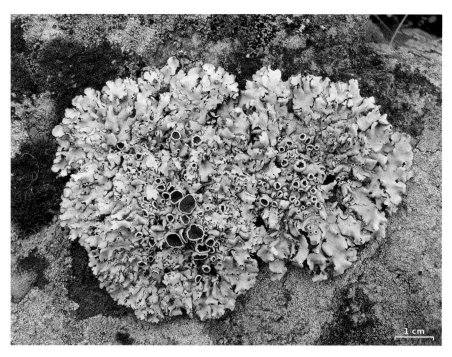

Xanthoparmelia cumberlandia (Cumberland Rock Shield Lichen)

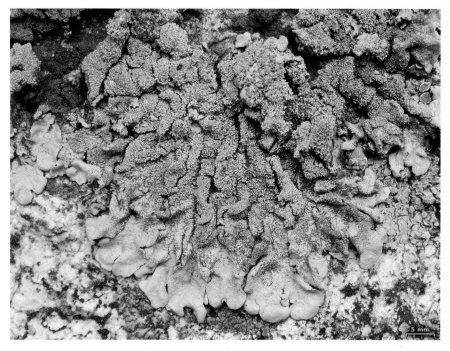

Xanthoparmelia mexicana (Salted Rock Shield Lichen)

turn into blood clots, and lichens can unblock the arterial plaque. Perhaps they are right.

In the study by Baustista-González et al. (2022), one person reported to the authors the use of tight rock shield lichen (*Xanthoparmelia lineola*) and salted rock shield lichen (*Xanthoparmelia mexicana*) decoctions to treat cancer. Lichen tea is prepared in a pewter or clay pot, with "three fingers" of lichen to one liter of water. The lichens are wrapped in cloth, or strained after placing them in hot water. The tea is taken up to three times daily.

Biomedicine would suggest that only a double-blind, placebo-controlled trial would lend further insight into their hypothesis. Smith and Pell (2003) wrote a tongue-in-cheek article in the *British Medical Journal* suggesting the need for such a trial to determine the effectiveness of parachutes in preventing major trauma related to gravitational challenge. They concluded that advocates of evidence-based medicine (the gold standard) have criticized the adoption of interventions evaluated by using only observational data: "We think that everyone might benefit if the most radical protagonists of evidence-based medicine organised and participated in a double blind, randomized, placebo controlled, crossover trial of the parachute."

Tarnished Gold: The Sickness of Evidence-Based Medicine is an excellent critique of evidence-based medicine (Hickey and Roberts 2011).

I am not suggesting a disbanding of scientific inquiry. However, the dismissive attitude of biomedicine and pharmaceutical companies toward natural products is impeding the search for, and development of, effective, less expensive compounds with predictable or fewer side effects.

Extracts from New Mexican rock shield were tested against FemX (melanoma), LS174 (colorectal), A549 (lung), and K562 (human chronic myeologenous leukemia) cell lines (Kosanic et al. 2014). Strong anticancer action was noted for all tested cell lines.

Plitt's rock shield lichen (*Xanthoparmelia plitti*) methanol extracts show weak antibacterial activity (Bate et al. 2020).

Shingled rock shield lichen (*Xanthoparmelia somloënsis* syn. *Xanthoparmelia stenophylla*) grows on exposed boulders, mainly in the eastern and parts of the southeastern United States. The lichen is also found in southwestern Alberta and down the Great Western Basin, and in the western Northwest Territories. In parts of Montana, collections of up to 126 kilograms per hectare have been obtained.

The Navajo use the dry powder of this lichen for impetigo (*Streptococcus* sp.).

The lichen is known as *tschétláat* (rock covering) (Elmore, 1943). It contains 2% usnic acid, as well as salazinic and norstitic acids. Known to the Navajo as ground lichen, it is also boiled for a range of colors—red, brown, or orange—to dye leather, baskets, and wool.

Ozturk et al. (2021) examined both these lichens for their effect on breast cancer cells. The usnea species exhibited strong antigrowth activity and was especially cytotoxic against MDA-MB-231 and H1299 cells.

The related *Xanthoparmelia taractica*, found in Mexico, is a hyperaccumulator of zinc.

Ethanol extracts of another peppered rock shield (*Xanthoparmelia tinctina* ssp. *conspersa*) show antiviral activity against HPIV-2 (Karagoz and Aslan 2005). This virus accounts for about 60% of influenza cases in children aged 1–2 years.

Tucson shield lichen (*Xanthoparmelia tucsonensis* syn. *Parmelia tucsonensis*) contains 2-O-methyllobtusatic acid.

The lichen *Xanthoparmelia verrucilifera* (*Neofuscelia verrucilifera* syn. *Parmelia verrucilifera*) contains glomellic and glomelliferic acid.

Variable rock frog or shingled rock shield lichen (*Xanthoparmelia wyomingica* syn. *Parmelia wyomingica*) grows on rocks or mossy soil from central British Columbia and Alberta, in alpine regions, south to New Mexico. It contains salazinic acid and traces of norstictic acid.

XANTHORIA
Sunburst Lichens

Geographic Range: from Alaska to Georgia

Habitat: rocks, wood, bone, bark

Medicinal Applications: antifungal, antibacterial, anti-tumor, intermittent fevers, menstrual problems, substitute for quinone

Notable Chemicals: parietin, salazinic and norstictic acids, xanthorin

Elegant sunburst lichen (*Xanthoria elegans* syn. *Rusavskia elegans*) is usually bright orange but can vary from pale yellow-orange to dark red-orange in color. It is widely found on rocks, wood, bone, or on nutrient-rich bird or animal deposits. Due to its presence, Inuit hunters use this information to locate burrows of hoary marmots. Poachers, unfortunately, use this knowledge to find nests of peregrine falcons.

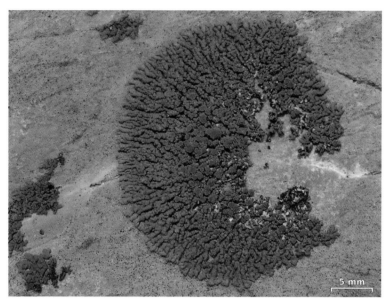

Xanthoria elegans syn. *Rusavskia elegans*
(Elegant Sunburst Lichen)

Medical Uses

It contains salazinic and norstictic acids, as well as xanthorin and erythro-glaucin, which possesses moderate antioxidant activity (Wang et al. 2006). However, it also prevents the final step of mitochondrial oxidative phosphory-lation necessary for the production of ATP (Betina and Kuzela 1987).

Extracts were tested against 12 cancer cell lines, and this lichen, as well as *Alectoria nigricans*, proved most antiproliferative (Ingolfsdottir et al. 2000). In this research, the lichen showed significant induction of quinone reductase against hepatoma cells.

Water extracts and chemotherapy drug mitomycin C were studied together, and separately, on human lymphocytes. The lichen extract had no genotoxic effect, and in fact showed a protective role toward cells injured by mitomycin C. The authors (Turkez et al. 2012b) suggest the extract is a potential source of natural anti-genotoxicants.

Wall lichens are bright yellow orange in sunny regions, and gray in the shade. According to the doctrine of signatures by John Moore, the yellow-orange color suggests benefit in jaundice and other liver disease.

Hooded sunburst lichen (*Xanthoria fallax* syn. *Xanthomendoza fallax*) is found on oak, elm, and poplar tree bark, and rarely on rocks. It is, like other

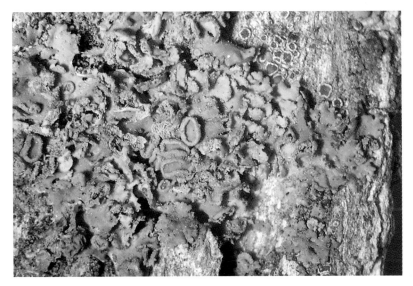

Xanthoria fallax syn. *Xanthomendoza fallax*
(Hooded Sunburst Lichen)

Xanthoria, a beautiful orange color. It contains the compounds fallacinal and erythroglaucinic acid. Methanol extracts of this lichen inhibit Epstein–Barr virus activation induced by teleocidin B-4, a tumor-promoting pathway (Yamamoto et al. 1998).

Maritime sunburst or wall lichen (*Xanthoria parietina* syn. *Teloschistes parietinus*) has been tested for antimicrobial activity (Mendili et al. 2021). This beautiful lichen is found close to ocean shorelines, often on the bark of elm or poplar, and sometimes on rocks. It contains parietin, also found in *Caloplaca* species, and the anthraquinone citreorosein, as well as teloschistin acetate (monoacetylfallacinol). Its yellow color has led to its use in Europe and elsewhere for the treatment of jaundice (Llano 1951).

It has also been used as a substitute for quinone, and to treat intermittent fevers (Schneider 1904; Lindley 1849). Methanol extracts of this lichen exhibit chemopreventive and cytotoxic activity (Ingólfsdóttir et al. 2000). Work by Yamamoto et al. (1998) found extracts inhibited Epstein–Barr virus activation induced by teleocidin B-4 tumor promotion.

While in Spain, I found this lichen was slowly simmered in wine, cooled, and then given to women for menstrual problems. It is known as *flor de piedra* (stone flower) or *rompiedra* (stone breaker), referring to use in kidney disorders, including stones. (These names apply to both *Xanthoparmelia* and *Xanthoria* interchangeably.)

Parietin and various lichen extracts were found active against the bacterium *Staphylococcus aureus* and the fungi *Rhizoctonia solani*. An extract inhibited proliferation and induced apoptosis in breast cancer cells (Basile et al. 2015), and ovarian cancer cells (Backorova et al. 2011

As in many lichens, hot-water-soluble polysaccharides are found but largely ignored by science. The presence of 1,4- and 1,6-alpha-D-glucans exerts significantly increased phagocytosis and TNF-alpha and IL-1B secretion. Work by Rashid et al. (2019) determined the effects were due to an interaction of the galactomannan with the transmembrane pattern-recognition protein Dectin-2 of the macrophages.

This lichen contains parietin, which inhibits tau protein. Both beta-amyloid plaque and tau tangles are implicated in Alzheimer's disease and other neurological/brain disorders (Cornejo et al. 2016).

Parietinic acid is also found in this lichen. Work by Pant et al. (2021) found the acid to be a potential inhibitor of Ag85C, a target for multiple-drug-resistant and extensively drug-resistant tuberculosis. It may shorten the treatment time and alleviate the various side effects associated with current antitubercular medications.

Parietin (also known as physcion) derived from this species displays varying degrees of antitumor activity (Dias and Urban 2009). When prepared in liposomes, to overcome bioavailability, parietin exhibited photodynamic and anti-angiogenic activity in triple negative breast cancer cell lines. Clathrin-mediated endocytosis predominated (Ayoub et al. 2022).

Physcion also exhibits antifungal activity. Work by Qi et al. (2022) used *Aspergillus terreus* in a lab setting to produce the compound in a highly efficient and economic manner.

This lichen showed benefit in complications of diabetes in a rat study (Ouahiba et al. 2018). Control of blood glucose, lipid profile, and oxidative status was shown through activation of antioxidant enzymes and decreased lipid peroxidation in the liver.

Citreorosein, mentioned earlier as a component of this lichen, inhibits degranulation and leukotriene-4, suggesting benefit in the prevention of allergic inflammation (Lu et al. 2012). It strongly inhibits COX-2 prostaglandin generation in mast cells, suggesting potential therapeutic activity in treating inflammatory conditions (Lue et al. 2012a).

Xanthoria parietina essence facilitates an awakening, bringing wisdom and understanding. It can help to relieve fears, nervousness, and confusion. It is for those who walk around in circles. It helps balance the solar plexus, central nervous system, liver, lungs, and nerves according to Silvercord Essences.

XYLOPSORA

Clam Lichen

Fries's clam lichen (*Xylopsora friesii* syn. *Hypocenomyce friesii*) contains friesiic acid. The species is named in honor of Elias Magnus Fries (1794–1878). He is considered by many lichenologists to be the father of mushroom taxonomy. The related *Xylopsora canopeorum* is found on the crowns of the giant *Sequoia sempervirens* trees in California. It also contains friesiic acid, as well as thamnolic acid.

This brings us to the end of our journey on the traditional usage and health benefits of lichens.

I leave the final word to lichenologist Nastassja Noell:

In lichens, we can find a biological analog for how to build healthy communities, gravitate towards a deeper understanding of the sacredness of relationships, and listen to the dangling murmur of emergent potentialities that can only become whole if we delve into relationships the way that lichens do: fully dedicated to symbioses, fully present through all seasons of our experience, and always sharing the narratives of place (McCoy 2016).

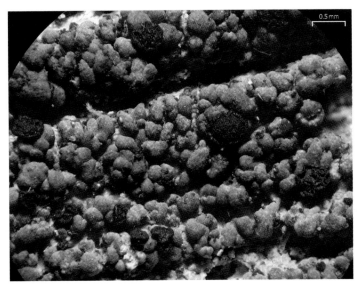

Xylopsora friesii (Fries's Clam Lichen)

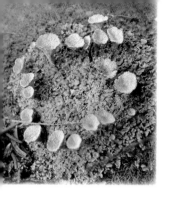

Lichen Chemistry

Atranorin to Zeorin

Lichen chemistry can vary widely, depending upon lichen location, the climate, the substrate, and time of year.

More than a thousand unique secondary metabolites have been identified to date, with fewer than two dozen assessed for effectiveness in various in vitro models, including cancer cells (Backorová et al. 2012). Many of the secondary metabolites develop along the polymalonate pathway.

Both water-soluble polysaccharides and alcohol-soluble compounds contribute to their medicinal benefit.

Lichen polysaccharides are immune modulating, enhancing the production of nitrous oxide and affecting production of pro- and anti-inflammatory cytokines (interleukins [IL]-10, IL-12, IL-1ß, tumor necrosis factor-alpha [TNF]-alpha, and interferon [IFN]-a/ß) by both macrophages and dendritic cells (Shrestha et al. 2015a).

It should be noted that in many cases the whole lichen extract is more efficacious than the isolated compound. Also, isolated compounds influence their activity on macrophage cells in different manners. Salazinic and fumarprotocetraric acids, for example, induce release of hydrogen peroxide, while usnic and diffractaic acids induce release of nitric oxide (Santos et al. 2004).

Extraction methods and toxic residues are an area of concern for human health. For home use, ethanol is probably the safest extraction for internal benefit, and fat or oil-based extractions for external application to various skin conditions. Many of the in vitro and in vivo studies, to date, involve acetone, methanol, and ethyl acetate extraction.

Work by Sepulveda et al. (2023) identified a green extraction using ultrasound and ethyl lactate. The isolation and detection of lichen substances was comparable to using methanol extraction, without the toxicity.

Another method that improves human health efficacy is liposomal formulation. This method shows substantial improvement in solubility, bioactivity, and cytotoxicity in animal studies (Tatipamula et al. 2022).

A few of the most important secondary metabolites in lichens are listed here.

ATRANORIN

Found in Lichens

Acarospora	Flavoparmelia	Megalaria	Ramalina
Asahinea	Gymnoderma	Melanelia	Rimelia
Biatora	Haematomma	Parmelia	Rinodina
Bryoria	Heterodermia	Parmotrema	Stereocaulon
Buellia	Hypogymnia	Phyllospora	Thamnolia
Cetrelia	Hypotrachyna	Physcia	Umbilicaria
Cladonia	Lecanora	Platismatia	Usnea
Diploicia	Lecidella	Pleurosticta	
Diploschistes	Lepraria	Pyxine	

Atranorin is found in numerous lichens.

A review of atranorin (ATR) by Studzinska-Sroka et al. (2017) looked at the various activities exhibited by this, one of the most studied lichen secondary metabolites. Various cancer studies involve bone and joint, colorectal, brain, cervical, breast, prostate, lung, melanoma, and ovarian cancer. The literature describes anti-inflammatory, analgesic, wound healing, antibacterial, antifungal, cytotoxic, antioxidant, antiviral, and immune-modulating activity. Atranorin's lack of toxicity was confirmed in several animal in vivo assays.

Work by Backorová et al. (2012) looked at the cytotoxicity of four secondary metabolites and found ATR activates programmed cell death (apoptosis) in A2780 (human ovarian) and HT-29 (human colon) cancer cell lines, probably through the mitochondrial pathway.

ATR was tested for its efficacy in antitumor and hepatoprotective activity in a mouse model of 4T1 triple negative induced breast cancer. Administration of ATR resulted in longer survival times, reduced tumor size and the number of apoptotic 4T1 cells.

Atranorin exhibits cytotoxicity against human breast cancer cells via interaction with Akt activity (Harikrishnan et al. 2021). It also shows cytotoxicity against MCF-7 breast cancer cell lines (Andania et al. 2019).

Results by Solár et al. (2016) suggest ATR is more proapoptotic than antiproliferative both in vitro and in vivo. Normal NMuMG (mammary epithelial) cells were less sensitive to ATR, and a protective effect against oxidative stress in livers of tumor-bearing mice was noted.

ATR was found cytotoxic against human breast, lung, epithelial, melanoma, prostate and murine leukemia cancer cell lines (Ureña-Vacas et al. 2023).

Both ATR and usnic acid are active against three strains of methicillin-resistant *Staphylococcus aureus* (MRSA) and biofilm extracted from cystic fibrosis patients (Pompilio et al. 2013).

Babesia parasites affect both humans and animals. The first human case was determined in Zagreb, Croatia, in 1957, and then in the Irish countryside in 1968. It is transmitted by white-footed mice in the eastern United States, where *Borrelia burgdorfei* (Lyme disease) is present and more common. Work by Beshbishy et al. (2020) found ATR effective against infected mice. More significant was the synergistic and additive efficacy when combined with existing drugs.

ATR induced apoptosis in HCT-116 colon cancer cell lines (Roser et al. 2022).

A study on Wistar rats suggests ATR acts as an antioxidant and markedly changes behavior. After one month of daily treatment with ATR, hippocampal neurogenesis increased in the hilus and subgranular zone, together with the number of NeuN mature neurons in hilus and CA1 regions. This suggests a potential antidepressant/anxiolytic effect associated with ATR (Urbanska et al. 2022).

ATR is neuroprotective and stimulates brain-derived neurotrophic factor and nerve growth factor expression (Reddy et al. 2016). A parallel study by Simko et al. (2022) found atranorin increased anabolic effect on skeletal muscles, with no toxicity at 10 mg/kg body weight.

ATR exhibits antiviral activity against the hepatitis C virus, inhibiting viral entry (Vu et al. 2015).

Mouse studies by Melo et al. (2008) suggest ATR exerts an analgesic and anti-inflammatory effect.

ATR inhibits COX-1 and COX-2 enyzmes, again suggestive of analgesic and anti-inflammatory activity (Bugni et al. 2009).

BARBATOLIC ACID

Found in Lichen

Bryoria

Barbatolic acid exhibits promising anti-angiogenic and anti-migratory potential in T-47D (human breast ductal carcinoma, and cisplatin-resistant BRCA2-mutated breast cancer cell lines (Varol 2018).

BAEOMYCESIC ACID

Found in Lichens

Chaenotheca	Flavocetraria	Rimelia
Cladonia	Parmelia	Thamnolia

Baeomycesic acid shows a slight antiproliferative potential against pancreas, ovary, and colorectal cancer cell lines (Haraldsdóttir et al. 2004).

CAPERATIC ACID

Found in Lichens

Flavoparmelia	Melanelia	Platismatia

Caperatic acid is a polycarboxylic fatty acid present in several lichen species. Work by Paluszczak et al. (2018) found it tended to reduce Axin2 expression in both HCT116 and DLD-1 colon cancer cell lines. It works by inhibiting Wnt signaling.

Caperatic acid crosses the blood–brain barrier and has potential for treatment of glioblastoma. It exerted cytotoxicity on T98G cells, inhibited the Wnt/ß-catenin pathway, and was even stronger in co-treatment with the drug temozolomide (Majchrzak-Celinska et al. 2022).

CHLOROATRANORIN

Found in Lichens

Acarospora	Candelaria	Heterodermia	Parmelia
Alectoria	Diploicia	Hypogymnia	Platismatia

Chloroatranorin found in *Parmotrema saccatilobum* exhbits partial inhibition of COX-1, suggesting analgesic and anti-inflammatory activity (Bugni et al., 2009).

CHRYSOPHANOL

Found in Lichen

Caloplaca

Chrysophanol exhibits anticancer, antioxidant, neuroprotectant, antibacterial, antiviral and regulation of blood lipids (Xie et al., 2019). PubMed has 755 listed research studies.

DIFFRACTAIC ACID

Found in Lichens

Alectoria	*Parmelia*	*Rimelia*
Hypogymnia	*Parmotrema*	*Usnea*

Thioredoxin reductase 1 (TrxR1) is a therapeutic target for breast cancer due to its overexpression in tumor cells. Relatedly, diffractaic acid (DA) induces cytotoxicity in both MCF-7 and MDA-MB-453 breast cancer cells. Work by Kalin et al. (2022) found upregulation of the BAX/BCL2 ratio and the P53 gene in MCF-7 cells, but only the P53 in MDA-MB-453 cells. The gene, protein, and enzyme of TrxR1 were suppressed by MCF-7 cells, whereas in the other breast cancer cell line only enzyme activity was suppressed.

DA induces cytotoxicity, apoptosis, and antimigration. The authors, Kalin et al. therefore conclude diffractaic acid may be an effective therapy for breast cancer treatment.

In a study by Truong et al. (2014), DA showed significant cytotoxic activity against human breast (MCF-7), human epithelial (HeLa), and human lung (NCI-H460) cancer cell lines, and Brisdelli et al. (2013) found DA to be cytotoxic to a colon (HCT-116) cancer cell line.

DA exhibited antitumor activity on Swiss albino mice with Ehrlich ascites carcinoma (Koragoz et al. 2014). DA derived from *Usnea longissima* protected rats from liver damage when the rats were exposed to carbon tetrachloride (Koragoz et al. 2015).

DA shows moderate cytotoxicity on glioblastoma multiforme cancer cell lines (Emsen et al. 2018).

DA was the most effective compound against the *Mycobacterium tuberculosis* cell line. Honda et al. (2010) tested four lichen species and 26 individual compounds. Both norstictic and usnic acids were the second most effective.

DA inhibited gastric lesions and reduced oxidative stress and neutrophil infiltration in a rat study (Bayir et al. 2006).

Dengue is a flavivirus, carried by mosquitoes, resulting in 21,000 deaths annually. Work by Loenurit et al. (2023) examined depsides and depsidones from two species each of *Usnea* and *Parmotrema*. DA showed the highest cytotoxicity, and similar efficacies were found in dengue serotypes 1-4, Zika, and chikungunya viruses. The authors suggest DA could become a mosquito-borne antiviral, targeting viral replication.

DIVARICATIC ACID

Found in Lichens

Canoparmelia	Dirinaria	Haematomma	Ramalina
Cladonia	Evernia	Niebla	

Divaricatic acid (DV) shows activity against *Bacillus subtilis*, *Staphylococcus aureus*, and MRSA, as well as anti-*Candida* activity (Oh et al. 2018).

DV exhibits strong activity against human UACC-62 and B16-F10 murine melanoma cancer cell lines, with more selectivity against melanoma cells than against 3T3 normal cells (Brandão et al. 2013).

EMODIN

Found in Lichens

Heterodermia	Nephroma	Oxneria

PubMed cites over 3,300 research studies on benefits of emodin. It is found in several lichen species, but is also present in several TCM (Traditional Chinese Medicine) herbs, including rhubarb root. Emodin possesses significant anti-cancer, neuroprotective, anti-diabetic activity, anti-pseudorabies and other viral infections, hepatoprotective, prevents cardiovascular calcification, and encourages gut microbiome regeneration.

EPANORIN

Found in Lichens

Acarospora	Lecanora

Epanorin inhibits the proliferation of MCF-7 breast cancer cell lines and induces cell cycle arrest at G0/G1. Work by Palacios-Moreno et al. (2019) confirmed the lack of cytototoxicity on normal cell line HEK-293 and human fibroblasts.

EUMELANIN

Found in Lichen

Lobaria

Eumelanin is a member of the melanin family helping block harmful UV or visible radiation. *EU* derives from the ancient Greek, meaning "good." Eumelanin exhibits protection against diethylnitrosamine-induced liver injury in a rat study by Altindag et al. (2022). A lack of eumelanin production by people with red hair makes them more susceptible to skin cancer (Nasti and Timares, 2015).

EVERNIC ACID

Found in Lichens

Evernia	*Pleurosticta*	*Umbilicaria*
Parmotrema	*Ramalina*	*Usnea*

Evernic acid (EA) protects primary cultured neurons against toxin-induced death, mitochondrial dysfunction, and oxidative stress. EA crosses the blood–brain barrier.

In vivo, EA ameliorated induced motor dysfunction, dopaminergic neuronal loss, and neuroinflammation in the nigrostriatal pathway. Lee et al. (2021) suggest EA is a potential therapeutic candidate for treatment of Parkinson's disease.

Earlier work found neuroprotective activity of EA, in part due to activation of the nuclear factor erythroid-2 pathway (Fernández-Moriano et al. 2017a).

EA exhibits cytotoxicity against glioblastoma multiforme and inhibits kynurenine pathway enzymes (Studzinska-Sroka et al. 2021).

Several studies have described its anticancer, antimicrobial, and antifungal effects.

EA showed strong cytotoxicity against HeLa (epithelial) cells and reduced proliferation of A549 (lung) cancer cells. Studies on healthy HUVEC cells resulted in no toxicity, with this contrast suggesting EA may be a good candidate for cancer treatment (Kizil et al. 2015).

One avenue of targeting cancer cells is via thioredoxin reductase, due to its overexpression in many human tumors. Work by Kalin et al. (2023) looked at the potential of evernic acid on its potential antiproliferative, anti-migratory, and apoptotic activity. The compound suppressed the proliferation of MCF-7 and MDA-MB-453 breast cancer cell lines, not through apoptosis but by inhibiting thioredoxin reductase.

Girardot et al. (2021) found that EA showed weak toxicity against HeLa cells but slowed the maturation of, and reduced already formed biofilms of, *Candida albicans*.

Cystic fibrosis affects the respiratory and digestive systems. Infections of *Pseudomonas aeruginosa* are a major cause of mortality and morbidity. EA inhibits this bacterium and its quorum sensing systems. That is, an individual bacterium is no great cause for concern, but large groupings and biofilm

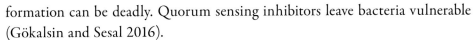

formation can be deadly. Quorum sensing inhibitors leave bacteria vulnerable (Gökalsin and Sesal 2016).

EA is a moderate inhibitor of tumor-promoter-induced Epstein–Barr virus activation (Yamamoto et al. 1995).

FUMARPROTOCETRARIC ACID

Found in Lichens

Bryoria	Cetraria	Cladonia	Melanelia

Fumarprotocetraric acid (FUM) inhibits tau protein covalently, avoiding cytotoxicity of aggregates in cells. Tau protein aggregation with misfolded structure is one aspect of neurodegenerative disorders (González et al. 2021).

Earlier work by Fernandez-Moriano et al. (2017) found FUM protects against oxidative damage in the mitochondrial membrane, and upregulates antioxidant enzymes. It mediates cytotoxicity in two models of neurons and astrocyte cells (SH-SY5Y and U373-MG).

This suggests potential therapy in oxidative stress disease, such as neurodegenerative disorders.

GYROPHORIC ACID

Found in Lichens

Acarospora	Dactylina	Menegazzia	Peltigera
Biatora	Hypogymnia	Micarea	Punctelia
Bryoria	Lasallia	Ocellularia	Rinodina
Cetraria	Lobaria	Parmelia	Solorina
Cladonia	Melanelia	Parmotrema	Umbilicaria

Gyrophoric acid (GA) is present in various lichens, particularly in various *Umbilicaria* species.

This depside shows cytotoxic and antiproliferative activity against several cancer cell lines and is a broad-spectrum antimicrobial (Singh et al. 2022).

GA exhibits antiproliferative and apoptosis activity against HeLa (human epithelial/cervical) cells and other tumor cells.

Work by Backorova et al. (2011) and Kosanic et al. (2014) found cytotoxicity of GA against A2780 (ovarian), HL60 (leukemia), Jurkat (T cell lymphocyte leukemia), Fem-X (melanoma), and K562 (chronic myelogenous leukemia) cancer cell lines. GA also reduced the percentage of Fem-X and K562 cells in the G0/G1 phase and s-G2/M phases of the cell cycle. It also inhibited the clonogenic abiity of breast SK-BR-3 cancer cell lines.

GA-treated cells showed a significant increase in caspase-3 activation, followed by PARP cleavage, PS externalization, and cell cycle changes mediated by oxidative stress (Goga et al. 2019).

GA not only causes cell cycle arrest, comprises cell survival, and promotes apoptosis, but it also impinges on topoisomerase-1 activity (Mohammadi et al. 2022). Its ability to treat inflammation and glycation in diabetes and cardiovascular disease requires further research.

Shim (2020) reports anti-aging effects of GA on UVA-irradiated normal human dermal fibroblasts. GA treatment favorably influenced both MMP1 (matrix metalloproteinases 1) and mRNA (messenger ribonucleic acid) expression levels, consistent with anti-aging. GA may be therapeutic as a psoriasis treatment, based on its inhibition of the human keratinocyte HaCaT cell line (Kumar and Müller 1999).

GA consists of three orsellenic acid units and is almost nine times more potent as an inhibitor of protein tyrosine phosphatase 1B (PTP1B) than lecanoric acid (described later), which has two orsellinic rings. Lecanoric acid in turn is almost nine times more potent than methylorselllinate. This is significant because PTP1B is a major negative regulator of insulin signaling and a possible target for type 2 diabetes and obesity (Seo et al. 2009).

GA possesses antihypertensive activity by acting as an angiotensin II type-1 receptor antagonist (Huo et al. 2019).

ISOLECANORIC ACID

Found in Lichen

Parmotrema

Isolecanoric acid has been investigated by de Pedro et al. (2016) for its protection in amyotrophic lateral sclerosis (ALS) and Parkinson's disease models. Pretreatment with this acid prevented mitochondrial dysfunction in SH-SY5Y cells, by decreasing membrane potential, reducing oxidative stress via ROS, attenuating early and late apoptosis, and inhibiting glycogen synthase kinase-2 beta and casein kinase I.

Recent work by Matias-Valiente et al. (2024) found isolecanoric acid modulates inflammation and muscle regeneration in a mice model of Duchenne muscular dystrophy.

LECANORIC ACID

Found in Lichens

Cladonia	*Hypocenomyce*	*Parmotrema*	*Umbilicaria*
Dactylina	*Melanelia*	*Punctelia*	*Usnea*
Diploschistes	*Lecanora*	*Roccella*	

Lecanoric acid (LA) is also present in numerous lichens.

It inhibited cell colony formation in HCT116 colon cancer cells and induced a G2 cell cycle block in several other lines. LA arrested cell cycle, presumably in the M phase, since expression of cyclin B1 and phosphorylated histone H3 was upregulated, and the inactive cyclin-dependent kinase 1 was reduced in colon cancer cells. Cell death by LA is prominent in cancer cells but does not affect primary immune cells (Roser et al. 2022).

Thioredoxin reductase (TrxR) helps protect our cells against oxidative stress. But the overexpression is often found in many aggressive tumors. Five lichen metabolites (diffractaic, evernic, lobaric, lecanoric, and vulpinic acids) were tested for inhibition of TrxR. All exhibited stronger inhibitory effect on TrxR than cisplatin and doxorubicin (chemotherapy drugs). Lecanoric acid was especially aggressive (Ozgencli et al. 2018).

LA exhibits activity against Hep2 (larynx), MCF-7 (breast), 786-0 (kidney), B16-F10 (murine melanoma), HeLa (epithelial/cervix), A549 (lung), and LS174 (colorectal) cancer cell lines (Ristic et al. 2016; Bogo et al. 2010).

LA also shows potential neuroprotective potential, based on mouse neuroblastoma (N2a) cells. Significant inhibitory activity against acetylcholinesterase and butyrylcholinesterase was noted (Mapari et al. 2021).

A number of bioactive derivatives have been obtained from lecanoric acid (Gomes et al. 2002).

LA shows antifungal activity against the pathogen *Aspergillus fumigatus*, which kills 600,000 people annually.

It also shows strong inhibition against *Rhizoctonia solani*, first identified on potato tubers by Julius Kühn in 1858. *Rhizoctonia solani* is present in both its anamorphic and teleomorphic forms, and causes widespread disease in commercial crops. It causes damping off of infected seeds, with failure of germination. Cereal crops in Canada are severely affected, but the fungus also causes crop failure in soybeans, sugar beets, tomatoes, potatoes, and the cabbage family (Paguirigan et al. 2022).

LUPEOL

Found in Lichens

Evernia	Flavocetraria	Parmotrema

Lupeol is a pentacyclic triterpenoid that shows promise against cancer, diabetes, obesity, cardiovascular disease, kidney and liver issues, skin disease and neurological disorders (Sohang et al. 2022).

Lupeol exhibits antioxidant and anti-inflammatory activity, and high blood-brain barrier permeability, suggesting reduction of oxidative stress in Alzheimer's disease (Park et al. 2023).

LOBARIC ACID

Found in Lichens

Bryoria	Heterodermia	Stereocaulon
Cladonia	Protoparmelia	Usnea

Lobaric acid and two other lichen metabolites were tested against 12 different human cancer cell lines. In work by Haraldsdóttir et al. (2004), lobaric acid showed the greatest inhibition against all cell lines. Three lines from pancreas and leukemia and single cells from breast, prostate, small cell lung, ovary, stomach, and colorectal cancer cell lines showed inhibition.

The Chikungunya virus is spread by mosquitoes, originally from Africa and Asia, and is now found in the Americas. The name translates roughly as "bends you up" or "stooped walk." Symptoms include high fever, fatigue, rash, red eyes, and nausea within two to five days of bite. There is neither vaccine nor cure. However, a study of 3,051 compounds discovered several small molecules capable of inhibiting the virus's nsP1 RNA capping enzyme. Lobaric acid was found to inhibit the binding and guanylation, as well as to attenuate viral growth, in hamster and human Huh7 cell lines (Feibelman et al. 2018).

Atopic dermatitis (AD) results from multiple factors associated with immune dysfunction and skin barrier disruption. Protease-activated receptor 2 (PAR2) is involved in epidermal permeability and epithelial inflammation. Work by Joo et al. (2016) found that lobaric acid applied topically is a PAR2 antagonist and may be a therapeutic solution.

Infertility in women is increasingly common. Some scientists believe that environmental factors, such as herbicides and pesticides, may be responsible for aberrant menstrual cycles. Tetramethrin (Tm) is a commonly used pesticide reported to exert estrogen antagonistic effects on female rats. Tm decreased levels of luteinizing hormone, follicular stimulating hormone, progesterone, estrone, and estradiol, while increasing testosterone levels. Work by Nguyen et al. (2022) examined the role of lobaric acid on the estrous cycle. Lobaric acid competes with Tm for gonadotropin-releasing hormone, and may be useful in management of insecticide-induced menstrual cycle issues.

Lobaric acid is cytotoxic against HSC-3 (human oral squamous carcinoma) cell lines (Andania et al. 2019).

Endocannabinoid receptors (CB1 and CB2) are found throughout the human body. CB1 is most common in the central nervous system, while CB2 is mainly concerned with the immune system. The increasing popularity and efficiency of cannabinoid products has led to a widespread search for compounds that influence these G-protein-coupled receptors. Selective CB2 agonists help reduce inflammation and neuropathy. Work by Mohamed et al. (2023) investigated 235 depsidones from various plant and lichen sources. Among these, lobaric acid was identified with a high binding score when screened against the CB2 receptor.

METHYL EVERNATE

Found in Lichens

Peltigera	Ramalina

Methyl evernate inhibits HeLa (human epithelial), A549 (lung) and LS174 (colon) cancer cell lines (Ristic et al. 2016a). In the same study, methyl evernate was found a stronger antimicrobial than evernic, obtusatic, sekikaic acid, and atranorin.

NORSTICTIC ACID

Found in Lichens

Acarospora	Heterodermia	Stereocaulon
Baeomyces	Lecanora	Thelomma
Buellia	Lobaria	Toninia
Cetraria	Parmotrema	Umbilicaria
Cladonia	Pleurosticta	Usnea
Dimelaena	Ramalina	Xanthoparmelia
Graphina	Rhizocarpon	Xanthoria

Norstictic acid (NA) is found in a number of lichen species. In a study of 4,000 compounds by McCullough et al. (2022), NA was the most potent inhibitor of protein histidine phosphatase. This protein is an important cellular regulator, involved in attenuating cancer cell proliferation, liver fibrosis and neuronal health. It plays a role in the cascade leading to nutrient-induced insulin secretion. Abnormalities in this signaling lead to impaired insulin in glucolipo-toxicity and type 2 diabetes (Kowluru et al. 2011; Kamath et al. 2010).

Norstictic acid (NA) inhibits MDA-MB-231 breast cancer cell lines, in terms of proliferation, migration, and invasion in a mouse xenograft model.

Triple negative breast cancers (TNBCs) have worse patient outcomes and higher mortality rates. The proto-oncogenic receptor tyrosine kinase c-Met is usually dysregulated in TNBCs, leading to aggressive cell invasion and tumor metastasis (Ebrahim et al. 2016). NA is a selective allosteric transcriptional regulator, in a patient-derived model of TNBC.

Inhibitors of transcriptional protein–protein interactions (PPIs) are valuable tools for therapeutic application. The PPI network, mediated by the co-activator Med25, regulates stress response and motility pathways. Dysregulation of the PPI network contributes to oncogenesis and metastasis. NA blocks this pathway (Garlick et al. 2021).

OLIVETORIC ACID

Found in Lichens

Cetrelia	Tuckermannopsis

Olivetoric acid (OA) possesses antimicrobial and antioxidant activity. It induced cytotoxicity and genotoxicity against the glioblastoma multiforme (U87MG) cell line and primary rat cerebral cortex (PRCC) cells, via lactate dehydrogenase and oxidative DNA damage. OA also showed activity against HepG2 (hepatic) carcinoma cells (Emsen et al. 2016; Emsen et al. 2021).

OA inhibits angiogenesis, which is the means by which cancer cells feed themselves by extending blood vessels. It disrupts microtubules and inhibits actin polymerization (Koparal et al. 2010).

PANNARIN

Found in Lichens

Dimelaena	Leprocaulon	Phyllospora	Rinodina
Lecanora	Pannaria	Psoroma	Sphaerophorus

Pannarin exhibits moderate synergistic activity with gentamicin against various strains of methicillin-resistant *Staphylococcus aureus* (MRSA). When combined with levofloxacin, the combination was antagonistic, and made no difference when combined with erythromycin (Celenza et al. 2012).

PERLATOLIC ACID

Found in Lichens

Canoparmelia	Cladonia	Melanelia
Cetrelia	Dimelaena	Stereocaulon

Perlatolic acid (PER) is active against MRSA strains, and is synergistic with gentamicin and antagonistic with levofloxacin (Bellio et al. 2015). This acid also exhibits activity against SARS-CoV-2 in recent work by Desmarets et al. (2023).

PHYSCION (PARIETIN)

Found in Lichens

Candelaria	Umbilicaria	Xanthoria

Physcion (parietin) provides the yellow, orange, and red pigmentation found in numerous lichen species.

Physcion exhibits activity against human breast (MCF-7) cancer cell lines in mice, via modulation of oxidative stress-mediated mitochondrial apoptosis and immune response (Zhang et al. 2021). Acute lymphoblastic leukemia is the most common form of malignancy in children and ranks as third most common cancer in adults. This relates to studies by Gao et al. (2017) that found physcion significantly suppressed cell growth, induced apoptosis, and blocked cell cycle progression in vitro; physcion downregulated the expression of HOXA5, which is responsible for antileukemia activity.

The compound also inhibits human colorectal (SW620) cancer cells in vitro, not by affecting cell viability but inhibiting cell adhesion, migration, and invasion. Suppression of SOX2 is involved (Han et al. 2016).

Physcion markedly induced apoptosis in human hepatocellular (Huh7 and Bel7402) carcinoma cell lines (Pan et al. 2018) and in human gastric (SGC-7901) cancer cell lines (Xiong et al. 2015).

Physcion induces apoptosis, oxidative stress, and autophagy in human cervical cancer cell lines (Trybus et al. 2021) and human nasopharyngeal (CNE2) carcinoma, due to downregulation of Sp1 and suppression of miR27a in tumor tissue (Pang et al. 2016). The compound is hydrophobic and thus poorly soluble. Prepared as a liposome, it becomes anti-angiogenic, and induces apoptosis in triple negative breast cancer cell lines (Ayoub et al. 2022).

Physcion may also be a good alternative to doxycycline to combat virulent *Chlamydia psittaci* infection, helping prevent transmission from animals to humans (Liu et al. 2023).

Homocysteine-induced vascular endothelial dysfunction is common in cardiovascular disease. Work by Ji et al. (2021) found physcion prevents this condition by activating Ca^{2+} and Akt-eNOS-N signaling pathways, suggesting potential for prevention of cardiovascular disease. It also significantly increased levels of p38 and JNK.

Physcion has been found to have a neuroprotective effect against cerebral ischemia–reperfusion injury, based on in vivo study by Dong et al. (2021).

Parietin is poorly water soluble, but combined with a cyclodextrin complex it may help treat infections associated with multi-drug-resistant bacteria (Ayoub et al. 2022a).

Parietin (another name for physcion) inhibited the aggregation process of tau, a protein involved in Alzheimer's disease (Cornejo et al. 2016).

It also heals wounds, and is an alternative to zinc in skin healing, as it induces cell proliferation at low doses in cases of dermal fibroblast loss (Gundogdu et al. 2019).

PHYSCIOSPORIN

Found in Lichens

Pseudocyphellaria

Physciosporin was investigated by Tas et al. (2021) for its effects on energy metabolism and antitumor activity on human breast MCF-7 (estrogen and progesterone positive) and MDA-MB-231 (triple negative) cancer cell lines. Tas et al. found physciosporin significantly decreased the mRNA level of PGCl-*a* genes in both types of breast cancer cells. In vivo work suggests the compound may hold promise to treat the hormone-insensitive triple-negative cells by targeting energy metabolism.

PHYSODIC ACID

Found in Lichens

Alectoria	Dactylina	Hypogymnia	Usnea
Candelariella	Evernia	Hypotrachyna	

Physodic acid is not competitive with ATP, and is more soluble than another lichen derivative, norlobaridone. It exhibits weak inhibition of various tumor cell lines, but could be studied for its unique molecular structure in terms of improved activity against MPP1 (M-phase phosphoprotein 1) (Talapatra et al. 2016), which is upregulated in various kinds of bladder cancer.

Physodic acid and perlatolic acid, derived from lichens, are potent inhibitors, suggesting novel approaches to inflammatory disorders (Bauer et al. 20120). This could be applicable to managing microsomal prostaglandin E2 synthase-1 (mPGES-1), which is a target of many nonsteroidal anti-inflammatory drugs (NSAIDs) such as ibuprofen, acetaminophen, and the like.

Physodic acid is found in many lichens. In terms of cancer treatement, the isolated compound was found effective against the acute lymphoblastic leukemia Jurkat cells. Physodic acid induced cell death, DNA damage, and cell cycle arrest, with minimal cytotoxicity to normal cells (Kelio et al. 2021). Also, physodic acid activated apoptosis in A375 melanoma cancer cells, probably involving the reduction of Hsp70 expression (Cardile et al. 2017).

It may also be useful in treating prostate cancer. Work by Cardile et al. (2022) confirmed the apoptotic activity of physodic acid on LNCaP (prostate) cancer cells. In addition, physodic acid sensitized the cells to tumor necrosis factor (TNF)-related apoptosis-inducing ligand (TRAIL), suggesting adjuvant therapy combinations. Physodic acid also exhibits activity against human breast cancer cell lines (Studzinska-Sroka et al. 2016).

PROTOCETRARIC ACID

Found in Lichens

Bryoria	Flavoparmelia	Parmelia	Ramalina
Cetraria	Graphina	Parmotrema	Usnea
Cladonia	Hypogymnia	Pleurosticta	

Protocetraric acid (PCA) shows inhibitory activity against the SARS-CoV2 virus (Fagnani et al. 2022).

PCA shows significant antimicrobial activity against *Salmonella typhi* and significant antifungal activity against *Trichophyton rubrum*, better than standard antifungal drugs (Nishanth et al. 2015).

PCA is also cytotoxic and highly selective against UACC-62 melanoma cancer cells. This suggests more study of its potential (Brandão et al. 2013).

PROTOLICHESTERINIC ACID

Found in Lichens

Cetraria	Gymnoderma	Ramalina
Flavocetraria	Parmelia	Stereocaulon
Flavoparmelia	Punctelia	Tuckermannopsis

Protolichesterinic acid (PA) is found in Iceland moss and related lichens. The chemical structure is similar to the fatty acid synthase (FASN) inhibitor C75.

Work by Bessadóttir et al. (2014) found its primary effect is inhibition of FASN activity, with secondary effects on human epidermal growth factor receptor 2 (HER2) expression and signaling. It increased FASN expression in SK-BR-3 breast cancer cells, and is synergistic with lapatinib, suggesting its use alone or in a combination treatment for HER2-overexpressing breast cancer.

PA enhances doxorubicin-induced apoptosis in HeLa (cervical) cancer cell lines in vitro. This was associated with caspase-3, -8, and -9 activation, and an increase in Bim protein expression, suggesting a useful combination with chemotherapy drugs (Briscelli et al. 2016).

An in vitro study on two cancer cell lines, T-47D (breast) and AsPC-1 (pancreas), found PA exhibited antiproliferative activity. Both cell lines showed structural changes in mitochondria. The authors of the study believe PA is metabolically processed and expelled from cells, leading indirectly to increased glutathione levels, with minimal effects on redox balance (Jóhannsson et al. 2022).

PA inhibits multiple melanoma (RPM I8226 and U266) and pancreatic (AsPC-1) cancer cell lines. In fact, the acid entered the pancreatic cancer cells. The antiproliferative and pro-apoptotic effects of PA are not mediated through inhibition of LOX (lipoxygenase) activity (Bessadóttir et al. 2015).

PA isolated from Iceland moss (*Cetraria islandica*) reduces LRRC8A expression and volume-sensitive release of organic osmolytes in human lung epithelial cancer cells. (Thorsteinsdottir et al. 2016).

PA and other lichen constituents were tested for antiproliferative activity against 12 human cancer cell lines (Haraldsdóttir et al. 2004).

PA isolated from *Usnea* species showed antifungal properties against

Candida tropicalis, through the accumulation of intracellular ROS, and mitochondria-mediated cell death due to apoptosis (Kumar and Mohandas 2017).

PA is an inhibitor of *Candida albicans*, neutralizing its virulence, and exhibits therapeutic efficacy in a murine candidiasis model. It does so through inhibition of cystathionine ß-synthase, which is the major enzyme that synthesizes hydrogen sulfide in the pathogenic fungus (Chang et al. 2022).

Protolichesterinic acid is also active against *Aspergillus flavus*, a common food mold (fungus).

PSOROMIC ACID

Found in Lichens

Cladonia	Lepraria	Rhizocarpon	Squamarina
Graphina	Ocellularia	Rhizoplaca	Usnea
Lecanora	Psoroma	Sarcogyne	

Psoromic acid (PSA) is present in many lichens, including *Cladonia mitis* and *Psoroma* species.

Hassan et al. (2018) found that PSA showed profound inhibitory effect against all *Mycobacterium tuberculosis* strains tests, comparable to the drug isoniazid but without its side effects. The extract also showed inhibition against arylamine *N*-acetyltransferase comparable to the drug's effect.

Rab geranylgeranyl transferase inhibitors have potential to treat cancer and osteoporosis. Psoromic acid potently and selectively inhibits this process (Deraeve et al. 2012).

Psoromic acid inhibits the replication of herpes simplex 1 and herpes simplex 2, and inactivates HSV-1 DNA polymerase (Hassan et al. 2019).

Usnea complanata, under submerged fermentation, produces psoromic acid, which shows inhibition of angiotensin-converting enzyme, suggestive of benefit in cardiovascular conditions (Behera et al. 2012).

A study from Chile (Sepulveda et al. 2013) found psoromic acid reduced gastric ulcer lesions in mice by 65%. Other lichen compounds also were found effective, including lobaric acid (76%), atranorin (63%), and perlatolic acid (45%).

RAMALIC ACID

Found in Lichen

Ramalina

Ramalic acid possesses antimicrobial and antifungal activity, as well as moderate antioxidative potential.

It shows weak to moderate cytotoxicity against HeLa (cervical/epilthelial), A549 (lung), and LS174 (colon) human cancer cell lines (Ristic et al. 2016).

RHIZOCARPIC ACID

Found in Lichens

Acarospora	Psilolechia	Rhizocarpon

Rhizocarpic acid exhibits weak activity against *Bacillus subtilis*, and modest but selective antitumor activity against NS-1 (murine myeloma) cells with more than tenfold potency relative to its enantiomer, *ent*-rhizocarpic acid (James et al. 2023).

Rhizocarpic acid shows potential antiviral activity against SARS-CoV-2 (Joshi et al. 2021).

SALAZINIC ACID

Found in Lichens

Flavocetraria	Pseudoparmelia	Usnea
Heterodermia	Ramalina	Xanthoparmelia
Parmelia	Rimelia	Xanthoria
Parmotrema	Thelomma	
Pleurosticta	Umbilicaria	

Salazinic acid is a potent modulator of nuclear factor erythroid 2-related factor (Nrf2), nuclear factor-kappa B (NF-kB), and STAT3 signaling pathways. Salazinic acid and physodic acid showed the highest activity against colorectal cancer cells (Papierska et al. 2021)

Nrf2 and NF-kappaB signaling pathways play a central role in suppressing or inducing inflammation and angiogenesis. Targeting both transcription factors simultaneously may be an important strategy for cancer chemoprevention and therapy.

Nrf2 is involved in expression of antioxidant and phase 2 metabolizing enzymes, which have direct antiproliferative activity. Its cross-talk with NF-kB has great anti-inflammatory potential that can be used in inflammation-induced/-associated cancers. STAT3, on the other hand, is involved in multiple pathways of cancer initiation and progression (Ahsan et al. 2022).

While activation of Nrf2 and inhibition of NF-kB may protect normal cells against cancer initiation and promotion, enhanced expression and activation of cancer cells may lead to resistance in chemotherapy and radiation (Krajka-Kuzniak and Baer-Dubowska 2021).

Salazinic acid is a potential inhibitor of SARS-CoV-2 3CL (3-chymotrypsin-like) cysteine protease (Fagnani et al. 2022).

SEKIKAIC ACID

Found in Lichens

Niebla	Ramalina

Sekikaic acid (SE) is a potent antiviral, showing activity against both a recombinant strain A2 strain respiratory syncytial virus. It appears to interfere with replication at a viral postentry step. Note that virus replication is a two-step process: First the virus reprograms the cell to produce virions, and then the virions escape the infected cell and move into the body.

SE activity is higher than that of ribavirin (Lai et al. 2013).

SQUAMATIC ACID

Found in Lichens

Alectoria	Cladonia	Sphaerophorus
Chaenotheca	Flavocetraria	Thamnolia

Squamatic acid derived by an acetone extract exhibits activity against methicillin-resistant *Staphylococcus aureus* (MRSA), and reference strain of SA, comparable to chloramphenicol (Studzinska-Sroka et al. 2015).

STICTIC ACID

Found in Lichens

Acarospora	Lepraria	Pseudocyphellaria
Baeomyces	Lobaria	Rinodina
Bryoria	Menegazzia	Stereocaulon
Dimelaena	Parmelia	Umbilicaria
Graphina	Parmotrema	Usnea
Hypotrachyna	Porpidia	Xanthoparmelia

Stictic acid is a potential reactivation compound. This can be aimed at the tumor suppressor p53, which is the most frequently mutated gene associated with human cancer. There is a transiently open binding pocket between loop L1 and sheet S3 of the p53 core domain. Mutation of residue Cys124, located at the center of the pocket, abolishes p53 reactivation by PRIMA-1, a known reactivation compound. Work by Wassman et al. (2013) on human osteosarcoma cells found that stictic acid is a potential reactivator.

Later work by Omar and Tuszynski (2015) docked 12 known activators to p53 into the open pocket just mentioned. They predicted the absorption, distribution, metabolism, excretion, and toxicity of these compounds, and found that the non-alkylating ligand of stictic acid exhibits great potential as a p53 activator. It has less adverse effect, but poorer pharmacokinetic properties, than other treatments.

Bacteria fatty acid biosynthesis (FAS) contains several enzymes that make it an excellent target for antimicrobial compounds. The purified ß-hydroxyacyl-acyl carrier protein dehydratase, obtained from *Francisella tularensis* and *Yersinia pestis*, was inhibited by stictic acid. This suggests a benefit for stictic acid in a natural approach to bacterial infections (McGillick et al. 2016). Both of these bacteria are gram-negative *Coccobacilli* that are lethal if untreated. The former causes tularemia, and the pneumonic phase is lethal without treatment. The latter is source of the Black Death or bubonic plague that killed millions of people, a disease associated with fleas and rodents. About one to two thousand cases are reported annually to the World Health Organization (WHO).

Stictic acid derived from *Xanthoparmelia* species protects U373 MG cells from hydrogen peroxide-induced damage, suggesting its use for antioxidative protection in neurodegenerative disorders such as Alzheimer's and Parkinson's disease (de Paz et al. 2010).

TARAXEROL

Found in Lichen

Evernia

Taraxerol exhibits activity in a molecular receptor-docking study against SARS-Cov-2 proteins (Joshi et al. 2022). The compound induced apoptosis in HeLa (epithelial/cervical) cancer cell lines (Yaoi et al. 2017). Taraxerol also significantly inhibited acetylcholinesterase and anti-amnesic activity in animal studies, suggesting possible therapeutic activity in memory impairment associated with Alzheimer's disease (Berté et al. 2018).

TENUIORIN ACID

Found in Lichens

Peltigera	*Pseudocyphellaria*

Tenuiorin acid exhibits weak to moderate antiproliferative activity against T-47D (breast), WIDR (colon), and PANC-1 (pancreas) cancer cell lines (Ingólfdóttir et al. 2002).

Tenuiorin acid appears to be a potent neuroprotective compound, acting as a tau inhibitor (Salgado et al. 2020).

TINCTORINONE

Found in Lichens

Parmelia	*Parmotrema*

Tinctorinone exhibits strong inhibition of alpha-glucosidase, suggestive of possible benefit in blood sugar dysregulation (Bui et al. 2022).

TRIVARIC ACID

Found in Lichen

Ramalina

Trivaric acid may have use in the development of antidiabetic compounds. In vitro studies reveal it inhibits protein tyrosine phosphatase 1B (PTP1B) by blocking its active site. It also improves insulin-stimulated glucose uptake via the insulin receptor pathway in liver HepG2 cell line. In vivo mouse studies show benefits of trivaric acid through significant improvement of lipid and glycemic profiles (Sun et al. 2017; 2017a).

Trivaric acid is a potent human neutrophil and pancreatic elastase inhibitor (Zheng et al. 2012). Pancreatic elastase assists production of enzymes, and low levels of it in stool suggest insufficient pancreas function. On the other hand, high levels may be associated with chronic pancreatitis, diabetes, Crohn's disease, ulcerative colitis, and cystic fibrosis.

Recent work by Marinaccio et al. (2022) suggests neutrophil elastase inhibitors may be useful in treating respiratory symptoms associated with COVID-19.

USNIC ACID

Found in Lichens

Acarospora	Dimelaena	Lecanora	Ramalina
Alectoria	Evernia	Lobaria	Rhizoplaca
Asahinea	Flavocetraria	Melanelia	Squamarina
Bryoria	Flavoparmelia	Niebla	Stereocaulon
Cetraria	Haematomma	Parmelia	Umbilicaria
Cladina	Hypotrachyna	Parmotrema	Usnea
Cladonia	Lasallia	Punctelia	Vulpicida

Usnic acid (UA) is common to many lichen genera. The levels present vary widely, from 0.04 to 6.49% dry weight.

It is not soluble in water or glycerine, is more soluble in ethanol, and is most soluble in ether, acetone, and other risky or unpleasant chemicals. Research has found usnic acid is most soluble in one hour of heat reflux with acetone. This yellow pigment is decently soluble in oils and fats, with the application of moderate heat.

Usnic acid isomers are both right-handed (+) and left-handed (–) enantiomers. Between 1948 and 2018 only about 20 papers were published on the subject (Galanty et al. 2019). Lichens tend to contain one or the other isomer of UA. For example, *Alectoria ochroleuca* and *Flavocetraria nivalis* contain (–)-usnic acid, and some *Usnea* species tend to contain more (+)-usnic acid. Others contain both.

Both usnic acids show strong larvicidal activity and induced 100% mortality on third–fourth larval stages of the house mosquito, *Culex pipiens* (Cetin et al. 2008).

Most of the studies to date have been on the right-handed isomer. These numerous studies suggest antibacterial, antifungal, anti-biofilm, antioxidant, cytotoxic, photoprotective, antiviral, antiprotozoal, anti-inflammatory, analgesic, antiproliferative, antimitotic and hepatoxic activity.

Usnic acid exhibited the highest liver state activity against *Plasmodium berghei*, the malaria parasite (Lauinger et al. 2013).

Usnic acid may be useful in the treatment of osteoporosis. In work by Kim et al. (2018) it significantly inhibited RANKL-mediated osteoclast formation, and prevented lipopolysaccharide-induced bone erosion in mice. Osteoclasts are the only cells in our body that can resorb bone, and are produced by monocytes/macrophages in the presence of RANKL and then activated by response from the immune system.

Usnic acid inhibits growth, induces cell cycle arrest, and induces apoptosis in human lung carcinoma (A549) cells (Singh et al. 2013).

It induces cell cycle arrest, apoptosis, and autophagy in gastric cancer cells, both in vitro and in vivo. In research by Geng et al. (2018), usnic acid treatment was more effective in treating cancer in mice than the chemotherapy drug 5-FU (fluorouracil) alone.

Work by Kilic et al. (2019) found usnic acid possesses antiproliferative activity against three lines of breast cancer cells.

Also, it was found to stimulate apoptosis and autophagy in HEPG2 and SNU-449 hepatocellular carcinoma cell lines, without damaging normal cells (Yurdacan et al. 2019).

Work by Kumer et al. (2020a) investigated anticancer activity of UA against the human gastric adenocarcinoma AGS and SNU-1 gastric carcinoma cell lines. It caused a significant increase in mitochondrial membrane depolarization and apoptosis induced by an increase in the ratio of Bax:Bcl-2 expression and cleaved PARP.

Usnic acid is an effective anti-biofilm agent against Group A *Streptococci* bacteria. It reduced the cellular components (protein and fatty acids) of the biofilm (Nithyanand et al. 2015). This is no real surprise, as a gargle of usnea tincture in water is extremely effective for strep throat.

(+)-Usnic acid inhibits glutathione reductase and glutathione *S*-transferase, suggestive of benefit against free radical damage (Ceylan et al. 2019).

Both enantiomers of usnic acid inhibit the influenza (swine) virus H1N1 (Sokolov et al. 2012).

Usnic acid seems to be more stable and effective against SARS-CoV-2 main protease, out of 26 lichen compounds tested. Variolaric and gyrophoric acids also have potential to inhibit the virus (Gupta et al. 2022).

UA blocks virus activity through a mechanical barrier effect as a nasal spray. Work by Galla et al. (2023) found usnic acid creates a branch capable of forming a protective barrier at 37°C. It blocks virus activity without altering physiological nasal homeostasis.

Usnic acid modulates mammalian cell circadian rhythms. Work on fibroblast cells by Srimani et al. (2022) noted the usnic acid cells showed shorter period lengths, through amplitude reduction and increased rhythm dampening. Human implications are unknown.

Usnic acid is somewhat toxic but coating it with seaweed (fucoidan) liposomes may be an effective way to treat tuberculosis (Salviano et al. 2021; Vasarri et al. 2023). In clinical practice I recommended usnea tincture to treat the disease in a 16-year-old female, after two years of no success with various antibiotics. It worked.

Usnic acid inhibits both acetylcholinesterase and butyrylcholinesterase associated with neurodegenerative disease. Inhibitors have been used in clinical trials for myasthenia gravis, glaucoma, postural tachycardia syndrome, and dementia (Cakmak and Gülcin 2019).

The wide use of over the counter and prescription anticholinergic medications may be contributing to the rapid rise of Alzheimer's disease and other neurological conditions. The brain neurons fire with the help of acetylcholine, and inhibition with an anticholinergic drugs reduces the ability to transmit. Antianxiety medications, tricyclic antidepressants, sleeping pills, cough syrups, treatments for motion sickness, nausea, and sinus congestion, antihistamines, and numerous other medications are included in this long list of drugs. Think R(espiratory), U(rological), N(ausea), and G(astrointestinal) and research the issue for you and your family.

On the other hand, the interaction of usnic acid enantiomers with acetylcholinesterase inhibition was researched by Cazarin et al. (2021). The effects were measured in the hippocampus and cortex of mice, and the usnic acid enantiomers evoked a receptor interaction with acetylcholinesterase-like galantamine. Usnic acid improved learning and memory, and reduced the IL-1ß levels in the hippocampus.

The drug bleomycin is used to treat malignant ascites tumors but can cause pulmonary fibrosis. A mouse study found that combining usnic acid with the drug was more effective in reducing tumor growth and toxicity (Su et al. 2017).

Earlier work by Sarak et al. (2009) found usnic acid and clarithromycin synergistic in the treatment of *Helicobacter pylori* bacteria, implicated in gastric and duodenal ulcers.

Usnic acid combines well with some well-known antibiotics for methicillin-resistant *Staphylococcus aureus* (MRSA), first reported in 1945. The first reports of vancomycin-resistant SA came in 2002.

Segatore et al. (2012) evaluated usnic acid in combination with five antibiotics. Synergism was found with clindamycin, gentamycin, and oxacillin. Work by Tozatti et al. (2015) found a combination of usnic acid with penicillin and tetracycline showed no synergistic antimicrobial benefit.

Bioadhesive polymeric films based on usnic acid show benefit in burn wound treatment. A preparation of usnic acid and PVP K90 (0.1%) provided the highest concentration, and was effective against *Staphylococcus epidermis*, *Enterococcus faecalis*, *Bacillus cereus*, and *Streptococcus pyogenes*. Normal cell viability is not compromised (Pagano et al. 2019).

Usnic acid has been extracted from *Usnea longissima* by supercritical carbon dioxide. Optimal conditions for deriving the highest amount of UA are 42°C, 4.3% ethanol for 7.48 hours (Dincer et al. 2021).

Several other studies are noted in the *Usnea* section on pages 239–54.

VULPINIC ACID

Found in Lichens

Bryoria	*Chaenotheca*	*Letharia*
Candelaria	*Chrysothrix*	*Vulpicida*

Thioredoxin reductase (TrxR) helps protect our cells against oxidative stress. However, its overexpression is often found in many aggressive tumors. Five lichen metabolites (diffractaic, evernic, lobaric, lecanoric and vulpinic acid) were tested for inhibition of TrxR. All exhibited stronger inhibitory effect on TrxR than did cisplatin and doxorubicin (chemotherapy drugs). Vulpinic acid was especially aggressive (Ozgencli et al. 2018).

In atherosclerosis, the endothelial damage is the basis for disease. Vulpinic acid decreased hydrogen peroxide-induced oxidative stress on human tissue, suggesting benefit in cardiovascular conditions (Sahin et al. 2019).

Vulpinic acid was examined for its effect on MCF-7 (breast) cancer and MCF-12A (breast epithelial) cells. A study by Cansaran-Duman et al. (2021a) involved the regulation of microRNA, and vulpinic acid was specifically inhibitory, suppressing breast cancer cell proliferation, and it may downregulate the expression of 12 microRNAs by repressing the FOXO-3 gene. In turn, it regulates apoptosis signaling pathways.

Vulpinic acid is cytotoxic to HepG2 (hepatic), NS20Y (neuroblastoma), and HUVEC (endothelial) cell lines (Koparal 2015).

Vulpinic acid induces apoptosis in MCF-7 and SK-BR-3 breast cancer cell lines (Kilic et al. 2018). The latter estrogen-positive cancer is resistant to treatment by chemotherapy drug doxorubicin. Vulpinic acid also suppresses the proliferation and migration of both MCF-7 and MDA-MB-453 breast cancer cells. The activity was stronger than with the chemotherapy drugs carboplatin and docetaxel (Kalin et al. 2022a). It induced the gene expression of thioredoxin reductase, while inhibiting its protein expression and enzymatic activity in both cell lines.

Vulpinic acid induces apoptosis in melanoma (A375) cells, without damaging normal human epidermal cells. This suggests a use in topical or transdermal treatment of maligned melanoma cancer (Yangin et al. 2022).

Both usnic acid and vulpinic acid show antimicrobial and antifungal activity against common agricultural pathogens. Strong antibacterial activity was shown in work by Paguirigan et al. (2022) against the plant pathogen *Clavibacter michiganensis* subsp. *Michiganensis.* The bacteria cause ring rot, or wilt and cankers, on tomato plants. One present practice is to spray the seed bed with streptomycin, another problematic agricultural practice associated with the spread of antibiotic resistance. Usnic acid and vulpinic acid also reduce the growth of fungal *Diaporthe eres* associated with disease in apples, peaches, and hazelnut crops, and *D. actinidiae*, a pathogen of kiwi. The two acids also show strong inhibition of *Sclerotinia sclerotiorum*, a white mold pathogen destructive to various legume and pulse crops, as well as to sunflowers.

XANTHONES

Found in Lichens	
Buellia	*Pseudoparmelia*
Lecanora	*Usnea*

Lichens account for only 5% of the xanthones found in nature. Plants account for about 80%, and nonlichenized fungi the remaining 15%.

Xanthones are mainly created by a polyketide intermediate, with a structure exhibiting a methyl group at position 8. A few xanthones are created via a pathway leading to a ravenlin skeletion (methyl group position 3) and the anthroquinone emodin (Pogam and Boustie 2016).

Examples include umbilicaxanthones A and B, derived from *Umibicaria proboscidea* (Rezanka et al. 2003), and *hirtusneanoside*, found in *Usnea hirta* (Rezanka et al. 2007).

Thus far, about 72 xanthones containing one to 4 chlorine atoms have been found in lichens.

A few examples include 7-chlorolichexanthone derived from *Lecanora schofieldii* syn. *Myriolecis schofieldii* and 2,4,7-trichloro-3-O-methylnorlichexanthone found in *Calopadia perpallida*.

ZEORIN

Found in Lichens

Cladonia	Lecanora	Parmotrema	Rinodina
Haematomma	Lecidella	Phyllospora	Usnea
Heterodermia	Megalaria	Physcia	

Zeorin is a triterpenoid found in a number of lichens. The compound inhibits alpha-glucosidase, 700-fold more potently than acarbose. The number of type 2 diabetics and related complications in society is skyrocketing. Work by Thadhani and Karunaratne (2017) reviewed 10 lichen compounds for their antidiabetic activity.

More than 27 triterpenoids, from various isolated sources, are reported to be PTP1B (protein tyrosine phosphatase IB) inhibitors. This is a major negative regulator of insulin signaling, and inhibition may be useful in treating type 2 diabetes. Of all tested, zeorin was the most inhibitory (Jiang et al. 2012).

Zeorin inhibits butyrylcholinesterase, associated with neurodegenerative conditions such as Alzheimer's disease (Mapari et al. 2021).

Resources

Consortium of Lichen Herbaria, Lichen Portal (website)

Entangled Life by Merlin Sheldrake (New York: Random House, 2020). Brillant book!

Field Guide to the Lichens of White Rocks (Boulder, Colorado) by Erin Tripp (Denver: University Press of Colorado, 2017). Excellent overview of regional lichens.

The Hidden Kingdom of Fungi by Keith Seifert (Vancouver BC: Greystone Books, 2022). Full of interesting personal stories.

Keys to Lichens of North America by Irwin M. Brodo (New Haven, CT: Yale University Press, 2016). Nice addition to keying out lichens.

Lichen Songs: New and Selected Poems by George Venu (American Fork, UT: Kelsay Books, 2017).

Lichens by Vincent Zonca (Hoboken, NJ: Polity Press, 2023). A beautifully crafted book, weaving lichens, people, art, and politics.

Lichens of North America by Irwin M. Brodo, S.D. Sharnoff, S. Sharnoff (New Haven, CT: Yale University Press, 2001). THE definitive book on the lichens subject, with incredible photos and descriptions.

Lichens of the North Woods by Joe Walewski (Duluth, MN: Kollath-Stensaas, 2007). Great regional information with good pictures.

The Lives of Lichens: A Natural History by Robert Lücking and Toby Spribille (Princeton University Press 2024).

Macrolichens of the Pacific Northwest by Bruce McCune and Linda Geiser (Corvallis: Oregon State University Press, 1997). A classic for everyone's library shelf.

Mushroom and Lichen Dyers United on Facebook, hosted by Alissa Allen

North Dakota State University: North American Lichen Checklist by Theodore L. Esslinger

Rocky Mountain Lichen Primer by James N. Corbridge Jr. and William A. Weber (Denver: University Press of Colorado, 1998). Useful for identification.

The Secret Book of Lichens by Kristupas Sabolius and Aiste Ambrazeviciute (Lithuania: Kivarpa).

The Secret World of Lichens by Troy McMullin, (Richmond Hill, ON: Firefly Books, 2022). Great introduction to 40 lichen species from the chief mycologist of the Canadian Museum of Nature.

Trouble with Lichen [fiction] by John Wyndham (New York: Ballantine Books/Penguin Random House, 1960). A take on women and aging by a great science fiction writer.

Urban Lichens by Jessica L. Allen and James C. Lendemer (New Haven, CT: Yale University Press, 2021). For lichen enthusiasts of 60 species found in larger cities.

Ways of Enlichenment (website)

Bibliography

Abdallah, E. M. 2019. "Evaluation of Antimicrobial Activity of a Lichen Used as a Spice (*Platismatia glauca*)." *Advancements in Life Sciences* 6 (3): 110–15.

Abdolmaleki, H., and M. Sohrabi. 2016. "Biosynthesis of Silver Nanoparticles by Two Lichens *Usnea articulata* and *Ramalina sinensis* and Investigation of Their Antibacterial Activity against Some Pathogenic Bacteria." *Ebnesina Journal* 17 (4): 33–42.

Abdullah, S. M., K. Kolo, and S. M. Sajadi. 2020. "Greener Pathway toward the Synthesis of Lichen-Based $ZnO@TiO_2@SiO_2$ and $Fe_3O_4@SiO_2$ Nanocomposites and Investigation of Their Biological Activities." *Food Science and Nutrition* 8 (8): 4044–54.

Abdullah, S. T., H. Hamid, M. Ali, S. H. Ansari, and M. S. Alam. 2007. "Two New Terpenes from the Lichen *Parmelia perlata*." *Indian Journal of Chemistry, Section B, Organic and Medicinal Chemistry* 46 (1): 173–76.

Acikgöz, B., I. Karalti, M. Ersöz, Z. M. Coskun, et al. 2013. "Screening of Antimicrobial and Cytotoxic Effects of Two *Cladonia* Species." *Zeitschrift für Naturforschung Section C Journal of Bioscience* 68: 191–97.

Adams III, W. W., B. Demming-Adams, and O. L. Lange. 1993. "Carotenoid Composition and Metabolism in Green and Blue-Green Algal Lichens in the Field." *Oecologia* 94 (4): 576–84.

Ahmed, K. S. Z., S. S. Z. Ahmed, A. Thangakumar, and R. Krishnaveni. 2019. "Therapeutic Effect of *Parmotrema tinctorum* against Complete Freund's Adjuvant-Induced Arthritis in Rats and Identification of Novel Isophthalic Ester Derivative." *Biomedicine and Pharmacotherapy* 112: 108646.

Ahsan, H., S. U. Islam, M. B. B. Ahmed, and Y. S. Lee. 2022. "Role of Nrf2, STAT3, and Src as Molecular Targets for Cancer Chemoprevention." *Pharmaceutics* 14 (9): 1775.

Akpinar, A., A. Cansev, and M. Isleyen. 2021. "Effects of the Lichen *Peltigera canina* on *Cucurbita pepo* spp. *pepo* Grown in Soil Contaminated by DDTs." *Environmental Science and Pollution Research International* 28 (12): 14576–85.

Alexandrino, C. A. F., N. K. Honda, M. D. Matos, et al. 2019. "Antitumor Effect of Depsidones from Lichens on Tumor Cell Lines and Experimental Murine Melanoma." *Revista Brasileira de Farmacognosia* 29: 449–56.

Allen, J. L., R. T. McMullin, Y. F. Wiersma, and C. Scheidegger. 2021. "Population Genetics and Biogeography of the Lungwort Lichen in North America Support Distinct Eastern and Western Gene Pools." *American Journal of Botany* 108 (12): 2416–24.

Almer, J., P. Resi, H. Gudmundsson, D. Warshan, O. S. Andrésson, and S. Werth. 2023.

"Symbiont-Specific Responses to Environmental Cues in a Threesome Lichen Symbiosis." *Molecular Ecology* 32 (5): 1045–61.

Alqahtani, M. A., M. R. A. Othman, and A. E. Mohammed. 2020. "Bio Fabrication of Silver Nanoparticles with Antibacterial and Cytotoxic Abilities Using Lichens." *Scientific Reports* 10 (1): 16781.

Altindag, F., S. Bogoksayan, and S. Bayram. 2022. "Eumelanin Protects the Liver against Diethylnitrosamine-Induced Liver Injury." *Toxicology* 480: 153311.

Amssayef, A., M. Ajebli, and M. Eddouks. 2021. "Aqueous Extract of Oakmoss Produces Antihypertensive Activity in L-NAME-Induced Hypertensive Rats through sGC-cGMP Pathway." *Clinical and Experimental Hypertension* 43 (1): 49–55.

Amssayef, A., I. Bouadid, and M. Eddouks. 2022. "Oakmoss Exhibits Antihyperglycemic Activity in Streptozotocin-Induced Diabetic Rats." *Cardiovascular and Hematology Disorders - Drug Targets*, March 16, 2022.

Andania, M. M., F. Ismed, M. Taher, S. J. A Ichwan, A. Bakhtiar, and D. Arbain. 2019. "Cytotoxic Activities of Extracts and Isolated Compounds of Some Potential Sumatran Medicinal Plants against MCF-7 and HSC-3 Cell Lines." *Journal of Mathematical and Fundamental Sciences* 51 (3): 225–42.

Andrade, J. C., M. F. B. Morais Braga, G. M. M. Guedes, S. R. Tintino, et al. 2018. "Cholecalciferol, Ergosterol, and Cholesterol Enhance the Antibiotic Activity of Drugs." *International Journal of Vitamin and Nutrition Research* 88 (5–6): 244–50.

Andre, A., and A. Fehr. 2001. *Gwich'in Ethnobotany: Plants Used by the Gwich'in for Food, Medicine, Shelter and Tools.* Inuvik, NWT: Gwich'in Social and Cultural Institute and Aurora Research Institute.

Araújo, R. V. S., M. R. Melo-Júnior, E. I. C. Beltrão, L. A. Mello, M. Iacomini, A. M. A. Carneiro-Leão, et al. 2011. "Evaluation of the Antischistosomal Activity of Sulfated a-D-glucan from the Lichen *Ramalina celastri* Free and Encapsulated into Liposomes." *Brazilian Journal of Medical and Biological Research* 44 (4): 311–18.

Ari, F., S. Celikler, S. Oran, N. Balikci, S. Ozturk, M. Z. Ozei, D. Ozyurt, and E. Ulukaya. 2014. "Genotoxic, Cytotoxic, and Apoptotic Effects of *Hypogymnia physodes* (L.) Nyl. on Breast Cancer Cells." *Environmental Toxicology* 29 (7): 804–13.

Ari, F., N. Aztopal, S. Oran, S. Bozdemir, S. Celikler, S. Ozturk, and E. Ulukaya. 2014a. "*Parmelia sulcata* Taylor and *Usnea filipendula* Stirt Induce Apoptosis-Like Cell Death and DNA Damage in Cancer Cells." *Cell Proliferation* 47 (5): 457–64.

Ari, F., E. Ulukaya, S. Oran, S. Celikler, S. Ozturk, and M. Z. Ozel. 2015. "Promising Anticancer Activity of a Lichen, *Parmelia sulcata* Taylor, against Breast Cancer Cell Lines and Genotoxic Effect on Human Lymphocytes." *Cytotechnology* 67 (3): 531–43.

Aslan, A., M. Güllüce, M. Sökmen, A. Adigüzel, F. Sahin, and H. Özkan. 2006. "Antioxidant and Antimicrobial Properties of the Lichens *Cladonia foliacea, Dermatocarpon miniatum, Everinia divaricate, Evernia prunastri,* and *Neofuscella pulla.*" *Pharmaceutical Biology* 44 (4): 247–52.

Aslan, A., G. Agar, L. Alpsoy, E. Kotan, and S. Ceker. 2012. "Protective Role of Methanol

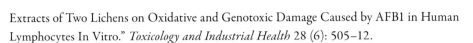

Extracts of Two Lichens on Oxidative and Genotoxic Damage Caused by AFB1 in Human Lymphocytes In Vitro." *Toxicology and Industrial Health* 28 (6): 505–12.

Asplund, J., K. A. Solhaug, and Y. Gausiaa. 2010. "Optimal Defense: Snails Avoid Reproductive Parts of the Lichen *Lobaria scrobiculata* Due to Internal Defense Allocation." *Ecology* 91 (10): 3100–3105.

Atlay, F., F. Odabasoglu, M. Halici, A. Cakir, E. Cadirci, A. Aslan, O. A. Berktas, and C. Kazaz. 2015. "Gastroprotective and Antioxidant Effects of *Lobaria pulmonaria* and Its Metabolite Rhizonyl Alcohol on Indomethacin-Induced Gastric Ulcer." *Chemistry and Biodiversity* 12 (11): 1756–67.

Augusto, S., J. Sierra. M. Nadal, and M. Schuhmacher. 2015. "Tracking Polycyclic Aromatic Hydrocarbons in Lichens: It's All about the Algae." *Environmental Pollution* 207: 441–45.

Avonto, C., A. G. Chittiboyina, S. I. Khan, O. R. Dale, J. F. Parcher, M. Wang, and I. A. Khan. 2021. "Are Atranols the Only Skin Sensitizers in Oakmoss? A Systematic Investigation Using Non-animal Methods." *Toxicology In Vitro* 70: 105053.

Ayoub, A. M., M. U. Amin, G. Ambreen, A. A. Dayyih, et al. 2022. "Photodynamic and Antiangiogenic Activities of Parietin Liposomes in Triple Negative Breast Cancer." *Biomaterial Advances* 134: 112543.

Ayoub, A. M., B. Gutberiet, E. Preis, A. M. Abdelsalam, et al. 2022a. "Parietin Cyclodextrin-Inclusion Complex as an Effective Formulation for Bacterial Photoinactivation." *Pharmaceutics* 14 (2): 357.

Azizuddin, S. Imran, and M. I. Choudhary. 2017. "In Vivo Anti-inflammatory and Anti-platelet Aggregation Activities of Longissiminone A, Isolated from *Usnea longissima*." *Pakistan Journal of Pharmaceutical Sciences* 30 (4): 1213–17.

Backorová, M., M. Backor, J. Mikes, R. Jendzelovsky, and P. Fedorocko. 2011. "Variable Responses of Different Human Cancer Cells to the Lichen Compounds Parietin, Atranorin, Usnic and Gyrophoric Acid." *Toxicology in Vitro* 25 (1): 37–44.

Backorová, M., R. Jendzelovsky, M. Kello, M. Backor, et al. 2012. "Lichen Secondary Metabolites Are Responsible for Induction of Apoptosis in HT-29 and A2780 Human Cancer Cell lines." *Toxicology in Vitro* 26: 462–68.

Bajpai, R., R. Srivastava, and D. K. Upreti. 2023. "Unraveling the Ameliorative Potentials of Native Lichen *Pyxine cocoes* (Sw.) Nyl., During COVID 19 Phase." *International Journal of Biometeorology* 67 (1): 67–77.

Balaji, P., and G. N. Hariharan. 2007. "In Vitro Antimicrobial Activity of *Parmotrema praesorediosum* Thallus Extracts." *Research Journal of Botany* 2 (1): 54–59.

Bank, T. H., II. 1953. "Botanical and Ethnobotanical Studies in the Aleutian Islands: II. Health and Medical Lore of the Aleuts." *Papers of the Michigan Academy of Science, Arts and Letters* 38: 415–31.

Barry, V. C., and D. Twomey. 1950. "Anti-Tubercular Substances VI. Derivatives of Diploicin." *Proceedings of the Royal Irish Academy Section B: Biological, Geological, and Chemical Science* 53: 55–59.

Barti, S., S. Nayaka, and R. Kumar. 2022. "Evaluation of Some Traditional Therapeutic

Properties of *Usnea longissima* (Ascomycota, Lichenized Fungi): Antimicrobial, Antiquorum and Antioxidant." *Journal of Microbiology, Biotechnology and Food Sciences* 11 (4): e3163.

Basile, A., D. Rigano, S. Loppi, A. Di Santi, A. Nebbioso, S. Sorbo, B. Conte, et al. 2015. "Antiproliferative, Antibacterial and Antifungal Activity of the Lichen *Xanthoria parietina* and Its Secondary Metabolite Parietin." *International Journal of Molecular Sciences* 16 (4): 7861–75.

Basnet, B. B., L. Liu, W. Zhao, R. X. Liu, K. Ma, L. Bao, et al. 2019. "New 1, 2- Naphthoquinone-Derived Pigments from the Mycobiont of Lichen *Trypethelium eluteriae* Sprengel." *Natural Product Research* 33 (14): 2044–50.

Bastien, J. W. 1983. "Pharmacopoeia of the Qollahuaya Andeans." *Journal of Ethnopharmacology* 8: 97–111.

Bauer, J., B. Waitenberger, S. M. Noha, D. Schuster, J. M. Rollinger, J. Boustie, et al. 2012. "Discovery of Depsides and Depsidone from Lichen as Potent Inhibitors of Microsomal Prostaglandin E2 Synthase-1 Using Pharmacophore Models." *ChemMedChem* 7 (12): 2077–81.

Baur, A., B. Baur, and L. Fröberg. 1994. "Herbivory on Calcicolous Lichens: Different Food Preferences and Growth Rates in Two Co-existing Land Snails." *Oecologia* 98 (3–4): 313–19.

Bautista-González, J. A., A. Montoya, R. Bye, M. Esqueda, and M. Herrera-Campos. 2022. "Traditional Knowledge of Medicinal Mushrooms and Lichens of Yuman Peoples in Northern Mexico." *Journal of Ethnobiology and Ethnomedicine* 8 (1): 52.

Bayir, Y., F. Odabasoglu, A. Cakir, et al. 2006. "The Inhibition of Gastric Mucosal Lesion, Oxidative Stress and Neutrophil-Infiltration in Rats by the Lichen Constituent Diffractaic Acid." *Phytomedicine* 13: 584–90.

Behera, B. C., B. Adawadkar, and U. Makhija. 2004. "Capacity of Some Graphidaceous Lichens to Scavenge Superoxide and Inhibition of Tyrosinase and Xanthine Oxidase Activities." *Current Science* 87 (1): 83–87.

Behera, B. C., N. Mahadik, and M. Morey. 2012. "Antioxidative and Cardiovascular Protective Activities of Metabolic Usnic Acid and Psoromic Acid Produced by Lichen Species *Usnea complanata* under Submerged Fermentation." *Pharmaceutical Biology* 50 (8): 968–79.

Bellio, P., B. Segatore, A. Mancini, L. Di Pietro, et al. 2015. "Interaction between Lichen Secondary Metabolites and Antibiotics against Clinical Isolates Methicillin-Resistant *Staphylococcus aureus* Strains." *Phytomedicine* 22 (2): 223–30.

Benedik, E. 2022. "Sources of Vitamin D for Humans." *International Journal of Vitamin and Nutrition Research* 92 (2): 118–25.

Bennet, D., and T. Tiner. 1993. *Up North: A Guide to Ontario's Wilderness from Blackflies to the Northern Lights.* Markham, ON: Reed Books.

Berté, T. E., A. P. Dalmagro, P. L. Zimath, A. E. Goncalves, C. Meyre-Silva, et al. 2018. "Taraxerol as a Possible Therapeutic Agent on Memory Impairments and Alzheimer's Disease: Effects against Scopolamine and Streptozotocin-Induced Cognitive Dysfunctions." *Steroids* 132: 5–11.

Beshbishy, A. M., G. Batiha, L. Alkazmi, E. Nadwa, E. Rashwan, et al. 2020. "Therapeutic Effects of Atranorin towards the Proliferation of *Babesia* and *Theilera* Parasites." *Pathogens* 9 (2): 127.

Bessadóttir, M., E. Á. Skúladóttir, S. Gowan, S. Eccles, et al. 2014. "Effects of Anti-proliferative Lichen Metabolite, Protolichesterinic Acid on Fatty Acid Synthase, Cell Signaling and Drug Response in Breast Cancer Cells." *Phytomedicine* 21: 1717–24.

Bessadóttir, M., F. F. Eiriksson, S. Becker, M. H. Ögmundsdóttir, et al. 2015. "Anti-proliferative and Pro-apoptotic Effects of Lichen-Derived Compound Protolichesterinic Acid Are Not Mediated by its Lipoxygenase-Inhibitory Activity." *Prostaglandins Leukotrienes and Essential Fatty Acids* 98: 39–47.

Betina, V., and S. Kuzela. 1987. "Uncoupling Effect of Fungal Hydroxyanthraquinones on Mitochrondrial Oxidative Phosphorylation." *Chemico-Biological Interactions* 62 (2): 179–89.

Bézivin, C., S. Tomasi, F. Lohézic-Le-Dévéhat, and J. Boustie. 2003. "Cytotoxic Activity of Some Lichen Extracts on Murine and Human Cancer Cell Lines." *Phytomedicine* 10: 499–503.

Bhat, N. B., S. Das, B. V. S. Sridevi, et al. 2023. "Molecular Docking and Dynamics Supported Investigation of Antiviral Activity of Lichen Metabolites of *Roccella montagnei*: An *In Silico* and *In Vitro* Study." *Journal of Biomolecular and Structural Dynamics* 41 (21): 11484–97.

Black, P. L., J. T. Arneson, and A. Cuerrier. 2008. "Medicinal Plants Used by the Inuit of Qikiqtaaluk (Baffin Island, Nunavut)." *Botany* 86: 15763.

Boas, F. 1921. "Ethnology of the Kwakiutl." *Thirty-Fifth Annual Report of the Bureau of American Ethnology*, 1913–1914: 743–94.

Bogo, D., M. F. C. de Matos, N. K. Honda, E. C. Pontes, et al. 2010. "In Vitro Antitumour Activity of Orsellinates." *Zeitschrift fur Naturforschung C Journal of Bioscience* 65 (1–2): 43–48.

Bone, E. 2011. *Mycophilia*: *Revelations from the Weird World of Mushrooms*. New York: Rodale.

Bouchard, R., and D. Kennedy. 1979. *Shuswap Stories: Collected 1971–5*. Vancouver: CommCept Publishing.

Brandäo, L. F. G., G. B. Alcantara, M. Matos, D. Bogo, et al. 2013. "Cytotoxic Evaluation of Phenolic Compounds from Lichens against Melanoma Cells." *Chemical and Pharmaceutical Bulletin* (Tokyo) 61 (2): 176–83.

Bray, P., J. Ferlay, I. Soerjomataram, et al. "Global Cancer Statistics 2018. GLOBOCAN Estimates of Incidence and Mortality Worldwide for 36 Cancers in 185 Countries." *CA: A Cancer Journal for Clinicians* 68 (6): 394–424.

Brisdelli, F., M. Perilli, D. Sellitri, et al. 2013. "Cytotoxic Activity and Antioxidant Capacity of Purified Lichen Metabolites: An In Vitro Study." *Phytotherapy Research* 27: 431–37.

Brisdelli, F., M. Perilli, D. Sellitri, P. Bellio, A. Bozzi, G. Amicosante, M. Nicoletti, M. Piovano, and G. Celenza. 2016. "Protolichesterinic Acid Enhances Doxorubicin-Induced Apoptosis in HeLa Cells In Vitro." *Life Sciences* 158: 89–97.

Brodo, I. M., S. D. Sharnoff, and S. Sharnoff. 2001. *Lichens of North America*. New Haven, CT: Yale University Press.

Bugni, T. S., C. D. Andjelic, A. R. Pole, P. Rai, C. M. Ireland, and L. R. Barrows. 2009. "Biologically Active Components of a Papua New Guinea Analgesic and Anti-inflammatory Lichen Preparation." *Fitoterapia* 80 (5): 270–73.

Bui, V. M., T. H. Duong, T. A. M. Nguyen, T. N. V. Nguyen, N. H. Nguyen, et al. 2022. "Two New Phenolic Compounds from the Vietnamese Lichen *Parmotrema tinctorum*." *Natural Product Research* 36 (13): 3429–34.

Bui, V. M., T. H. Duong, W. Chavasiri, K. P. P. Nguyen, and B. L. C. Huynh. 2022. "A New Depsidone from the Lichen *Usnea ceratina* Arch." *Natural Products Research* 36 (9): 2263–69.

Bui, V. M., B. L. C. Huynh, N. K. T. Pham, et al. 2022a. "Usneaceratins A and B, Two New Secondary Metabolites from the Lichen *Usnea ceratina*." *Natural Product Research* 36 (15): 3945–50.

Burkholder, P. R., and A. W. Evans. 1945. "Further Studies of the Antibiotic Activity of Lichens." *Bulletin of the Torrey Botanical Club* 72 (2): 157–64.

Burlando, B., E. Ranzato, A. Volante, et al. 2009. "Antiproliferative Effects on Tumor Cells and Promotion of Keratinocyte Wound Healing by Different Lichen Compounds." *Planta Medica* 75: 607–13.

Burlingame, B. 2000. "Wild Nutrition." *Journal of Food Composition and Analysis* 2: 99–100.

Burt, S. R., J. K. Harper, and L. G. Cool. 2022. "A New Depsidone from the Neotricone-Rich Chemotype of the Lichenized Fungus *Usnea fulvoreagens*." *Natural Product Research* 14: 1–7.

Bustinza, F. 1952. "Antibacterial Substances from Lichens." *Economic Botany* 64 (4): 402–6.

Cakmak, K. C., and I. Gülgin. 2019 "Anticholinergic and Antioxidant Activities of Usnic Acid-an Activity-Structure Insight." *Toxicology Reports* 6: 1273–80.

Calcott, M. J., D. F. Ackerley, A. Knight, R. A. Keyzers, and J. G. Owen. 2018. "Secondary Metabolism in the Lichen Symbiosis." *Chemical Society Review* 47 (5): 1730–60.

Camerio-Leão, A. M. A., D. F. Buchi, M. Iacomini, P. A. J. Gorin, and M. B. M. Oliveria. 1997. "Cytotoxic Effect against HeLa Cells of Polysaccharides from the Lichen *Ramalina celastri*." *Journal of Submicroscopic Cytology and Pathology* 29 (4): 503–9.

Campanella, L., M. Delfini, P. Ercole, A. Iacoangeli, and G. Risuleo. 2002. "Molecular Characterization and Action of Usnic Acid: A Drug That Inhibits Proliferation of Mouse Polyomavirus In Vitro and Whose Main Target Is RNA Transcription." *Biochemie* 84: 329–34.

Candan, M., M. Yilmaz, T. Tay, M. Kivanc, and H. Türk. 2006. "Antimicrobial Activity of Extracts of the Lichen *Xanthoparmelia pokornyi* and Its Gyrophoric and Stenosporic Acid Constituents." *Zeitschrift für Naturforschung Section C Journal of Biosciences* 61 (5–6): 319–23.

Candan, M., M. Yilmaz, T. Tay, M. Erdem, and A. O. Turk. 2007. "Antimicrobial Activity of Extracts of the Lichen *Parmelia sulcata* and Its Salazinic Acid Constituent." *Zeitschrift für Naturforschung C: A Journal of Biosciences* 62 (7): 619–21.

Cansaran, D., D. Cetin, M. G. Halici, and O. Atakol. 2006. "Determination of Usnic Acid in Some *Rhizoplaca* Species from Middle Anatolia and Their Antimicrobial Activities." *Zeitschrift fur Naturforschung Section C Journal of Bioscience* 61 (1–2): 47–51.

Cansaran, D., D. Kahya, E. Yurdakuloi, and O. Atakol. 2006a. "Identification and Quantitation of Usnic Acid from the Lichen *Usnea* Species of Anatolia and Antimicrobial Activity." *Zeitschrift für Naturforschung C Journal of Bioscience* 61 (11–12): 773–76.

Cansaran, D., O. Atakol, M. G. Halici, and A. Aksoy. 2007. "HPLC Analysis of Usnic Acid in Some *Ramalina* Species from Anatolia and Investigation of Their Antimicrobial Activities." *Pharmaceutical Biology* 45 (1): 77–81.

Cansaran-Duman, D., G. G. Eskiler, B. Colak, and E. S. Kucukkara. 2021. "Vulpinic Acid as a Natural Compound Inhibits the Proliferation of Metastatic Prostate Cancer Cells by Inducing Apoptosis." *Molecular Biology Reports* 48 (8): 6025–34.

Cansaran-Duman, D., S. Yangin, and B. Colak. 2021a. "The Role of Vulpinic Acid as a Natural Compound in the Regulation of Breast Cancer-Associated miRNAs." *Biological Research* 54 (1): 37.

Carbonero, E. R., A. V. Montai, S. M. Woranovicz-Barreira, et al. 2002. "Polysaccharides of Lichenized Fungi of Three *Cladina* spp.: Significance as Chemotypes." *Phytochemistry* 61 (6): 681–86.

Cardile, V., A. C. E. Graziano, R. Avola, M. Piovano, and A. Russo. 2017. "Potential Anticancer Activity of Lichen Secondary Metabolite Physodic Acid." *Chemico-Biologica Interactions* 263: 36–45.

Cardile, V., A. C. E. Graziano, R. Avola, A. Madrid, and A. Russo. 2022. "Physodic Acid Sensitizes LNCaP Prostate Cancer Cells to TRAIL-Induced Apoptosis." *Toxicology in Vitro* 84: 105432.

Carpentier, C., E. F. Queiroz, L. Marcourt, J. L. Wolfender, J. Azelmat, D. Grenier, S. Boudreau, N. Voyer, et al. 2017. "Dibenzofurans and Pseudodepsidones from the Lichen *Stereocaulon paschale* Collected in Northern Quebec." *Journal of Natural Products* 80 (1): 210–14.

Carpentier, C., X. Barbeau, J. Azelmat, K. Vaillancourt, D. Grenier, P. Lague, and N. Voyer. 2018. "Lobaric Acid and Pseudodepsidones Inhibit NF-kB Signaling Pathway by Activation of PPAR-y." *Bioorganic and Medicinal Chemistry* 26 (22): 5845–51.

Casano, L. M., E. M del Campo, F. J. Garcia-Breijo, J. Reig-Armiñana, et al. 2011. "Two *Trebouxia* Algae with Different Physiological Performances Are Ever-Present in Lichen Thalli of *Ramalina farinacea*. Coexistence versus Competition?" *Environmental Microbiology* 13 (3): 806–18.

Casselman, K. D. 2011. *Lichen dyes: The New Source Book*. 2nd rev. ed. Dover Publications.

Cazarin, C. A., A. P. Dalmagro, A. E. Gonçalves, et al. 2021. "Usnic Acid Enantiomers Restore Cognitive Deficits and Neurochemical Alterations Induced by aß(1-42) in Mice." *Behavioral Brain Research* 397: 112945.

Ceker, S., F. Orhan, S. Sezen, M. Gulluce, H. Ozkan, A. Aslan, and G. Agar. 2018. "Anti-mutagenic and Anti-oxidant Potencies of *Cetraria Aculeata* (Schreb.) Fr., *Cladonia Chlorophaea* (Flörke ex Sommerf.) Spreng. and *Cetrelia olivetorum* (Nyl.) W. L. Culb. and C. F. Culb)." *Iranian Journal of Pharmaceutical Research* 17 (1): 326–35.

Celenza, G., B. Segatore, D. Setacci, P. Bellio, et al. 2012. "In Vitro Antimicrobial Activity of Pannarin Alone and in Combination with Antibiotics against Methicillin-Resistant *Staphylococcus aureus* Clinical Isolates." *Phytomedicine* 19 (7): 596–602.

Cetin, H., O. Tufan-Cetin, A. O. Turk, T. Tay, M. Candan, A. Yanikoglu, and H. Sumbul. 2008. "Insecticidal Activity of Major Lichen Compounds, (-)-Usnic and (+)-Usnic Acid, against the Larvae of House Mosquito, *Culex pipiens* L." *Parasitology Research* 102 (6): 1277–79.

Ceylan, H., Y. Demir, and S. Beydemir. 2019. "Inhibitory Effects of Usnic and Carnosic Acid on Some Metabolic Enzymes: An In Vitro Study." *Protein and Peptide Letters* 26 (5): 364–70.

Chakor, N., G. Patil, D. Writer, G. Periyasamy, et al. 2012. "First Total Synthesis of Prasinic Acid and Its Anticancer Activity." *Bioorganic and Medicinal Chemistry Letters* 22 (21): 6608–10.

Chang, W. Q., Y. Li, L. Zhang, A. X. Cheng, and H. X. Lou. 2012. "Retigeric Acid B Attenuates the Virulence of *Candida albicans* via Inhibiting Adenylyl Cyclase Activity Targeted by Enhanced Farnesol Production." *PLoS ONE* 7 (7): e41624.

Chang, W. Q., M. Zhang, X. Y. Jin, H. J. Zhang, et al. 2022. "Inhibition of Fungal Pathogenicity by Targeting the H_2S-Synthesizing Enzyme Cystathionine B-synthase." *Science Advances* 8 (50): eadd5366.

Chavarria-Pizarro, T., P. Resl, T. Kuhl-Nagel, et al. 2022. "Antibiotic-Induced Treatments Reveal Stress-Responsive Gene Expression in the Endangered Lichen *Lobariapulmonaria*." *Journal of Fungi* (Basel) 8 (6): 625.

Chen, Y. Y., and J. Li. 2021. "Glutinol Inhibits the Proliferation of Human Ovarian Cancer Cells via P13K/AKT Signaling Pathway." *Tropical Journal of Pharmaceutical Research* 20 (7).

Cheng, B., S. G. Cao, V. Vasquez, T. Annamalai, G. Tamayo-Castillo, J. Clardy, and Y. C. Tse-Dinh. 2013. "Identification of Anziaic Acid, a Lichen Depside from *Hypotrachyna* sp., as a New Topoisomerase Poison Inhibitor." *PLoS ONE* 8 (4): e60770.

Chestnut, V. K. 1902. *Plants Used by the Indians of Mendocino County, California. Systematic and Geographic Botany, and Aboriginal Uses of Plants.* Washington, DC: Government Printing Office, 295–408.

Cho, E., K. J. Youn, H. Y. Kwon, J. Jeon, W. S. Cho, et al. 2022. "Eugenitol Ameliorates Memory Impairments in 5XFAD Mice by Reducing Aß Plaques and Neuroinflammation." *Biomedicine and Pharmacotherapy* 148: 112763.

Choi, R. Y., J. R. Ham, J. Yeo, et al. 2017. "Anti-obesity Property of Lichen *Thamnolia vermicularis* Extract in 3T3-L1 Cells and Diet-Induced Obese Mice." *Preventive Nutrition and Food Science* 22 (4): 285–92.

Chon, S. H., E. J. Yang, T. H. Lee, and K. S. Song. 2016. "ß-Secretase (BACE1) Inhibitory and Neuroprotective Effects of p-terphenyls from Polyzellus Multiplex." *Food and Function* 7 (9): 3834–42.

Choudhary, M., Azizuddin, S. Jalil, and A-ur-Rahman. 2005. "Bioactive Phenolic Compounds from a Medicinal Lichen, *Usnea longissima*." *Phytochemistry* 66 (19): 2346–50.

Chrysayi-Tokousbalies, M., and M. A. Kastanias. 2003. "Cynodontin: A Fungal Metabolite with Antifungal Properties." *Journal of Agricultural and Food Chemistry* 51 (17): 4920–23.

Clement, D. 1990. *L'ethnobotanique montagnaise de Mingan.* Collection Nordicana 53, Quebec: Université Laval.

Cobanoglu, G., C. Sesal, B. Gökmen, and S. Cakar. 2010. "Evaluation of the Antimicrobial Properties of Some Lichens." *South-Western Journal of Horticulture Biology and Environment* 1 (2): 153–58.

Cogno, I. S., P. Gilardi, L. Comini, S. C. Núñez-Montoya, J. L. Cabrera, and V. A. Rivarola. 2020. "Natural Photosensitizers in Photodynamic Therapy: In Vitro Activity against Monolayers and Spheroids of Human Colorectal Adenocarcinoma SW480 Cells." *Photodiagnosis and Photodynamic Therapy* 31: 101852.

Cohen, P., and G. H. N. Towers. 2004. "Anthraquinones and Phenanthroperylenequinones from *Nephroma laevigatum*." *Journal of Natural Products* 58 (4).

Colak, S., F. Geyikoglu, T. O. Bakir, H. Türkez, and A. Aslan. 2016. "Evaluating the Toxic and Beneficial Effects of Lichen Extracts in Normal and Diabetic Rats." *Toxicology and Industrial Health* 32 (8): 1495–504.

Cometto, A., S. D. Leavitt, A. N. Millanes, M. Wedin, M. Grube, and L. Muggia. 2022. "The Yeast Lichenosphere: High Diversity of Basidiomycetes from the Lichens *Tephromela atra* and *Rhizoplaca melanophthalma*." *Fungal Biology* 126 (9): 587–608.

Compton, B. D. 1993. "Upper North Wakashan and Southern Tsimshian Ethnobotany: The Knowledge and Usage of Plants and Fungi among the Oweekeno, Hanaksiala (Kitlope and Kemano), Haisla (Kitamaat) and Kitasoo Peoples of the Central and North Coasts of British Columbia." Ph.D. thesis, University of British Columbia.

Cook, W. E., M. F. Raisbeck, T. E. Cornish, E. S. Williams, B. Brown, G. Hiatt, and T. J. Kreeger. 2007. "Paresis and Death in Elk (*Cervus elaphus*) Due to Lichen Intoxication in Wyoming." *Journal of Wildlife Diseases* 43 (3): 498–503.

Cooke, M. C. 1893. *Romance of Life amongst Plants: Facts and Phenomena of Cryptogamic Vegetation*. London: Society for Promoting Christian Knowledge.

Cordova, M. M., D. F. Martins, M. D. Silva, C. H. Baggio, E. R. Carbonero, A. C. Ruthes, M. Iacomini, and A. R. S. Santos. 2013. "Polysaccharide Glucomannan Isolated from *Heterodermia obscurata* Attenuates Acute and Chronic Pain in Mice." *Carbohydrate Polymers* 92 (2): 2058–64.

Cornejo, A., F. Salgado, J. Caballero, R. Vargas, M. Simirgiotis, and C. Areche. 2016. "Secondary Metabolites in *Ramalina terebrata* Detected by UHPLC/ESI/MS/MS and Identification of Parietin as Tau Protein Inhibitor." *International Journal of Molecular Science* 17 (8): 1303.

Coskun, Z. M., M. Ersoz, B. Acikgoz, I. Karalti, et al. 2015. "Anti-proliferative and Apoptotic Effects of Methanolic Extracts from Different *Cladonia* Species on Human Breast Cancer Cells." *Folia Biologica* (*Praha*) 61: 97–103.

Crawford, S. 2001. "Ethnolichenology of *Bryoria fremontii*: Wisdom of Elders, Population Ecology, and Nutritional Chemistry." UK: University of Lethbridge.

Crockett, M., S. Kageyama, D. Homen, C. Lewis, J. Osborn, and L. Sander. 2003. "Antibacterial Properties of Four Pacific Northwest Lichens." *Botany 465 Lichenology* at Oregon State University.

Cui, C. B., H. Kakeya, and H. Osada. 1996. "Spirotryprostatin B, a Novel Mammalian Cell Cycle Inhibitor, Produced by *Aspergillus fumigatus*." *Journal of Antibiotics* 49 (8): 832–35.

Curtin, L. S. M. 1949. *By the Prophet of the Earth: Ethnobotany of the Pima*. Tucson: University of Arizona Press.

Da Silva, M de L., P. A. Gorin, and M. Iacomini. 1993. "Unusual Carbohydrates from the Lichen, *Parmotrema cetratum*." *Phytochemistry* 34 (3): 715–17.

Daminova, A. G., A. M. Rogov, A. E. Rassabina, R. P. Beckett, and F. V. Minibayeva. 2022. "Effect of Melanization on Thallus Microstructure in the Lichen *Lobaria pulmonaria*." *Journal of Fungi* (Basel) 8 (8): 791.

Darwin, E. 1791. *The Loves of Plants*. Canto 1: 349–50.

Das, S. K., D. Chatterjee, and M. Uddin. 2002. "Induction of Pro-renin Converting Enzyme mk9 by Thyroid Hormone in the Guinea-Pig Liver." *Biochemistry and Biophysical Research Communications* 293 (1): 412–15.

Davies, J., H. Wang, T. Taylor, K. Warabi, X. H. Huang, and R. J. Andersen. 2005. "Uncialmycin, a New Enediyne Antibiotic." *Organic Letters* 7 (23): 5233–36.

Davis, E. W., and J. A. Yost. 1983. *Novel Hallucinogens from Eastern Ecuador*. Botanical Museum Leaflets, Cambridge, MA: Harvard University 29 (3): 291–95.

Dawoud, T. M., N. S. Alharbi, A. M. Theruvinthalakal, A. Thekkangil, S. Kadaikunnan, et al. 2020. "Characterization and Antifungal Activity of the Yellow Pigment Produced by a *Bacillus* sp. DBS4 Isolated from the Lichen *Dirinaria agealita*." *Saudi Journal of Biological Sciences* 27 (5): 1403–11.

De Barros Alves, G. M., M. B. de Sousa Maia, E. de Sousa Franco, et al. 2014. "Expectorant and Antioxidant Activities of Purified Fumarprotocetraric Acid from *Cladonia verticillaris* Lichen in Mice." *Pulmonary Pharmacology and Therapeutics* 27: 139–43.

Delebassée, S., L. Mambu, E. Pinault, et al. 2017. "Cytochalasin E in the Lichen *Pleurosticta acetabulum*. Anti-proliferative Activity against Human HT-29 Colorectal Cancer Cells and Quantitative Variability." *Fitoterapia* 121: 146–51.

de Paz, G. A., J. Raggio, M. P. Gómez-Serranillos, O. M. Palomino, et al. 2010. "HPLC Isolation of Antioxidant Constituents from *Xanthoparmelia* spp." *Journal of Pharmacology and Biomedical Analysis* 53 (2): 165–71.

de Pedro, N., J. Cantizani, F. J. Ortiz-López, et al. 2016. "Protective Effects of Isolecanoric Acid on Neurodegenerative In Vitro Models." *Neuropharmacology* 101: 538–48.

Deraeve, C., Z. Guo, R. S. Bon, W. Blankenfeldt, et al. 2012. "Psoromic Acid Is a Selective and Covalent Rab-Prenylation Inhibitor Targeting Autoinhibited RabGGTase." *ACS Publications* 134 (17): 7384–91.

Desmarets, L., M. Millot, M. Chollet-Krugler, J. Boustie, et al. 2023. "Lichen or Associated Micro-Organism Compounds Are Active against Human Coronaviruses." *Viruses* 15 (9): 1859.

Devi, A. P., T. H. Duong, S. Ferron, M. A. Beniddir, M. H. Dinh, Y. K. Nguyen, N. K. T. Pham, et al. 2020. "Salazinic Acid-Derived Depsidones and Diphenylethers with a-Glucosidase Inhibitory Activity from the Lichen *Parmotrema dilatatum*." *Planta Medica* 85 (16): 1216–24.

Dias, D., J. M. White, and S. Urban. 2007. "Pinastric Acid Revisited: A Complete NMR and X-ray Structure Assignment." *Natural Product Research* 21 (4): 366–76.

Dias, D. A., and S. Urban. 2009. "Phytochemical Investigation of the Australian Lichens *Ramalina glaucescens* and *Xanthoria parietina*." *Natural Product Communications* 4 (7): 959–64.

Diaz-Allen, C., R. W. Spjut, A. D. Kinghorn, and H. L. Rakotondraibe. 2021. "Prioritizing Natural Product Compounds Using 1D-TOCSY NMR Spectroscopy." *Trends in Organic Chemistry* 22: 99–114.

Dieu, A., M. Millot, Y. Champavier, L. Mambu, V. Chaleix, V. Sol, and V. Gloaguen. 2014. "Uncommon Chlorinated Xanthone and Other Antibacterial Compounds from the Lichen *Cladonia incrassata*." *Planta Medica* 80 (11): 931–35.

Dieu, A., L. Mambu, Y. Champavier, V. Chaleix, V. Sol, V. Gloaguen, and M. Millot. 2020. "Antibacterial Activity of the Lichens *Usnea florida* and *Flavoparmelia caperata* (Parmeliaceae)." *Natural Products Research* 34 (23): 3358–62.

Dincer, C. A., C. Gökalp, B. Getiren, A. Yildiz, and N. Yildiz. 2021. "Supercritical Carbon Dioxide Extraction of *Usnea longissima* (L.) Ach.: Optimization by Box-Behnken design (BBD)." *Turkish Journal of Chemistry* 45 (4): 1249–56.

Ding, C., P. X. Tian W. Xue, et al. 2011. "Efficacy of *Cordyceps sinensis* in Long Term Treatment of Renal Transplant Patients." *Frontiers in Bioscience* (Elite Ed) 3: 301–7.

Ding, G., Y. Li, S. Fu, S. C. Liu, J. C. Wei, and Y. S. Che. 2009. "Ambuic Acid and Torreyanic Acid Derivatives from the Endolichenic Fungus *Pestalotiopsis* sp." *Journal of Natural Products* 72 (1): 182–86.

Do, T. H., T. H. Duong, T. N. M. An, et al. 2023. "Two New a-glucosidase Inhibitory Depsidones from the Lichen *Parmotrema cristiferum* (Taylor) Hale." *Chemistry and Biodiversity* 20 (3).

Dong, X. B., L. Wang, G. Song, W. X. Wang, and J. Q. Chen. 2021. "Physcion Protects Rats against Cerebral Ischemia-Reperfusion Injury via Inhibition of TLR4/NF-kB Signaling Pathway." *Drug Design Development and Therapy* 15: 277–87.

Dragana, S. V., M. A. Pushilin, V. P. Glazunov, V. A. Denisenko, and V. P. Anufriev. 2014. "Total Synthesis of Hybocarpone, a Cytotoxic Naphthazarin Derivative from the Lichen *Lecanora hybocarpa*, and Related Compounds." *Natural Product Communications* 9 (12): 1765–68.

Duffin, C. J. 2022. "'The Periwig of a Dead Cranium': Medicinal Skull Moss." *Pharmaceutical Historian* 52 (3): 75–85.

Duong, T. H., V. K. Nguyen, J. Sichaem, T. N. Tran, et al. 2022. "Reticulin, a Novel C_{43}-spiroterpenoid from the Lichen *Parmotrema reticulatum* Growing in Vietnam." *Natural Products Research* 36 (14): 3705–12.

Duong, T. H., T. N. M. An, T. K. D. Le, et al. 2023. "Parmoferone A, a New Depsidone from the Lichen *Parmotrema cristiferum*." *Natural Product Research*, 1–6.

Ebrahim, H. Y., H. E. Elsayed, M. M. Mohyeldin, et al. 2016. "Norstictic Acid Inhibits Breast Cancer Cell Proliferation, Migration, Invasion and In Vivo Invasive Growth Through Targeting C-Met." *Phytotherapy Research* 30 (4): 557–66.

Ebrahim, H. Y., M. R. Aki, H. E. Elsayed, R. A. Hill, and K. A. El Sayed. 2017. "Usnic Acid Benzylidene Analogues as Potent Mechanistic Target of Rapamycin Inhibitors for the Control of Breast Malignancies." *Journal of Natural Products* 80 (4): 932–52.

EDI Environmental Dynamics Inc. 2005. *Mt. Nansen Terrestrial and Aquatic Effects Study—Summary of Community Survey*. Whitehorse, Yukon: Government of Yukon, Abandoned Mines Branch.

Edwards, H. G. M., M. R. D. Seaward, and S. J. Attwood. 2003. "FT-Raman Spectroscopy of Lichens on Dolomitic Rocks: An Assessment of Metal Oxalate Formation." *Analyst* 128 (10): 1218–21.

Edwards, H. G. M., E. M. Newton, D. L. Dickensheets, and D. D. Wynn-Williams. 2003a. "Raman Spectroscopic Detection of Biomolecular Markers from Antarctic Materials: Evaluation for Putative Martian Habitats." *Spectrochima Acta A: Molecular and Biomolecular Spectroscopy* 59 (10): 2277–90.

Ehsani, M., S. Bartsch, S. M. M. Rasa, J. Dittmann, et al. 2022. "The Natural Compound Atraric Acid Suppresses Androgen-Regulated Neo-angiogenesis of Castration-Resistant Prostate Cancer through Angiopoietin 2." *Oncogene* 41 (23): 3263–77.

Einarsdóttir, E., J. Groeneweg, G. G. Björnsdóttir, G. Harethardottir, et al. 2010. "Cellular Mechanisms of the Anticancer Effects of the Lichen Compound Usnic Acid." *Planta Medica* 76 (10): 969–74.

Eisenbert, T., M. Adellatif, S. Schroeder, et al. 2016. "Cardioprotection and Lifespan Extension by the Natural Polyamine Spermidine." *Nature Medicine* 22: 1428.

Elecko, J., M. Vilková, R. Frenák, D. Routray, D. Rucová, M. Backor, and M. Goga. 2022. "A Comparative Study of Isolated Secondary Metabolites from Lichens and Their Antioxidative Properties." *Plants* (Basel) 11 (8): 1077.

El-Garawani, I. M., W. A. Elkhateeb, G. M. Zaghiol, R. S. Almeer, E. F. Ahmed, M. E. Rateb, and A. E. A. Moneim. 2019. "*Candelariella vitellina* Extract Triggers In Vitro and In Vivo Cell Death through Induction of Apoptosis: A Novel Anticancer Agent." *Food and Chemical Toxicology* 127: 110–19.

El-Garawani, I. M. Emam, W. Elkhateeb, H. El-Seedi, S. Khalifa, S. Oshiba, S. Abou-Ghanima, and G. Daba. 2020. "In Vitro Antigenotoxic, Antithelminthic and Antioxidant Potentials Based on the Extracted Metabolites from Lichen, *Candelariella vitellina*." *Pharmaceutics* 12 (5): 477.

Elix, J. A. 2018. *A Catalogue of Standardized Chromatographic Data and Biosynthetic Relationships for Lichen Substances*. 4th ed. Canberra: Published by the author.

Elkhateeb, W. A., G. M. Daba, A. N. El-Dein, W. Fayad, M. N. Shaheen, E. M. Elmabdy, and T. C. Wen. 2020. "Insights into the In-Vitro Hypochloesterolemic, Antioxidant, Anti-rotavirus, and Anti-colon Activities of the Methanolic Extracts of a Japanese Lichen, *Candelariella vitellina*, and a Japanese Mushroom, *Ganoderma applanatum*." *Egyptian Pharmaceutical Journal* 19 (1): 67–73.

Elmore, F. H. 1943. *Ethnobotany of the Navajo, Monographs of the School of American Research* 8. Santa Fe: University of New Mexico Press.

Emsen, B., A. Aslan, B. Togar, and H. Turkez. 2016. "In Vitro Antitumor Activities of the Lichen Compounds Olivetoric, Physodic and Psoromic Acid in Rat Neuron and Glioblastoma Cells." *Pharmaceutical Biology* 54 (9): 1748–62.

Emsen, B., A. Aslan, H. Turkez, et al. 2018. The Anti-cancer Efficacies of Diffractaic, Lobaric and Usnic Acid: In Vitro Inhibition of Glioma." *Journal of Cancer Research and Therapeutics* 14: 941–51.

Emsen, B., O. Ozdemir, T. Engin, B. Togar, S. Cavusoglu, and H. Turkez. 2019. "Inhibition of Growth of U87MG Human Glioblastoma Cells by *Usnea longissima* Ach." *Anais de Academia Brasileira de Ciencias* 91 (3): 20180994.

Emsen, B., and A. L. Kolukisa. 2020. "Cytogenic and Oxidative Effects of Three Lichen Extracts on Human Peripheral Lymphocytes." *Zeitschrift fur Naturforschchung Section C Journal of Biosciences* 76 (7–8): 291–99.

Emsen, B., G. Sadi, A. Bostanci, N. Gursoy, et al. 2021. "Evaluation of the Biological Activities of Olivetoric Acid, a Lichen-Derived Molecule, in Human Hepatocellular Carcinoma Cells." *Rendiconti Lincei. Scienze Fisiche e Naturali* 32: 135–48.

Endo, Y., H. Hayashi, T. Sato, M. Maruno, T. Ohta, and S. Nozoe. 1994. "Confluentic Acid and 2'-O-methylperlatolic Acid, Monoamine Oxidase B Inhibitors in a Brazilian Plant, *Himatanthus sucuuba.*" *Chemical and Pharmaceutical Bulletin* (Tokyo) 42 (6): 1198–201.

Enzensberger, H. M. 1965. "Lichenology." In *Blindenschrift*. Frankfurt, Germany: Surhkamp.

Ernst-Russell, M. A., J. A. Elix, C. L. L. Chai, A. C. Willis, N. Harnada, and T. H. Nash III. 1999. "Hybocarpone, a Novel Cytotoxic Naphthazarin Derivative from Mycobiont Cultures of the Lichen *Lecanora hybocarpa.*" *Tetrahedron Letters* 40 (34): 6321–24.

Esimone, C. O., K. C. Ofokansi, M. U. Adikwu, E. C. Ibezim, D. O. Abonyi, et al. 2007. "In Vitro Evaluation of the Antiviral Activity of Extracts from the Lichen *Parmelia perlata* (L.) Ach. against Three RNA Viruses." *Journal of Infections in Developing Countries* 1 (3): 315–20.

Esimone, C. O., T. Grunwald, C. S. Nworu, S. Kuate, P. Proksch, and K. Uberta. 2009. "Broad Spectrum Antiviral Fractions from the Lichen *Ramalina farinacea* (L.) Ach." *Chemotherapy* 55 (2): 119–26.

European Scientific Cooperative on Phytotherapy. 2003. *ESCOP Monographs*. 2nd ed. Stuttgart, Germany: Georg Thieme Verlag.

Fagnani, L., L Nazzicone, P. Bellio, N. Franceschini, D. Tondi, A. Verri, et al. 2022. "Protocetraric and Salazinic Acids as Potential Inhibitors of SARS-CoV-2 3CL Protease: Biochemical, Cytotoxic, and Computational Characterization of Depsidones as Slow-Binding Inactivators." *Pharmaceuticals* (Basel) 15 (6): 714.

Fang, B., Z. J. Li, Y. Qiu, N. Cho, and H. M. Yoo. 2021. "Inhibition of UBA5 Expression and Induction of Autophagy in Breast Cancer Cells by Usenamine A." *Biomolecules* 11 (9): 1348.

Farber, L., K. A. Sølhaug, P. A. Esseen, W. Bilger, and Y. Gauslaa. 2014. "Sunscreening Fungal Pigments Influence the Vertical Gradient of Pendulous Lichens in Boreal Forest Canopies." *Ecology* 95 (6): 1464–71.

Fazio, A. T., M. T. Adler, M. D. Bertoni, C. S. Sepulveda, E. B. Damonte, and M. S. Maier. 2007 "Lichen Secondary Metabolites from the Cultured Lichen Mycobionts of *Teloschistes chrysophthalmus* and *Ramalina celastri* and Their Anti-viral Activities." *Zeitschrift fur Naturforschung Section C Journal of Bioscience* 62 (7–8): 543–49.

Feazel, L. M., L. K. Baumgartner, K. L. Peterson, D. N. Frank, J. K. Harris, and N. R. Pace. 2009. "Opportunistic Pathogens Enriched in Showerhead Biofilms." *Proceedings of the National Academy of Science USA* 106 (38): 16393–99.

Feibelman, K. M., B. P. Fuller, L. F. Li, D. V. LaBarbera, and B. J. Geiss. 2018. "Identification of Small Molecule Inhibitors of the Chikungunya Virus nsP1 RNA Capping Enzyme." *Antiviral Research* 154: 124–31.

Felcykowska, A., A. Pastuszak-Skrzypczak, A. Pawlik, K. Bogucka, A. Herman-Antosiewicz, and B. Guzow-Krzeminska. 2017. "Antibacterial and Anticancer Activities of Acetone Extracts from In Vitro Cultured Lichen-Forming Fungi." *BMC Complementary and Alternative Medicine* 17 (1): 300.

Fernández-Moriano, C., P. K. Divakar, A. Crespo, and M. P. Gómez-Serranillos. 2015. "Neuroprotective Activity and Cytotoxic Potential of Two Parmeliaceae Lichens: Identification of Active Compounds." *Phytomedicine* 22 (9): 847–55.

Fernández-Moriano, C., P. K. Divakar, A. Crespo, and M. P. Gómez-Serranillos. 2017. "In Vitro Neuroprotective Potential of Lichen Metabolite Fumarprotocetraric Acid via Intracellular Redox Modulation." *Toxicology and Applied Pharmacology* 316: 83–94.

Fernández-Moriano, C., P. K Divakar, A. Crespo, and M. P. Gómez-Serranillos. 2017a. "Protective Effects of Lichen Metabolites Evernic and Usnic Acids against Redox Impairment-Mediated Cytotoxicity in Central Nervous System-Like Cells." *Food and Chemical Toxicology* 105: 262–77.

Fournet, A., M. E. Ferreira, A. R. de Arias, S. T. de Ortiz, et al. 1997. "Activity of Compounds Isolated from Chilean Lichens against Experimental Cutaneous Leishmaniasis." *Comparative Biochemistry and Physiology C Pharmacology Toxicology and Endocrinology* 116 (1): 51–54.

Francolini, I., P. Norris, A. Piozzi, G. Donelli, and P. Stoodley. 2004. "Usnic Acid, a Natural Antimicrobial Agent Able to Inhibit Bacterial Biofilm Formation on Polymer Surfaces." *Antimicrobial Agents and Chemotherapy* 48 (11): 4360–65.

Fraser, M. H. 2006. "Ethnobotanical Investigation of Plants Used for the Treatment of Type 2 Diabetes by Two Cree Communities in Quebec: Quantitative Comparisons and Antioxidant Evaluation." MSc thesis, Montreal: McGill University.

Freysdottir, J., S. Omarsdottir, K. Ingólfsdóttir, A. Vikingsson, and E. S. Olafsdóttir. 2008. "In Vitro and In Vivo Immunomodulating Effects of Traditionally Prepared Extract and Purified Compounds from *Cetraria islandica*." *International Immunopharmacology* 8 (3): 423–30.

Furmanek, L., P. Czarnota, and M. R. D. Seaward. 2019. "Antifungal Activity of Lichen Compounds against Dermatophytes: A Review." *Journal of Applied Microbiology* 127 (2): 308–25.

Furmanek, L., P. Czarnota, and M. R. D. Seaward. 2021. "The Effect of Lichen Secondary Metabolites on *Aspergillus* Fungi." *Archives of Microbiology* 204 (100).

Gabriel, L., and H. E. White. 1954. "Food and Medicines of the Okanakanes." *Report of the Okanagan Historical Society* 18: 24–29. Vernon, BC.

Gaikwad, S., N. Verma, B. O. Sharma, and B. C. Behera. 2014. "Growth Promoting Effects of Some Lichen Metabolites on Probiotic Bacteria." *Journal of Food Science Technology* 51: 2624–31.

Galanty, A., P. Koczurkiewicz, D. Wnuk, M. Paw, E. Karnas, I. Podolak, et al. 2017. "Usnic Acid and Atranorin Exert Selective Cytostatic and Anti-invasive Effects on Human Prostate and Melanoma Cancer Cells." *Toxicology in Vitro* 40: 161–69.

Galanty, A., P. Pasko, and I. Podolak. 2019. "Enantioselective Activity of Usnic Acid: A Comprehensive Review and Future Perspectives." *Phytochemistry Reviews* 18: 527–48.

Galla, R., S. Ferrari, S. Ruga, B. Mantuano, G. Rosso, et al. 2023. "Effects of Usnic Acid to Prevent Infections by Creating a Protective Barrier in an In Vitro Study." *International Journal of Molecular Sciences* 24 (4): 3695.

Gandhi, A. D., P. A. Miraclin, D. Abilash, S. Sathiyaraj, R. Velmurugan, et al. 2021. "Nanosilver Reinforced *Parmelia sulcata* Extract Efficiently Induces Apoptosis and Inhibits Proliferative Signalling in MCF-7 Cells." *Environmental Research* 199: 111375.

Gandhi, A. D., K. Umamahesh, S. Sathiyaraj, G. Suriyakata, R. Velmurugan, et al. 2022. "Isolation of Bioactive Compounds from Lichen *Parmelia sulcata* and Evaluation of Antimicrobial Property." *Journal of Infection and Public Health* 15 (4): 491–97.

Ganesan, A., A. Mahesh, J. P. Sundararaj, K. Mani, and P. Ponnusamy. 2016. "Antihyperglycemic and Antioxidant Activity of Various Fractions of *Parmotrema hababianum* in Streptozotocin-Induced Diabetic Rat." *Bangladesh Journal of Pharmacology* 11 (4): 935–39.

Gao, F., W. J. Liu, Q. J. Guo, Y. Q. Bai, H. Yang, and H. Y. Chen. 2017a. "Physcion Blocks Cell Cycle and Induces Apoptosis in Human B Cell Precursor Acute Lymphoblastic Leukemia Cells by Downregulating HOXA5." *Biomedicine and Pharmacotherapy* 94: 850–57.

Gao, X., H. L. Sun, D. S. Liu, J. R. Zhang, J. Zhang, M. M. Yan, and X. H. Pan. 2017. "Secalonic Acid-F Inhibited Cell Growth More Effectively Than 5-fluorouracil on Hepatocellular Carcinoma In Vitro and In Vivo." *Neoplasma* 64 (3): 344–50.

Garibaldi, A. 1999. *Medicinal Flora of the Alaska Natives*. Anchorage: University of Alaska.

Garlick, J. M., S. M. Sturlis, P. A. Bruno, J. A. Yates, A. L. Peiffer, et al. 2021. "Norstictic Acid Is a Selective Allosteric Transcriptional Regulator." *Journal of the American Chemical Society* 143 (25): 9297–302.

Garrett, J. T. 2003. *The Cherokee Herbal: Native Plant Medicine from the Four Directions*. Rochester, VT: Bear & Company.

Garrido-Huéscar, E., E. González-Burgos, P. M. Kirika, J. Boustie, S. Ferron, et al. 2022. "A New Cryptic Lineage in Parmeliaceae (Ascomycota) with Pharmacological Properties." *Journal of Fungi* (Basel) 8 (8): 826.

Garth, T. R. 1953. *Atsugewi Ethnobotany*. Anthropological Records [University of California] 14: 129–212.

GBD 2019. "Global Mortality Associated with 33 Bacterial Pathogens in 2019: A Systematic Analysis for the Global Burden of Disease Study 2019." *Lancet* 400 (10369): 2221–48.

Geng, X. G., X. Zhang, B. Zhou, C. J. Zhang, et al. 2018. "Usnic Acid Induces Cycle Arrest, Apoptosis, and Autophagy in Gastric Cancer Cells in Vitro and In Vivo." *Medical Science Monitor* 24: 556–66.

Ghate, N. B., D. Chaudhuri, R. Sarker, A. L. Sajem, S. Panja, J. Rout, and N. Mandal. 2013. "An Antioxidant Extract of Tropical Lichen, *Parmotrema reticulatum*, Induces Cell Cycle Arrest and Apoptosis in Breast Carcinoma Cell Line MCF-7." *PLoS ONE* 8 (12): e82293.

Gilmore, M. R. 1977. *Uses of Plants by the Indians of the Missouri River Region*. Lincoln: University of Nebraska Press.

Girardot, M., M. Millot, G. Hamion, J. L. Billard, C. Juin, G. Ntoutoume, V. Sol, L. Mambu, and C. Imbert. 2021. "Lichen Polyphenolic Compounds for the Eradication of *Candida albicans* Biofilms." *Frontier Cellular Infection Microbiology* 11: 698883.

Glew, R. S., D. J. Vanderjagt, L. T. Chuang, Y. S. Huang, et al. 2005. "Nutrient Content of Four Edible Wild Plants from West Africa." *Plant Foods for Human Nutrition* 60 (4): 187–93.

Godinez, J. C., and M. M. Ortega. 1989. *Liquenologia de Mexico. Historia y bibliografia. Cuadernos 3*. Mexico City: Instituto de Biologica UNAM.

Goel, M., P. Dureja, A. Rani, P. L. Uniyal, and H. Laatsch. 2011. "Isolation, Characterization and Antifungal Activity of Major Constituents of the Himalayan Lichen *Parmelia reticulata* Tayl." *Journal of Agricultural and Food Chemistry* 59 (6): 2299–307.

Goel, M., R. Kaira, P. Ponnan, J. A. A. S. Jayaweera, and W. W. Kumbukgolla. 2021. "Inhibition of Penicillin-Binding Proteins 2a (PBP2a) in Methicillin Resistant *Staphylococcus aureus* (MRSA) by Combination of Oxacillin and a Bioactive Compound from *Ramalina roesleri*." *Microbial Pathogenesis* 150: 104676.

Goga, M., M. Kello, M. Vilkova, K. Petrova, M. Backor, W. Adlassnig, and I. Lang. 2019. "Oxidative Stress Mediated by Gyrophoric Acid from the Lichen *Umbilicaria hirsuta* Affected Apoptosis and Stress/Survival Pathways in HeLa Cells." *BMC Complementary and Alternative Medicine* 19 (1): 221.

Gökalsin, B., and N. C. Sesal. 2016. "Lichen Secondary Metabolite Evernic Acid as Potential Quorum Sensing Inhibitor against *Pseudomonas aeruginosa*." *World Journal of Microbiology and Biotechnology* 32 (9): 150.

Gollapudi, S. R., H. Telikepalli, H. B. Jampani, et al. 1994. "Alectosarmentin, a New Antimicrobial Dibenzofuranoid Lactol from the Lichen *Alectoria sarmentosa*." *Journal of Natural Products* 57 (7): 934–38.

Golzadeh, N., B. D. Barst, N. Basu, J. M. Baker, J. C. Auger, and M. A. McKinney. 2020. "Evaluating the Concentrations of Total Mercury, Methylmercury, Selenium and Selenium:Mercury Molar Ratios in Traditional Foods of the Bigstone Cree in Alberta, Canada." *Chemosphere* 250: 126285.

Golzadeh, N., B. D. Barst, J. M. Baker, J. C. Auger, and M. A. McKinney. 2021. "Alkylated Polycyclic Aromatic Hydrocarbons Are the Largest Contributor to Polycyclic Aromatic Compound Concentrations in Traditional Foods of the Bigstone Cree Nation in Alberta, Canada." *Environmental Pollution* 275: 116625.

Gomes, A. T., N. Honda, F. M. Roese, R. M. Muzzi, and M. R. Marques. 2002. "Bioactive Derivatives Obtained from Lecanoric Acid, a Constituent of the Lichen *Parmotrema tinctorum* (Nyl.) Hale (Parmeliaceae)." *Revista Brasileira de Farmacognosia* 12: 74–75.

Goncu, B., E. Sevgi, C. K. Hancer, G. Gokay, and N. Ozten. 2020. "Differential Antiproliferative and Apoptotic Effects of Lichen Species on Human Prostate Carcinoma Cells." *PLOS ONE* 15 (9): e0238303.

Gong, F. Y., T. Ge, J. Liu, J. Xiao, X. C. Wu, et al. 2022. "Trehalose Inhibits Ferroptosis via NRF2/HO-1 Pathway and Promotes Functional Recovery in Mice with Spinal Cord Injury." *Aging* (Albany NY) 14 (7): 3216–32.

González, C., C. Cartagena, L. Caballero, F. Melo, C. Areche, and A. Cornejo. 2021. "The Fumarprotocetraric Acid Inhibits Tau Covalently, Avoiding Cytotoxicity of Aggregates in Cells." *Molecules* 26 (12): 3760.

Gordien, A. Y., A. L. Gray, and K. Ingleby. 2009. "Activity of Scottish Plant, Lichen and Fungal Endophyte Extracts against *Mycobacterium aurum* and *Mycobacterium tuberculosis*." *Phytotherapy Research* 24: 692–98.

Graney, J. R., M. S. Landis, K. J. Puckett, W. B. Studabaker, E. S. Edgerton, A. H. Legge, and K. E. Percy. 2017. "Differential Accumulation of PAHs, Elements and Pb Isotopes by Five Lichen Species from the Athabasca Oil Sands Region in Alberta, Canada." *Chemosphere* 184: 700–710.

Grudzinska, M., P. Pasko, D. Wrobel-Biedrawa, et al. 2022. "Antimelanoma Potential of *Cladonia mitis* Acetone Extracts—Comparative In Vitro Studies in Relation to Usnic Acid Content." *Chemistry and Biodiversity* 19 (7): e202200408.

Guerrero, R., L. Margulis, and M. Berlanga. 2013. "Symbioogeneis: The Holobiont as a Unit of Evolution." *International Microbiology* 16 (3): 133–43.

Güllüce, M., A. Aslan, M. Sokmen, F. Sahin, A. Adiguzel, et al. 2006. "Screening the Antioxidant and Antimicrobial Properties of the Lichens *Parmelia saxatilis, Platismatia glauca, Ramalina pollinaria, Ramalina polymorpha* and *Umbilicaria nylanderiana*." *Phytomedicine* 13 (7): 515–21.

Güllüce, M., G. Agar, A. Aslan, M. Karadayi, S. Bozari, and F. Orhan. 2021. "Protective Effects of Methanol Extracts from *Cladonia rangiformis* and *Umbilicaria vellea* against Known Mutagens Sodium Azide and 9-aminoacridine." *Toxicology and Industrial Health* 27 (8): 675–82.

Gundogdu, G., K. Gundogdu, K. A. Nalci, A. K. Demirkaya, et al. 2019. "The Effect of Parietin Isolated from *Rheum ribes* L. on In Vitro Wound Model Using Human Dermal Fibroblast Cells." *International Journal of Lower Extremity Wounds* 18 (1): 56–64.

Gunther, E. 1988. *Ethnobotany of Western Washington. The Knowledge and Use of Indigenous Plants by Native Americans.* Rev. ed. Seattle: University of Washington Press.

Guo, J., Z. L. Li, A. L. Wang, X. Q. Liu, J. Wang, X. Guo, Y. K. Jing, and H. M. Hua. 2011. "Three New Phenolic Compounds from the Lichen *Thamnolia vermicularis* and Their Antiproliferative Effects in Prostate Cancer Cells." *Planta Medica* 77 (18): 2042–46.

Gupta, A., N. Sahu, A. P. Singh, V. K. Singh, S. C. Singh, et al. 2022. "Exploration of Novel Lichen Compounds as Inhibitors of SARS-CoV-2 Mpro: Ligand-Based Design, Molecular

Dynamics, and ADMET Analyses." *Applied Biochemistry and Biotechnology* 194 (12): 6386–406.

Gupta, V. K., et al. 2007. "Antimycobacterial Activity of Lichens." *Pharmaceutical Biology* 45 (3): 200–204.

Gupta, V. K., S. Verma, S. Gupta, A. Singh, A. Pal, et al. 2012. "Membrane-Damaging Potential of Natural L-(-)-Usnic Acid in *Staphylococcus aureus*." *European Journal of Microbiology and Infectious Diseases* 31 (12): 3375–83.

Guzman, G. 2008. "Diversity and Use of Traditional Mexican Medicinal Fungi. A Review." *International Journal of Medicinal Mushrooms* 10 (3): 209–17.

Haiyuan, J. U., X. Q. Shen, D. Liu, M. H. Hong, and Y. H. Lu. 2019. "The Protective Effects of B-sitosterol and Vermicularin from *Thamnolia vermicularis* (Sw.) Ach. against Skin Aging In Vitro." *Anais da Academia Brasileirade Ciencias* 91 (4): e20181088.

Halama, P., and C. Van Haluwin. 2004. "Antifungal Activity of Lichen Extracts and Lichenic Acids." *Biocontrol* 49 (1): 95–107.

Halici, M., F. Odabasoglu, H. Suleyman, A. Cakir, A. Aslan, and Y. Bayir. 2005. "Effects of Water Extract of *Usnea longissima* on Antioxidant Enzyme Activity and Mucosal Damage Caused by Indomethacin in Rats." *Phytomedicine* 12: 656–62.

Hamida, R. S., M. A. Ali, N. E. Abdelmeguid, M. I. Al-Zaban, L. Baz, and M. M. Bin-Meferij. 2021. "Lichens—A Potential Source of Nanoparticles Fabrication: A Review on Nanoparticles Biosynthesis and Their Prospective Applications." *Journal of Fungi* (Basel) 7 (4): 291.

Han, Y. T., X. H. Chen, H. Gao, J. L. Ye, and C. B. Wang. 2016. "Physcion Inhibits the Metastatic Potential of Human Colorectal Cancer SW620 Cells In Vitro by Suppressing the Transcription Factor SOX2." *Acta Pharmacologica Sinica* 37 (2): 264–75.

Hannaoui, S., I. Zemlyankina, S. C. Chung, et al. 2022. "Transmission of Cervid Prions to Humanized Mice Demonstrates the Zoonotic Potential of CWD." *Acta Neuropathologica* 144: 767–84.

Haraldsdóttir, S., E. Guolaugsdóttir, K. Ingólfsdóttir, and H. M. Ogmundsdóttir. 2004. "Antiproliferative Effects of Lichen-Derived Lipoxygenase Inhibitors on Twelve Human Cancer Cell Lines of Different Tissue Origin In Vitro." *Planta Medica* 70 (11): 1098–1100.

Harikrishnan, A., V. Veena, B. Lakshmi, et al. 2021. "Atranorin, an Antimicrobial Metabolite from Lichen *Parmotrema rampoddense* Exhibited In Vitro Anti-breast Cancer Activity through Interaction with Akt Activity." *Journal of Biomolecular Structure and Dynamics* 39: 1248–58.

Haritha, P., S. K. Patnaik, and V. B. Tatipamula. 2019. "Chemical and Pharmacological Evaluation of Manglicolous Lichen *Graphis ajarekarii* Patw. & C.R. Kulk." *Vietnam Journal of Science and Technology* 57 (3): 300–308.

Harmon, D. W. 1904. *A Journal of Voyages and Travels in the Interior of North America: Between the 47th and 58th Degrees of N. Lat., Extending from Montréal Nearly to the Pacific, a Distance of about 5,000 Miles: Including an Account of the Principal Occurrences During a Residence of Nineteen Years in Different Parts of the Country*. Toronto: George N. Morang.

Hart, J. 1974. "Plant Taxonomy of the Salish and Kootenai Indians of Western Montana." MA thesis, University of Montana.

Hart, J. 1976. *Montana—Native Plants and Early Peoples.* Helena: Montana Historical Society.

Hassan, S. T. S., M. Sudomová, K. Berchová-Bimová, et al. 2018. "Antimycobacterial, Enzyme Inhibition, and Molecular Interaction Studies of Psoromic Acid in *Mycobacterium tuberculosis*: Efficacy and Safety Investigations." *Journal of Clinical Medicine* 7 (8): 226.

Hassan, S. T. S., M. Sudomova, K. Berchova-Bimova, K. Smejkal, and J. Echeverria. 2019. "Psoromic Acid, a Lichen-Derived Molecule, Inhibits the Replication of HSV-1 and HSV-2, and Inactivates HSV-1 DNA Polymerase: Shedding Light on Antiherpetic Properties." *Molecules* 24 (16): 2912.

Hawksworth, D. L. 2003. "Hallucinogenic and Toxic Lichens." *International Lichenological Newsletter* 36: 33–35.

Hawksworth, D. L., and M. Grube. 2020. "Lichens Redefined as Complete Ecosystems." *New Phytologist* 227 (5): 1281–83.

Hawryl, A., M. Hawryl, A. Hajnos-Stolarz, et al. 2020. "HPLC Fingerprint Analysis with the Antioxidant and Cytotoxic Activities of Selected Lichens Combined with the Chemometric Calculations." *Molecules* 25 (18): 4301.

Hebda, R. J., N. J. Turner, S. Birchwater, et al. 1996. *Ulkatcho Food and Medicine Plants.* Anahim Lake, BC: Ulkatcho Indian Band.

Hellson, J. C., and M. Gadd. 1974. *Ethnobotany of the Blackfoot Indians.* Ottawa: National Museum of Man Mercury Series 19.

Hengameh, P., R. Shivanna, H. G. Rajkumar. 2016. "In Vitro Inhibitory Activity of Some Lichen Extracts against A-amylase Enzyme." *European Journal of Biomedical and Pharmaceutical Sciences* 3 (5): 315–18.

Herrick, J. W. 1995. *Iroquois Medical Botany.* Syracuse, NY: Syracuse University Press.

Hesbacher, S., B. Baur, A. Baur, and P. Proksch. 1995. "Sequestration of Lichen Compounds by Three Species of Terrestrial Snails." *Journal of Chemical Ecology* 21 (2): 233–46.

Hesse, A., M. Frick, H. Orzekowsky, K. Failing, and R. Neiger. 2018. "Canine Calcium Oxalate Urolithiasis: Frequency of Whewelllite and Weddellite Stones from 1979 to 2015." *Canadian Veterinary Journal* 59 (12): 1305–10.

Hickey, S., and H. Roberts. 2011. *Tarnished Gold: The Sickness of Evidence-based Medicine.* CreateSpace Independent Publishing.

Hirano, E., H. Saito, Y. Ito, K. Ishige, Y. Edagawa, et al. 2003. "PB-2, a Polysaccharide Fraction from Lichen *Flavoparmelia baltimorensis*, Peripherally Promotes the Induction of Long-Term Potentiation in the Rat Dentate Gyrus In Vivo." *Brain Research* 963 (1–2): 307–11.

Ho, X. Q., L. S. Qiao, Y. K. Chen, X. Chen, Y. S. He, and Y. L. Zhang. 2019. "Discovery of Novel Multi-target Inhibitor of Angiotensin Type I Receptor and Neprilysin Inhibitors from Traditional Chinese Medicine." *Scientific Reports* 9 (1): 16205.

Honda, N. K., F. R. Pavan, R. G. Coelho, S. R. de Andrade Leite, A. C. Micheletti, et al. 2010. "Antimycobacterial Activity of Lichen Substances." *Phytomedicine* 17 (5): 328–32.

Hong, J. M., S. S. Suh, T. K. Kim, J. E. Kim, S. J. Han, et al. 2018. "Anti-cancer Activity of Lobaric Acid and Lobarstin Extracted from the Antarctic Lichen *Stereocaulon alpinum*." *Molecules* 23 (3): 658.

Hosoya, M., J. Balzarini, S. Shigeta, and E. De Clercq. 1991. "Differential Inhibitory Effects of Sulfated Polysaccharides and Polymers on the Replication of Various Myxoviruses and Retroviruses, Depending on the Composition of the Target Amino Acid Sequences of the Viral Envelope Glycoproteins." *Antimicrobial Agents and Chemotherapy* 35 (12): 2515–20.

Huang, C. H. 2020. "Extensively Drug-Resistant *Alcaligenes faecalis* Infection." *BMC Infectious Diseases* 20: 833.

Huang, H. L., P. L. Lu, C. H. Lee, and I. W. Chong. 2020. "Treatment of Pulmonary Disease Caused by *Mycobacterium kansasii*." *Journal of the Formosan Medical Association* Suppl 1: S51–57.

Huang, X. J., J. B. Ma, L. X. Wei, J. Y. Song, C. Li, et al. 2018. "An Antioxidant Alpha-glucan from *Cladina rangiferina* (L.) Nyl. and Its Protective Effect on Alveolar Epithelial Cells from Pb^{2+}-Induced Oxidative Damage." *International Journal of Biological Macromolecules* 112: 101–9.

Hunn, E. S. 1990. *Nch'i-Wana: "The Big River": Mid-Columbia Indians and Their Land*. Seattle: University of Washington Press.

Hunn, G. accessed in 2005. Unpublished 1976–1980 ethnobotany field notes.

Huovinen, K., and T. Ahti. 1986. "The Composition and Contents of Aromatic Lichen Substances in *Cladonia*, Section Unciales." *Annales Botanici Fennici* 23 (3): 173–88.

Huryn, D. M., D. J. P. Kornfilt, and P. Wipf. 2020. "P97: An Emerging Target for Cancer, Neurodegenerative Diseases, and Viral Infections." *Journal of Medicinal Chemistry* 63 (5): 1892–907.

Hussain, M., H. Bakhsh, S. K. Syed, M. S. Ullah, et al. 2021. "The Spasmolytic, Bronchodilator and Vasodilator Activities of *Parmotrema perlatum* Are Explained by Anti-muscarinic and Calcium Antagonistic Mechanisms." *Molecules* 26 (21): 5348.

Huyen, V. T., N. T. T. Tram, N. M. Cuong, N. P. Dam, L. Francoise, and B. Joël. 2017. "Phytochemical and Cytotoxic Investigations of the Lichen *Stereocaulon evolutum* Graewe." *Vietnam Journal of Chemistry* (International Edition) 55 (4): 429–32.

Huyen, V. T., O. Delalande, C. Lalli, S. Reider, S. Ferron, J. Boustie, B. Waltenberger, and F. L. Le Dévéhat. 2021. "Inhibitory Effects of Secondary Metabolites from the Lichen *Stereocaulon evolutum* on Protein Tyrosine Phosphatase 1B." *Planta Medica* 87 (9): 701–8.

Huynh, B. L. C., V. M. Bui, K. P. P. Nguyen, N. K. T. Pham, and T. P. Nguyen. 2022. "Three New Diphenyl Ethers from the Lichen *Parmotrema praesorediosum* (Nyl.) Hale (Parmeliaceae)." *Natural Products Research* 36 (8): 1934–40.

Huynh, B. L. C., N. K. T. Pham, and T. P. Nguyen. 2022a. "Paresordin A, a New Diphenyl Cyclic Peroxide from the Lichen *Parmotrema praesorediosum*." *Journal of Asian Natural Products Research* 24 (2): 190–95.

Huynh, B. L. C., T. T. L. Nguyen, V. K. Nguyen, et al. 2022b. "Three New Phenolic Compounds from the Lichen *Ramalina peruviana* Ach. (Ramalinaceae)." *Natural Product Research* 36 (8): 2009–14.

Hwang, Y. H., S. J. Lee, K. Y. Kang, J. S. Hur, and S. T. Yee. 2017. "Immunosuppressive Effects of *Bryoria* sp. (Lichen-Forming Fungus) Extracts via Inhibition of CD8+ T-Cell Proliferation and IL-2 Production in CD4+ T cells." *Journal of Microbiology and Biotechnology* 27 (6): 1189–97.

Igoli, J. O., A. I. Gray, C. J. Clements, P. Kantheti, and R. K. Singla. 2014. "Antitrypanosomal Activity and Docking Studies of Isolated Constituents from the Lichen *Cetraria islandica*: Possibly Multifunctional Scaffolds." *Current Topics in Medicinal Chemistry* 14 (8): 1014–21.

Ilbäck, N. G., and S. Källman. 1999. "The Lichen Rock Tripe (*Lasallia pustulata*) as Survival Food: Effects on Growth, Metabolism and Immune Function in Balb/c Mice." *Natural Toxins* 7 (6): 321–29.

Ingelfinger, R., M. Henke, L. Roser, T. Ulshofer, A. Calchera, G. Singh, M. J. Parnham, G. Geisslinger, R. Furst, I. Schmitt, and S. Schiffmann. 2020. "Unraveling the Pharmacological Potential of Lichen Extracts in the Context of Cancer and Inflammation with a Broad Screening Approach." *Frontiers in Pharmacology* 11: 1322.

Ingólfsdóttir, K., S. F. Bloomfield, and P. Hylands. 1985. "In Vitro Evaluation of the Antimicrobial Activity of Lichen Metabolites as Potential Preservatives." *Antimicrobial Agents and Chemotherapy* 28 (2): 289–92.

Ingólfsdóttir, K., M. A. Hjalmarsdottir, A. Sigurdsson, et al. 1997. "In Vitro Susceptibility of *Helicobacter pylori* to Protolichesterinic Acid from the Lichen *Cetraria islandica*." *Antimicrobial Agents and Chemotherapy* 41 (1): 215–17.

Ingólfsdóttir, K., B. Wiedemann, M. Birgisdóttir, A. Nenninger, S. Jónsdóttir, and H. Wagner 1997a. "Inhibitory Effects of Baeomycesic Acid from the Lichen *Thamnolia subuliformis* on 5-lipogenase In Vitro." *Phytomedicine* 4 (2): 125–28.

Ingólfsdóttir, K., G. A. Chung, V. G. Skulason, S. R. Gissurarson, and M. Vihelmsdottir. 1998. "Antimycobacterial Activity of Lichen Metabolite In Vitro." *European Journal of Pharmaceutical Sciences* 6 (2): 141–44.

Ingólfsdóttir, K., S. K. Lee, K. P. L. Bhat, K. J. Lee, H. B. Chai, and H. Kristinsson. 2000. "Evaluation of Selected Lichens from Iceland for Cancer Chemo-preventive and Cytotoxic Activity." *Pharmaceutical Biology* 38 (4): 313–17.

Ingólfsdóttir, K. 2002. "Usnic Acid." *Phytochemistry* 61 (7): 729–36.

Ingólfsdóttir, K., G. F. Gudmundsdóttir, H. M. Ogmundsdóttir, K. Paulus, S. Haraldsdóttir, H. Kristinsson, and R. Bauer. 2002. "Effects of Tenuiorin and Methyl Orsellinate from the Lichen *Peltigera leucophlebia* on 5-/15-lipoxygenases and Proliferation of Malignant Cell Lines In Vitro." *Phytomedicine* 9 (7): 654–58.

Ivanova, V., M. Backor, H. M. Dahse, and U. Graefe. 2010. "Molecular Structural Studies of Lichen Substances with Antimicrobial, Antiproliferative and Cytotoxic Effects from *Parmelia subrudecta*." *Preparative Biochemisty and Biotechnology* 40 (4): 377–88.

Jain, A. P., S. Bhandarkar, G. Rai, A. K. Yadav, and S. Lodhi. 2016. "Evaluation of *Parmotrema reticulatum* Taylor for Antibacterial and Antiinflammatory Activities." *Indian Journal of Pharmaceutical Science* 78 (1): 94–102.

James, P. J. C., D. Vuong, S. A. Moggach, E. Lacey, and M. J. Piggott. 2023. "Synthesis, Characterization, and Biodiversity of the Lichen Pigments Pulvinamide, Rhizocarpic Acid, and Epanorin and Congeners." *Journal Natural Products* 86 (3): 550–56.

Jayaprakasha, G. K., and L. J. Rao. 2000. "Phenolic Constituents from the Lichen *Parmotrema stuppeum* (Nyl.) Hale and Their Antioxidant Activity." *Zeitschrift für Naturforschung Section C Journal of Biosciences* 55 (11–12): 1018–22.

Jeong, G. S., P. F. Hillman, M. G. Kang, et al. 2021. "Potent and Selective Inhibitors of Human Monoamine Oxidase A from an Endogenous Lichen Fungus *Diaporthe mahothocarpus*." *Journal of Fungi* (Basel) 7 (10): 876.

Jeong, M. H., C. H. Park, J. A. Kim, E. D. Chou, et al. 2021a. "Production and Activity of Cristazarin in the Lichen-Forming Fungus *Cladonia metaborallifera*." *Journal of Fungi* (Basel) 7 (8): 601.

Jha, B. N., M. Shrestha, D. P. Pandey, et al. 2017. "Investigation of Antioxidant, Antimicrobial and Toxicity Activity of Lichens from High Altitude Regions of Nepal." *BMC Complementary and Alternative Medicine* 17 (1): 1–8.

Ji, X. W., H. J. Lyu, G. H. Zhou, B. Wu, Y. Y. Zhu, et al. 2021. "Physcion, a Tetra-Substituted 9,10-anthraquinone, Prevents Homocysteine-Induced Endothelial Dysfunction by Activating Ca^{2+} and Akt-eNOS-NO Signaling Pathways." *Phytomedicine* 81: 153410.

Jiang, C. S., L. F. Liang, and Y. W. Guo. 2012. "Natural Products Possessing Protein Tyrosine Phosphatase IB (PTP1B) Inhibitory Activity Found in the Last Decades." *Acta Pharmacologica Sinica* 33 (10): 1217–45.

Jin, J., X. Bian, P. Ge, H. Jing, L. Ding, and D. Ding. 2001. "The Effects of the Polysaccharides from *Dermatocarpon miniatum* on Oxygen Radicals and Lipid Peroxidation." *Zhong Yao Cai* 24 (9): 660–61.

Jóhannsson, F., P. Cherek, M. Xu, O. Rolfsson, and H. M. Ögmundsdóttir. 2022. "The Anti-proliferative Lichen-Compound Protolichesterinic Acid Inhibits Oxidative Phosphorylation and Is Processed via the Mercapturic Pathway in Cancer Cells." *Planta Medica* 88 (11): 891–98.

Johnson, C. J., J. P. Bennett, S. M. Biro, J. C. Duque-Velasquez, C. M. Rodriguez, R. A. Bessen, and T. E. Rocke. 2011. "Degradation of the Disease-Associated Prion Protein by a Serine Protease from Lichens." *PLoS ONE* 6 (5): e19836.

Johnson, L. M. 1997. "Health, Wholeness and the Land: Gitksan Traditional Plant Use and Healing." PhD thesis, University of Alberta.

Joo, Y. A., H. J. Chung, S. Y. Yoon, J. Park, J. E. Lee, C. H. Myung, and J. S. Hwang. 2016. "Skin Barrier Recovery by Protease-Activated Receptor-2 Antagonist Lobaric Acid." *Biomolecules and Therapeutics* (Seoul) 24 (5): 529–35.

Joshi, C., A. Chaudhari, C. Joshi, M. Joshi, and S. Bagatharia. 2022. "Repurposing of the Herbal Formulations: Molecular Docking and Molecular Dynamics Simulation Studies to Validate the Efficacy of Phytocompounds against SARS-CoV-2 Proteins." *Journal of Biomolecular Structure and Dynamics* 40 (18): 8405–19.

Joshi, T, P. Sharma, T. Joshi, H. Pundir, S. Mathpal, and S. Chandra. 2020. "Structure-Based Screening of Novel Lichen Compounds for SARS Coronavirus Main Protease (Mpro) and

Angiotensin-Converting Enzyme 2 (ACE2) Inhibitory Potentials as Multi-target Inhibitors of COVID-19." *Research Square* 25 (3): 1665–77.

Joshi, Y., K. Knudsen, X. Y. Wang, and J. S. Hur. 2010. "*Dactylospora glaucomariodes* (Ascomycetes, Dactylosporaceae): A Lichenicolous Fungus New to South Korea." *Mycobiology* 38 (4): 321–22.

Kaasalainen, U., D. P Fewer, J. Jokela, et al. 2012. "Cyanobacteria Produce a High Variety of Hepatotoxic Peptides in Lichen Symbiosis." *Proceedings of the National Academy of Sciences* 109 (15): 5886–91.

Kalin, S. N., A. Altay, and H. Budak. 2022. "Diffractaic Acid, a Novel TrxR1 Inhibitor, Induces Cytotoxicity, Apoptosis and Antimigration in Human Breast Cancer Cells." *Chemico-Biological Interactions* 361: 109984.

Kalin, S. N., A. Altay, and H. Budak. 2022a. "Inhibition of Thioredoxin Reductase 1 by Vulpinic Acid Suppresses the Proliferation and Migration of Human Breast Carcinoma." *Life Sciences* 310: 121093.

Kalin, S. N., A. Altay, and H. Budak. 2023. "Effect of Evernic Acid on Human Breast Cancer MCF-7 and MDA-MB-453 Cell Lines via Thioredoxin Reductase 1: A Molecular Approach." *Journal of Applied Toxicology.* 43 (8): 1148–58.

Kamath, V., C. N. Kyathanahalli, B. Jayaram, I. Syed, et al. 2010. "Regulation of Glucose and Mitochondrial Fuel-Induced Insulin Secretion by a Cytosolic Protein Histidine Phosphatase in Pancreatic ß-Cells." *American Journal of Physiology-Endocrinology Metabolism* 299 (2): E276–E286.

Kamei, H., T. Koide, Y. Hashimoto, T. Kojima, M. Hasegawa, and T. Umeda. 1997. "Effect of Allomelanin on Tumor Growth Suppression In Vivo and on the Cell Cycle Phase." *Cancer Biotherapy and Radiopharmaceuticals* 12 (4): 273–76.

Kang, T. R., J. N. Dinga, A. E. Orock, E. Monya, and M. N. Ngemenya. 2022. "Macrofilaricidal Activity, Acute and Biochemical Effects of Three Lichen Species Found on Mount Cameroon." *Journal of Parasitology Research* 2022: 1663330.

Karagoz, A., and A. Aslan. 2005. "Antiviral and Cytotoxic Activity of Some Lichen Extracts." *Biologica* 60 (3): 281–86.

Karagoz, I. D., M. Ozaslan, L. Guler, C. Uyar, and A. Cakir. 2014. "In Vivo Antitumoral Effect of Diffractaic Acid from Lichen Metabolites on Swiss Abino Mice with Ehrlich Ascites Carcinoma: An Experimental Study." *International Journal of Pharmacology* 10 (6): 307–14.

Karagoz, I. D., M. Ozaslan, I. H. Kilic, et al. 2015. "Hepatoprotective Effect of Diffractaic Acid on Carbon Tetrachloride-Induced Liver Damage in Rats." *Biotechnology and Biotechnological Equipment* 29 (5): 1011–16.

Karagoz, Y., K. Karagoz, F. Dadasoglu, and B. Ozturkkaragoz. 2018. "Extract Fractions Have Potent Antimicrobial Activity in Liquid—But Not in Solid Media." *Fresenius Environmental Bulletin and Advances in Food Sciences* 27 (6): 4293–97.

Karakus, B., F. Odabasoglu, A. Cakir, Z. Halici, et al. 2009. "The Effects of Methanol Extract of *Lobaria pulmonaria*, a Lichen Species, on Indomethacin-Induced Gastric Mucosal Damage, Oxidative Stress and Neutrophil Infiltration." *Phytotherapy Research* 23 (5): 635–39.

Kari, P. R. 1987. *Tanaina Plantlore*. Anchorage: US National Park Service.

Kathirgamanathar, S., W. D. Ratnasooriya, P. Baekstrom, R. J. Andersen, and V. Karunaratne. 2006. "Chemistry and Bioactivity of Physciaceae Lichens *Pyxine consocians* and *Heterodermia leucomelos*." *Pharmaceutical Biology* 44 (3): 217–20.

Katz, L., and R. H. Baltz. 2016. "Natural Product Discovery: Past, Present, and Future." *Journal of Industrial Microbiology and Biotechnology* 43 (2–3): 155–76.

Kay, M. S. 1995. "Environmental, Cultural, and Linguistic Factors Affecting Ulkatcho (Carrier) Botanical Knowledge." MSc thesis, University of Victoria.

Keane, K., and D. Howarth. 2003. *The Standing People*. Saskatoon, SK: The Root Woman and Dave.

Kello, M., T. Kuruc, K. Petrova, M. Goga, Z. Michalova, M. Coma, D. Rucova, and J. Mojzis. 2021. "Pro-Apoptotic Potential of *Pseudevernia furfuracea* (L.) *Zopf* Extract and Isolated Physodic Acid in Acute Lymphoblastic Leukemia Model In Vitro." *Pharmaceutics* 13 (12): 2173.

Kempe, C., H. Grüning, et al. 1997. "Iceland Moss Lozenges in the Prevention or Treatment of Oral Mucosa Irritation and Dried out Throat Mucosa." *Laryngorhinootologie* 76 (3): 186–88.

Kerik, J. 1981. *Living with the Land: Use of Plants by the Native People of Alberta*. Alberta Culture Circulating Exhibits Program, National Museums of Canada Fund, Provincial Museum of Alberta.

Kershengolts, B. M., L. A. Sydykova, V. V. Sharoyko, V. V. Anshakova, A. V. Stepanova, and N. A. Varofolomeeva. 2015. "Lichens' B-Oligosaccharides in the Correction of Metabolic Disorders in Type 2 Diabetes Mellitus." *Wiadomosci Lekarskie* 68 (4): 480–82.

Khanra, R., N. Bhattacharjee, T. K. Dua, A. Nandy, et al. 2017. "Taraxerol, a Pentacyclic Triterpenoid, from *Abroma augusta* Leaf Attenuates Diabetic Nephropathy in Type 2 Diabetic Rats." *Biomedicine and Pharmacotherapy* 94: 726–41.

Kharrazian, D. 2013. *Why Isn't My Brain Working?* Carlsbad, CA: Elephant Press.

Kilic, N., S. Aras, and D. Cansaran-Duman. 2018. "Determination of Vulpinic Acid Effect on Apoptosis and mRNA Expression Levels in Breast Cancer Cell Lines." *Anticancer Agents in Medicinal Chemistry* 18 (14): 2032–41.

Kilic, N., Y. O. Islakoglu, I. Büyük, B. Gur-Dedeoglu, and D. Cansaran-Duman. 2019. "Determination of Usnic Acid Responsive miRNAs in Breast Cancer Cell Lines." *Anticancer Agents in Medicinal Chemistry* 19 (12): 1463–72.

Kim, J. E., S. K. Min, J. M. Hong, K. H. Kim, S. J. Han, J. H. Yim, H. Park, and I. C. Kim. 2020. "Anti-inflammatory Effects of Methanol Extracts from the Antarctic Lichen, *Amandinea* sp. in LPS-Stimulated Raw 264.7 Macrophages and Zebrafish." *Fish and Shellfish Immunology* 107 (part A): 301–8.

Kim, K. J., M. H. Jeong, Y. J. Lee, S. J. Hwang, et al. 2018. "Effect of Usnic Acid on Osteoclastogenic Activity." *Journal of Clinical Medicine* 7 (10): 345.

Kim, K. J., Y. J. Lee, M. H. Jeong, J. S. Hur, and Y. J. Son. 2019. "Extracts of *Flavoparmelia* sp. Inhibit Receptor Activator of Nuclear Factor-$_k$B Ligand-Mediated Osteoclast Differentiation." *Journal of Bone Metabolism* 26 (2): 113–21.

Kim, M. K., H. Park, and T. J. Oh. 2014. "Antibacterial and Antioxidant Capacity of Polar Microorganisms Isolated from Arctic Lichen *Ochrolechia* sp." *Polish Journal of Microbiology* 63 (3): 317–22.

Kinoshita, K., M. Fukumaru. Y. Yamamot, K. Koyama, and K. Takahashi. 2015. "Biosynthesis of Panaefluoroline B from the Cultured Mycobiont of *Amygdalaria panaeola*." *Journal of Natural Products* 78 (7): 1745–47.

Kizil, H. E., G. Agar, and M. Anar. 2014. "Cytotoxic and Antiproliferative Effects of Evernic Acid on HeLa Cell Lines. A Candidate Anticancer Drug." *Journal of Biotechnology* 185: S29.

Kizil, H. E., G. Agar, and M. Anar. 2015. "Antiproliferative Effects of Evernic Acid on A549 and Healthy Human Cells: An In Vitro Study." *Journal of Biotechnology* 208: S28.

Koparal, A. T., G. Ulus, M. Zeytinoglu, T. Tay, and A. O. Türk. 2010. "Angiogenesis Inhibition by a Lichen Compound Olivetoric Acid." *Phytotherapy Research* 24 (5): 754–58.

Koparal, A. T. 2015. "Anti-angiogenic and Antiproliferative Properties of the Lichen Substances (-)-Usnic Acid and Vulpinic Acid." *Zeitschrift für Naturforschung Section C Journal of Biosciences* 70 (5–6): 159–64.

Kosanic, M., B. Rankovic, and J. Vukojevic. 2011. "Antioxidant Properties of Some Lichen Species." *Journal of Food Science and Technology* 48 (5): 584–90.

Kosanic, M. M., B. R. Rankovic, and T. P. Stanojkovic. 2012. "Antioxidant, Antimicrobial and Anticancer Activities of Three *Parmelia* Species." *Journal of the Science of Food and Agriculture* 92 (9): 1909–16.

Kosanic, M., N. Manojlovic, S. Jankovic, T. Stanojkovic, and B. Rankovic. 2013. "*Evernia prunastri* and *Pseudoevernia furfuraceae* Lichens and Their Major Metabolites as Antioxidant, Antimicrobial and Anticancer Agents." *Food and Chemistry Toxicology* 53: 112–18.

Kosanic, M., B. Rankovic, T. Stanojkovic, P. Vasiljevic, and N. Manojlovic. 2014. "Biological Activities and Chemical Composition of Lichens from Serbia." *Experimental and Clinical Services Journal* 13: 1226–38.

Kosanic, M., B. Rankovic, T. Stanojkovic, I. Stosic, D. Grujicic, and O. Milosevic-Djordjevic. 2016. "*Lasallia pustulata* Lichen as Possible Natural Antigenotoxic, Antioxidant, Antimicrobial and Anticancer Agent." *Cytotechnology* 68 (4): 999–1008.

Kosanic, M. 2018. "Extracts of Five *Cladonia* Lichens as Sources of Biologically Active Compounds." *Farmacia* 66: 644–51.

Kovácik, J., L. Husáková, M. Piroutková, and P. Babula. 2023. "Mercury Content and Amelioration of Its Toxicity by Nitric Oxide in Lichens." *Plants* (Basel) 12 (4): 727.

Kowluru, A., S. Klumpp, and J. Kriegistein. 2011. "Protein Histidine [De]phosphorylation in Insulin Secretion: Abnormalities in Models of Impaired Insulin Secretion." *Nauyn-Schmiedeberg's Archives of Pharmacology* 384 (4–5): 383–90.

Krajka-Kuzniak, V. and W. Baer-Dubowska. 2021. "Modulation of Nrf2 and NF-kB Signaling Pathways by Naturally Occurring Compounds in Relation to Cancer Prevention and Therapy. Are Combinations Better Than Single Compounds?" *International Journal of Molecular Sciences* 22 (15): 8223.

Kumar, J., P. Dhar, A. B. Tayade, D. Gupta, O. P. Chaurasia, D. K. Upreti, R. Arora, and R. B. Srivastava. 2014. "Antioxidant Capacities, Phenolic Profile and Cytotoxic Effects of Saxicolous Lichens from Trans-Himalayan Cold Desert of Ladakh." *PLos ONE* 9 (6): e98696.

Kumar, K., J. P. N. Mishra, and R. P. Singh. 2020a. "Usnic Acid Induces Apoptosis in Human Gastric Cancer Cells through ROS Generation and DNA Damage and Causes Up-Regulation of dna-pkcs and y-h2a. X Phosphorylation." *Chemico-Biologica Interaction* 315: 108898.

Kumar, K. C. S., and K. Müller. 1999. "Lichen Metabolites.2. Antiproliferative and Cytotoxic Activity of Gyrophoric, Usnic and Diffractaic Acid on Human Keratinocyte Growth." *Journal of Natural Products* 62 (6): 821–23.

Kumar, S. N., and C. Mohandas. 2017. "An Antifungal Mechanism of Protolichesterinic Acid from the Lichen *Usnea albopunctata* Lies in the Accumulation of Intracellular ROS and Mitochrondria-Mediated Cell Death Due to Apoptosis in *Candida tropicalis*." *Frontiers in Pharmacology* 8: 882.

Kumar, P. P., B. Siva, A. Anand, A. K. Tiwari, C. V. Rao, J. Boustie, and K. S. Babu. 2020. "Isolation, Semi-synthesis, Free-Radicals Scavenging, and Advanced Glycation End Products Formation Inhibitory Constituents from *Parmotrema tinctorum*." *Journal of Asian Natural Products Research* 22 (10): 976–88.

Kumari, M., S. Kamat, S. K. Singh, A. Kumar, and C. Jayabaskaran. 2023. "Inhibition of Autophagy Increases Cell Death in HeLa Cells through Usnic Acid Isolated from Lichens." *Plants* (Basel) 12 (3): 519.

Kurskaya, O., E. Prokopyeva, H. T. Bi, I. Sobolev, T. Murashkina, A. Shestopalov, L. X. Wei, and K. Sharshov. 2022. "Anti-influenza Activity of Medicinal Material Extracts from Qinghai-Tibet Plateau." *Viruses* 14 (2): 360.

Kwanlin Dün First Nation. 2017. *Kwanlin Dün First Nation Traditional Territory Land Vision*. Whitehorse, Yukon: Kwanlin Dün First Nation Lands and Resources Department.

Kwong, S. P., and C. H. Wang. 2020. "Review: Usnic Acid-Induced Hepatotoxicity and Cell Death." *Environmental Toxicology and Pharmacology* 80: 103493.

Lage, T. C. A., L. P. Horta, R. M. Montanari, J. G. Silva, A. de Fatima, S. A. Fernandes, and L. V. Modolo. 2016. "Structural Elucidation and Free Radical Scavenging Activity of a New o-Orsellinic Acid Derivative Isolated from the Lichen *Cladonia rappii*." *Natural Product Communications* 11 (9): 1311–12.

Lai, D., D. C. Odimegwu, C. Esimone, T. Grunwald, and P. Proksch. 2013. "Phenolic Compounds with In Vitro Activity against Respiratory Syncytial Virus from the Nigerian Lichen *Ramalina farinacea*." *Planta Medica* 79 (15): 1440–46.

Lamont, S. M. 1977. "The Fisherman Lake Slave and Their Environment: A Story of Floral and Faunal Resources." MSc thesis, University of Saskatchewan, Canada.

Lao, Z. H., Y. H. Fan, Y. H. Huo, F. Liao, et al. 2022. "Physcion, a Novel Inhibitor of 5a-Reductase That Promotes Hair Growth In Vitro and In Vivo." *Archives of Dermatological Research* 314 (1): 41–51.

Lauinger, I. L., L. Vivas, R. Perozzo, et al. 2013. "Potential of Lichen Secondary Metabolites against *Plasmodium* Liver Stage Parasites with FAS-II as the Potential Target." *Journal Natural Products* 76 (6): 1064–70.

Lawrence, S. 2022. *The Magic of Mushrooms: Fungi in Folklore, Superstition and Traditional Medicine.* London: Wellbeck Publishing Group.

Lawrey. 1986. "Biological Role of Lichen Substances." *Bryologist* 89 (2): 111–22.

Laxinamujila, H. Y. Bao, and T. Bau. 2013. "Advance in Studies on Chemical Constituents and Pharmacological Activity of Lichens in *Usnea* Genus." *Zhongguo Zhong Yao Za Zhi* 38 (4): 539–45.

Le, D. H., Y. Takenaka, N. Hamada, and T. Tanahasi. 2013. "Eremophilane-Type Sesquiterpenes from Cultured Lichen Mycobionts of *Sarcographa tricosa*." *Phytochemistry* 91: 242–48.

Leal, A., J. L. Rojas, N. A. Valencia-Islas, and L. Castellanos. 2018. "New ß-Orcinol Depsides from *Hypotrachyna caraccensis*, a Lichen from the Paramo Ecosystem and Their Free Radical Scavenging Activity." *Natural Product Research* 32 (12): 1375–82.

Lee, H. W., J. W. Kim, J. H. Yim, H. K. Lee, and S. Pyo. 2019. "Anti-inflammatory Activity of Lobaric Acid via Suppressing NF-kB/MAPK Pathways or NLRP3 Inflammasome Activation." *Planta Medica* 85 (4): 302–11.

Lee, K., J. H. Kim, H. K. Lee, and S. Pyo. 2016. "Inhibition of VCAM-1 Expression on Mouse Vascular Smooth Muscle Cells by Lobastin via Downregulation of p38, ERK ½ and NF-kB Signaling Pathways." *Archives of Pharmacal Research* 39 (1): 83–93.

Lee, M. S., E. Y. Cha, J. Y. Sul, I. S. Song, and J. Y. Kim. 2011. "Chrysophanic Acid Blocks Proliferation of Colon Cancer Cells by Inhibiting EGFR/mTOR Pathway." *Phytotherapy Research* 25 (6): 833–37.

Lee, M. Y., C. E. Haam, J. Y. Mun, G. Lim, B. H. Lee, and K. S. Oh. 2021a. "Development of a FOXM1-DBD Binding Assay for High-Throughput Screening Using TR-FRET Assay." *Biological and Pharmaceutical Bulletin* 44 (10): 1484–91.

Lee, S., Y. J. Suh, S. Yang, D. G. Hong, et al. 2021. "Neuroprotective and Anti-inflammatory Effects of Evernic Acid in an MPTP-Induced Parkinson's Disease Model." *International Journal of Molecular Science* 22: 2098.

Legarde, A., M. Millot, A. Pinon, M. Girardot, C. Imbert, T. S. Ouk, P. Jargeat, and L. Mambu. 2018. "Antiproliferative and Antibiofilm Potential of Endolichenic Fungi Associated with the Lichen *Nephroma laevigatum*." *Journal of Applied Microbiology* 126 (4): 1044–58.

Legarde, A., L. Mambu, P. Y. Mai, Y. Champavier, J. L. Stigliani, M. A. Beniddir, and M. Millot. 2021. "Chlorinated Bianthrones from the Cyanolichen *Nephroma laevigatum*." *Fitoterapia* 149: 104811.

Legouin, B., F. L. Le-Dévéhat, S. Ferron, I. Rouaud, P. Le Pogam, L. Cornevin, M. Bertrand, and J. Boustie. 2017. "Specialized Metabolites of the Lichen *Vulpicida pinastri* Act as Photoprotective Agents." *Molecules* 22 (7): 1162.

Leighton, A. L. 1985. *Wild Plant Use by the Woods Cree (Nihithawak) of East-Central Saskatchewan.* Ottawa: National Museum of Man Mercury Series 101.

Lendemer, J. C., K. G. Keepers, E. A. Tripp, C. S. Pogoda, C. M. McCain, and N. C. Kane. 2019. "A Taxonomically Broad Metagenomic Survey of 339 Species Spanning 57 Families Suggests Cystobasidiomycete Yeasts Are not Ubiquitous across All Lichens." *American Journal of Botany* 106 (8): 1090–96.

Le Pogam, P., A. C. Le Lamer, B. Siva, B. Legouin, A. Bondon, J. Graton, et al. 2016a. "Minor Pyranonaphthoquinones from the Apothecia of the Lichen *Ophioparma ventosa.*" *Journal of Natural Products* 79 (4): 1005–11.

Le Pogam, P., B. Leqouin, A. Geairon, H. Rogniaux, et al. 2016. "Spatial Mapping of Lichen Specialized Metabolites Using LDI-MSI: Chemical Ecology Issues for *Ophioparma ventosa.*" *Scientific Reports* 6: 37807.

Le Pogam, P., and J. Boustie. 2016b. "Xanthones of Lichen Source: A 2016 Update." *Molecules* 21 (3): 294.

Letwin, L. S. 2017. "Biological Activities of Select North American Lichens." MSc thesis, Lakehead University.

Letwin, L., L. Malek, Z. Suntres, and L. Christopher. 2020. "Cytotoxic and Antibiotic Potential of Secondary Metabolites from the Lichen *Umbilicaria muhlenbergii.*" *Current Pharmaceutical Biotechnol*ogy 21 (14): 1516–27.

Leudtke, R. R., R. A. Freeman, M. W. Martin, et al. 2002. "Pharmacological Survey of Medicinal Plants for Activity at Dopamine Receptor Subtypes I. Activation of DI-Like Receptor Linked Adenylyl Cyclase." *Pharmaceutical Biology* 40 (4): 315–25.

Li, C., X. D. Guo, M. Lei, J. Y. Wu, J. Z. Jin, X. F. Shi, et al. 2017. "*Thamnolia vermicularis* Extract Improves Learning Ability in APP/PS$_1$ Transgenic Mice by Ameliorating Both Aβ and Tau Pathologies." *Acta Pharmacologica Sinica* 38 (1): 9–28.

Li, J. W., R. Ding, H. Gao, L. D. Guo, X. S. Yao, Y. W. Zhang, and J. S. Tang. 2019. "New Spirobisnaphthalenes from an Endolichenic Fungus Strain CGMCC 3.15192 and Their Anticancer Effects Through the P53-P21 Pathway." *RSC Advances* 9 (67): 39082–89.

Li, J., S. P. Jiang, C. Y. Huang, and X. L. Yang. 2022. "Atraric Acid Ameliorates Hyperpigmentation through the Downregulation of the PKA/CREB/MITF Signaling Pathway." *International Journal of Molecular Science* 23 (24): 15952.

Li, X. B., Y. H. Zhou, R. X. Zhu, W. Q. Chang, et al. 2015. "Identification and Biological Evaluation of Secondary Metabolites from the Endolichenic Fungus *Aspergillus versicolor.*" *Chemistry and Biodiversity* 12 (4): 575–92.

Liang, Z. B., A. Sorribas, F. J. Sulzmaier, J. I. Jiménez, X. Wang, et al. 2011. "Stictamides A-C, MMP12 Inhibitors Containing 4-amino-3-hydroxy-5-phenylpentanoic Acid Subunits." *Journal of Organic Chemistry* 76 (10): 3635–43.

Liao, G. Z., J. Zhou, H. Wang, Z. G. Mao, et al. 2010. "The Cell Toxicity Effect of Secalonic Acid D on GH3 Cells and the Related Mechanisms." *Oncology Reports* 23 (2): 387–95.

Liba, C. M., F. I. S. Ferrara, G. P. Manfio, et al. 2006. "Nitrogen-Fixing Chemo-organotrophic Bacteria Isolated from Cyanobacteria-Deprived Lichens and Their Ability to Solubilize Phosphate and to Release Amino Acids and Phytohormones." *Journal of Applied Microbiology* 101 (5): 1076–86.

Liberman, D. F., F. L. Schaefer, R. C. Fink, M. Ramgopal, A. C. Ghosh, and R. Mulcahy. 1980. "Mutagenicity of Islandicin and Chrysophanol in the *Salmonella* Microsome System." *Applied and Environmental Microbiology* 40 (3): 476–79.

Liers, C., R. Ullrich, M. Hofrichter, F. V. Minibayeva, and R. P. Beckett. 2011. "A Heme Peroxidase of the Ascomyceteous Lichen *Leptogium saturninum* Oxidizes High-Redox Potential Substrates." *Fungal Genetics and Biology* 48 (12): 1139–45.

Lim, E. H., S. K. Mun, J. J. Kim, D. J. Chang, and S. T. Yee. 2022. "Anti-inflammatory Effects of *Phlebia* sp. Extract in Lipopolysaccharide-Stimulated RAW 264.7 Macrophages." *BioMed Research International* 2022: 2727296.

Lin, X., Y. J. Cai, Z. X. Li, et al. 2001. "*Cladonia furcate* Polysaccharide Induced Apoptosis in Human Leukemia K562 Cells." *Acta Pharmacologica Sinica* 22 (8): 716–20.

Lin, X., Y. J. Cai, Z. X. Li, et al. 2003. "Structure Determination, Apoptosis Induction, and Telomerase Inhibition of CFP-2, a Novel Lichenin from *Cladonia furcate*." *Biochimica et Biophysica Acta* 1622 (2): 99–108.

Liu, K., Y. K. Zheng, C. P. Miao, Z. J. Xiong, L. H. Xu, et al. 2014. "The Antifungal Metabolites Obtained from the Rhizospheric *Aspergillus* sp. YIM PH30001 against Pathogenic Fungi of *Panax notoginseng*." *Natural Product Research* 28 (24): 2334–37.

Liu, X. Y., H. L. Hu, J. Q. Liu, J. Q. Chen, et al. 2023. "Physcion, a Novel Anthraquinone Derivative against *Chlamydia psittaci* Infection." *Veterinary Microbiology* 279: 109664.

Liu, Y. Q., X. Y. Hu, T. Lu, et al. 2012. "Retigeric Acid B Exhibits Antitumor Activity through Suppression of Nuclear Factor-k_b Signaling in Prostate Cancer Cells In Vitro and In Vivo." *PLoS ONE* 7 (5): e38000.

Liu, Y. Q., Y. Ji, X. Z. Li, K. L. Tian, et al. 2013. "Retigeric Acid B-Induced Mitophagy by Oxidative Stress Attenuates Cell Death against Prostate Cancer Cells In Vitro." *Acta Pharmacologica Sinica* 34: 1183–91.

Liu, Y. Q., C. W. Yue, J. Li, J. Wu, S. K. Wang, D. Q. Sun, et al. 2018. "Enhancement of Cisplatin Cytotoxicity by Retigeric Acid B Involves Blocking DNA Repair and Activating DR5 in Prostate Cancer Cells." *Oncology Letters* 15 (3): 2871–80.

Liu, Y., S. Wu, Q. Zhao, Z. Yang, X. J. Yan, C. R. Li, W. L. Zha, and W. Yu. 2021. "Trehalose Ameliorates Diabetic Cardiomyopathy: Role of the PK2/PKR Pathway." *Oxidative Medicine and Cellular Longevity.* 2021: 6779559.

Liu, Z., B. Delavan, R. Roberts, and W. Tong. 2017. "Lessons Learned from Two Decades of Anticancer Drugs." *Trends in Pharmacological Sciences* 38 (10): 852–72.

Llano, G. A. 1951. *Economic Uses of Lichens*. Annual Report of the Smithsonian Institute Volume 385–422.

Loeanurit, N., T. L. Tuong, V. K. Nguyen, V. Vibulakhaophan, et al. 2023. "Lichen-Derived Diffractic Acid Inhibited Dengue Virus Replication in a Cell-Based System." *Molecules* 28 (3): 974.

Lohévic-Le Dévéhat, F., B. Legouin, C. Couteau, J. Boustie, and L. Coiffard. 2013. "Lichenic Extracts and Metabolites as UV Filters." *Journal of Photochemistry and Photobiology B* 120: 17–28.

Loosley, B. C., R. J. Andersen, and G. R. Dake. 2013. "Total Synthesis of Cladoniamide G." *Organic Letters* 15 (5): 1152–54.

Lopandic, K., O. Molnár, and H. Prillinger. 2005. "*Fellomyces mexicanus* sp. nov., a New Member of the Yeast Genus *Fellomyces* Isolated from Lichen *Cryptothecia rubrocincta* Collected in Mexico." *Microbiological Research* 160 (1): 1–11.

Lu, P., C. H. Zhang, L. M. Lifshitz, R. ZhuGe. 2017. "Extraoral Bitter Taste Receptors in Health and Disease." *Journal of General Physiology* 149 (2): 181–97.

Lu, Y., S. J. Suh, X. Li, S. L. Hwang, Y. Li, Y. Hwangbo, et al. 2012. "Citreorosein, a Naturally Occurring Anthraquinone Derivative Isolated from *Polygoni cuspidate radix*, Attenuates Cyclooxygenase-2-Dependent Prostaglandin D2 Generation by Blocking Akt and JNK Pathways in Mouse Bone Marrow-Derived Mast Cells." *Food and Chemical Toxicology* 50 (3–4): 913–19.

Lu. Y., Y. Li, Y. D. Jahng, J. K. Son, and H. W. Chang. 2012a. "Citreosein Inhibits Degranulation and Leukotriene C$_4$ Generation through Suppression of Syk Pathway in Mast Cells." *Molecular and Cellular Biochemistry* 365 (1–2): 333–41.

Lücking, R., and T. Spribille. 2024. *The Lives of Lichens.* Princeton University Press.

Lucarini, R., M. G. Tozatii, A. I. de Oliveira Salloum, et al. 2012. "Antimycobacterial Activity of *Usnea steineri* and Its Major Constituent (+)-Usnic Acid." *African Journal of Biotechnology* 11 (20): 4636–39.

Luo, H., C. T. Li, J. C. Kim, Y. P. Liu, J. S. Jung, et al. 2013. "Biruloquinone, an Acetylcholinesterase Inhibitor Produced by Lichen-Forming Fungus *Cladonia macilenta*." *Journal of Microbiology and Biotechnology* 23 (2): 161–66.

Luo, N., J. Fang, L. Q. Wei, M. Sahebkar, P. J. Little, et al. 2021. "Emodin in Atherosclerosis Prevention: Pharmacological Actions and Therapeutic Potential." *European Journal of Pharmacology* 890: 173617.

Mahrosh, H. S., and G. Mustafa. 2021. "An In Silico Approach to Target RNA-Dependent RNA Polymerase of COVID-19 with Naturally Occurring Phytochemicals." *Environment, Development and Sustainability* 23 (11): 16674–87.

Maier, M. S., M. L. Rosso, A. T. Fazio, M. T. Adler, and M. D. Bertoni. 2009. "Fernene Triterpenoids from the Lichen *Pyxine berteriana*." *Journal of Natural Products* 72 (10): 1902–4.

Majchrzak-Celinska, A., R. Kleszcz, E. Studzinska-Sroka, A. Kukaszyk, A. Szoszkiewicz, E. Stelcer, et al. 2022. "Lichen Secondary Metabolites Inhibit the Wnt/ß-Catenin Pathway in Glioblastoma Cells and Improve the Anticancer Effects of Temozolomide." *Cells* 11 (7): 1084.

Malekinejad, F., F. Kheradmand, M. H. Khadem-Ansari, and H. Malekinejad. 2022. "Lupeol Synergizes with Doxorubicin to Induce Anti-proliferative and Apoptotic Effects on Breast Cancer Cells." *DARU* 30 (1): 103–15.

Malo, M. E., C. Frank, E. Khokhoev, A. Gorbunov, A. Dontsov, et al. 2022. "Mitigating Effects of Sublethal and Lethal Whole-Body Gamma Irradiation in a Mouse Model with Soluble Melanin." *Journal of Radiological Protection* 42 (1).

Mammadov, R., B. Suleyman, D. Altuner, E. Demirci, et al. 2019. "Effect of Ethyl Acetate

Extract of *Usnea longissima* on Esophagogastric Adenocarcinoma in Rats." *Acta Cirugica Brasileira* 34 (3): e201900305.

Manojlovic, N. T., S. Solujic, and M. Milosev. 2005. "Antifungal activity of *Rubia tinctorum, Rhamnus frangula* and *Caloplaca cerina. Fitoterapia.*" 76 (2): 244–46.

Manojlovic, N. T., P. J. Vasiljevic, P. Z. Maskovic, M. Juskovic, and G. Bogdanovic-Dusanovic. 2012. "Chemical Composition, Antioxidant, and Antimicrobial Activities of Lichen *Umbilicaria cylindrica* (L.) Delise (Umbilicariaceae)." *Evidence Based Complementary and Alternative Medicine* 2021: 452431.

Manojlovic, N., A. B. Rancic, R. Décor, P. Vasiljevic, and J. Tomovic. 2021. "Determination of Chemical Composition and Antimicrobial, Antioxidant and Cytotoxic Activities of Lichens *Parmelia conspera* and *Parmelia perlata.*" *Journal of Food Measurement and Characterization* 15 (1): 686–96.

Mansour, A. G., E. Hariri, Y. Daaboul, S. Korjian, et al. 2017. "Vitamin K2 Supplementation and Arterial Stiffness among Renal Transplant Recipients—A Single-Arm, Single-Center Clinical Trial." *Journal of the American Society of Hypertension* 11 (9): 589–97.

Mapari, S., S. Gaikwad, R. Khare, M. Syed, P. Doshi, and B. C. Behera. 2021. "Neuroprotective Potential of Selected Lichen Compounds on Mouse Neuroblastoma (N2a) Cells." *EXCLI Journal* 20: 491–94.

Maqbul, M. S., H. M. B. Alhasel, and D. H. Majid. 2019. "Chemical Analysis (GC-FID-MS) and Antimicrobial Activity of *Parmotrema perlatum* Essential Oil against Clinical Specimens." *Oriental Journal of Chemistry* 35 (6): 1695–701.

Margesin, R., F. Schinner, J. C. Marx, and C. Gerday. eds. 2008. "Arctic lichens may be 3700–9000 years old while Antarctic crypto-endoliths and microbes trapped in glacial ice have carbon turn-over times of 10,000 and 100,000 years." *Psychophiles: From Biodiversity to Biotechnology.* Berlin: Springer-Verlag, 25.

Marinaccio, L., A. Stefanucci, G. Scioli, A. D. Valle, et al. 2022. "Peptide Human Neutrophil Elastase Inhibitors from Natural Sources: An Overview." *International Journal of Molecular Sciences* 23: 2924.

Marles, R. 2000. "The Ethnobotany of the Chipewyan of Northern Saskatchewan." MSc thesis, University of Saskatchewan.

Marles, R., C. Clavelle, L. Monteleone, N. Tays, and D. Burns. 2000. *Aboriginal Plant Use in Canada's Northwest Boreal Forest.* Natural Resources Canada. Vancouver: University of British Columbia Press.

Marque, J. M. M. 2019. *Anticancer Activity of Lichen Substances: A Systematic Review.* Porto: Faculdade de Ciências da Saúde, Universidade Fernando Pessoa.

Marshall, A. G. 1977. "Nez Perce Social Groups: An Ecological Interpretation." PhD thesis, Washington State University.

Martins, M. C., R. S. Lopes, P. S. Barbosa, et al. 2018. "Effects of Usnic, Barbatic and Fumarprotocetraric Acid on Survival of *Nasutitermes corniger* (Isoptera: Termitidae: Nasutitermitinae)." *Sociobiology* 65 (1): 79–87.

Mathey, A., P. Spiteller, and W. Steglich. 2002. "Draculone, a New Anthraquinone Pigment from the Tropical Lichen *Melanotheca cruenta*." *Zeitschrift fur Naturforschung Section C Journal of Bioscience* 57 (7–8): 565–67.

Matias-Valiente, L., C. Sanchez-Fernandez, L. Rodriguez-Outeiriño, et al. 2024. "Evaluation of Pro-regenerative and Anti-inflammatory Effects of Isolecanoric Acid in the Muscle: Potential Treatment of Duchenne Muscular Dystrophy." *Biomedicine and Pharmacotherapy* 170: 116056.

Mattoo, R. 2021. "Targeting Emerging *Mycobacterium avium* Infections: Perspectives into Pathways and Antimicrobials for Future Interventions." *Future Microbiology* 16: 753–64.

Maulidiyah, M., A. Darmawan, A. Hasan, et al. 2020. "Isolation, Structure Elucidation, and Antidiabetic Test of Vicanicin Compound from the Lichen *Teloschistes flavicans*." *Journal of Applied Pharmacology* 10 (11): 1–9.

Maulidiyah, M., A. Darmawan, W. Wahyu, A. Musdalifah, La O. A. Salim, and M. Nurdin. 2022. "Potential of Usnic Acid Compound from Lichen Genus *Usnea* sp. as Antidiabetic Agents." *Journal of Oleo Science* 71 (1): 127–34.

McClintock, W. 1910. *The Old North Trail.* London: MacMillan Publishers.

McCoy, P. 2016. *Radical Mycology: A Treatise on Seeing and Working with Fungi.* Portland, OR: Chthaeus Press. 139.

McDonald, S. J., B. N. VanderVeen, K. T. Velazquez, R. T. Enos, et al. 2022. "Therapeutic Potential of Emodin for Gastrointestinal Cancers." *Integrated Cancer Therapies* 21: e15347354211067469.

McGillick, B. E., D. Kumuran, C. Vieni, and S. Swaminathan. 2016. "ß-Hydroxyacl-acyl Carrier Protein Dehydratase (FabZ) from *Francisella tularensis* and *Yersinia pestis*: Structure Determination, Enzymatic Characterization, and Cross-Inhibition Studies." *Biochemistry* 55 (7): 1091–99.

McGinnis, M. W., Z. M. Parker, N. E. Walter, et al. 2009. "Spermidine Regulates *Vibrio cholera* Biofilm Formation via Transport and Signaling Pathways." *FEMS Microbiological Letters* 299: 166–74.

McKenna, R. A. 1959. "The Upper Tanana Indians." *Yale University Publications in Anthropology* 55: 1–226.

Mead, G. R. 1972. *The Ethnobotany of the California Indians: A Compendium of the Plants, Their Users and Their Uses.* Museum of Anthropology. Greenley, CO: University of Northern Colorado.

Melo, M. G., A. A. Araújo, C. P Rocha, et al. 2008. "Purification, Physiochemical Properties, Thermal Analysis and Antinociceptive Effect of Atranorin Extract from *Cladina kalbi*." *Biological and Pharmaceutical Bulletin* 31: 1977–80.

Mendili, M., B. Essghaier, M. R. D. Seaward, and A. Khadhri. 2021. "In Vitro Evaluation of Lysozyme Activity and Antimicrobial Effect of Extracts from Four Tunisian Lichens: *Diploschistes ocellatus*, *Flavoparmelia caperata*, *Squamarina cartilaginea* and *Xanthoria parietina*." *Archives of Microbiology* 203 (4): 1461–69.

Mendili, M., M. Bannour, M. E. M Araújo, M. R. D. Seaward, and A. Khadhri. 2021a.

"Lichenochemical Screening and Antioxidant Capacity of Four Tunisian Lichen Species." *Chemistry and Biodiversity* 18 (2): e2000735.

Merges, D., F. D. Grande, C. Greve, J. Otte, and I. Schmitt. 2021. "Virus Diversity in Metagenomes of a Lichen Symbiosis (*Umbilicaria phaea*): Complete Viral Genomes, Putative Hosts and Elevational Distributions." *Environmental Microbiology* 23 (11): 6637–50.

Merriam, C. H. 1966. *Ethnographic Notes on California Indian Tribes*. Berkeley: University of California Archeological Research Facility.

Meza-Menchaca, T., A. Ramos-Ligonio, A. López-Monteon, et al. 2019. "Insights into Ergosterol Peroxide's Trypanocidal Activity." *Biomolecules* 9 (9): 484.

Micheletti, A. N. Honda, F. Pavan, et al. 2013. "Increment of Antimycobacterial Activity of Lichexanthone Derivatives." *Medicinal Chemistry* 9 (7): 904–10.

Micheletti, A. C., N. K. Honda, I. M. Ravaglia, T. Matayoshi, and A. A. Spielmann. 2021. "Antibacterial Potential of 12 Lichen Species." *Anais da Academia Brasileira Ciências* 93 (4).

Millot, M., S. Tomasi, E. Studzinska, I. Rouaud, and J. Boustie. 2009. "Cytotoxic Constituents of the Lichen *Diploicia canescens*." *Journal of Natural Products* 72 (12): 2177–80.

Millot, M., F. Di Meo, S. Tomasi, J. Boustie, and P. Trouillas. 2012. "Photoprotective Capacities of Lichen Metabolites: A Joint Theoretical and Experimental Study." *Journal of Photochemistry and Photobiology B* 111: 17–26.

Miquez, F., U. Schiefelbein, U. Karsten, J. I. Garcia-Plazaola, and L. Gustavs. 2017. "Unraveling the Photoprotective Response of Lichenized and Free-Living Green Algae (Trebouxiophyceae, Chlorophyta) to Photochilling Stress." *Frontiers in Plant Science* 8: 1144.

Miral, A., A. Kautsky, S. Alves-Carvalho, L. Cottret, et al. 2022. "*Rhizocarpon geographicum* Lichen Discloses a Highly Diversified Microbiota Carrying Antibiotic Resistance and Persistent Organic Pollutant Tolerance." *Microorganisms* 10 (9): 1859.

Miral, A, P. Jargeat, L. Mambu, I. Rouard, S. Tranchimand, and S. Tomasi. 2022a. "Microbial Community Associated with the Crustose Lichen *Rhizocarpon geographicum* L. (DC.) Living on Oceanic Seashore: A Large Source of Diversity Revealed by Using Multiple Isolation Methods." *Environmental Microbiology Reports* 14 (6): 856–72.

Miyagawa, H., N. Hamada, M. Sato, and T. Ueno. 1994. "Pigments from the Cultured Lichen Mycobionts of *Graphis script* and *G. Desquamescens*." *Phytochemistry* 36 (5): 1319–22.

Moerman, D. E. 2010. *Native American Food Plants: An Ethnobotanical Dictionary*. Portland OR: Timber Press.

Mohamed, G. A., A. M. Omar, D. F. AlKharboush, M. A. Fallatah, et al. 2023. "Structure-Based Virtual Screening and Molecular Dynamics Simulation Assessments of Depsidones as Possible Selective Cannabinoid Receptor Type 2 Agonists." *Molecules* 28 (4): 1761.

Mohammadi, M. 2021. "Investigation on Anti-proliferative Effect of Gyrophoric Acid from the Lichen *Umbilicaria muhlenbergii* on Cancer Cells." Ph.D. diss., Lakehead University.

Mohammadi, M., L. Bagheri, A. Badreldin, P. Fatehi, et al. 2022. "Biological Effects of Gyrophoric Acid and Other Lichen Derived Metabolites, on Cell Proliferation, Apoptosis and Cell Signaling Pathways." *Chemico Biological Interactactions* 351: 109768.

Mohammed, G. 2002. *Catnip and Kerosene Grass: What Plants Teach Us about Life*. Sault Ste. Marie, Ontario: Candlenut Books.

Montoya, A., A. Estrada-Torres, and J. Caballero. "Comparative Ethnomycological Survey of Three Localities from La Malinche Vulcano, Mexico." *Journal of Ethnobiology and Ethnomedicine* 22 (1): 103–31.

Moreira, A. S. N., R. Braz-Filho, V. Mussi-Dias, and I. J. C. Vieira. 2015. "Chemistry and Biological Activity of *Ramalina* Lichenized Fungi." *Molecules* 20 (5): 8952–87.

Moreira, A. S. N., R. O. S. Fernandes, F. J. A. Lemos, et al. 2016. "Larvicidal Activity of *Ramalina usnea* Lichen against *Aedes aegypti*." *Revista Brasileira da Farmacognosia* 26: 530–32.

Moreno-Fuentes, A., E. Aguirre-Acosta, and L. Pérez-Ramírez. 2004. "Conocimientotradicional y cientifico de los hongos en el estado de Chihuahua." *México Etnobiologia* 4: 89–105.

Morita, H., T. Tsuchiya, K. Kishibe, S. Noya, M. Shiro, and Y. Hirasawa. 2009. "Antimitotic Activity of Lobaric Acid and a New Benzofuran, Sakisacaulon A from *Stereocaulon sasakii*." *Bioorganic and Medicinal Chemistry Letters* 19 (13): 3679–81.

Mourning Dove (Christine Quintasket). 1933. "How Coyote Happened to Make the Black Moss Food." In *Coyote Stories*, 119–25. Caldwell, ID: Caxton Press.

Mugas, M. L., G. Calvo, J. Marioni, M. Céspedes, F. Martinez, S. Vanzulli, et al. 2021. "Photosensitization of a Subcutaneous Tumour by the Natural Anthraquinone Parietin and Blue Light." *Scientific Reports* 11 (1): 23820.

Müh, U., M. Schuster, R. Heim, A. Singh, E. R. Olson, and E. P. Greenberg. 2006. "Novel *Pseudomonas aeruginosa* Quorum-Sensing Inhibitors Identified in an Ultra-High-Throughput Screen." *Antimicrobial Agents and Chemotherapy* 48: 4360–65.

Mun, S. K., K. Y. Kang, H. Y. Jang, Y. H. Hwang, S. G. Hong, S. J. Kim, H. W. Cho, D. J. Chang, J. S. Hur, and S. T. Yee. 2020. "Atratic Acid Exhibits Anti-inflammatory Effect in Lipopolysaccharide-Stimulated RAW264.7 Cells and Mouse Models." *International Journal of Molecular Sciences* 21 (19): 7070.

Murphey, E. V. A. 1959. *Indian Uses of Native Plants*. (3rd printing). Fort Bragg, CA: Mendocino County Historical Society.

Na-Cho Nyak Dun First Nation, J. Ritter, E. Hagar, and S. Peter. 2015. *Na-Cho Nyak Dun Northern Tutchone Dictionary*. Mayo, Yukon, Canada.

Nakayama, J., Y. Uemura, K. Nishiguchi, N. Yoshimura, Y. Igarashi, and K. Sonomoto. 2009. "Ambuic Acid Inhibits the Biosynthesis of Cyclic Peptide Quormones in Gram-Positive Bacteria." *Antimicrobial Agents and Chemotherapy* 53 (2): 580–86.

Nardemir, G., D. Yanmis, L. Alpsoy, M. Gulluce, G. Agar, and A. Aslan. 2015. "Genotoxic, Antigenotoxic and Antioxidant Properties of Methanol Extracts Obtained from *Peltigera horizontalis* and *Peltigera praetextata*." *Toxicology and Industrial Health* 31 (7): 602–13.

Nasti, T. H. and L. Timares. 2015. "MC1R, Eumelanin and Pheomelanin: Their Role in Determining the Susceptibility to Skin Cancer." *Photochemistry and Photobiology* 91 (1): 188–200.

Nayaka, S., D. K. Upreti, R. Khare. 2010. "*Acroscyphus*" (Singh, unpublished) in "Medicinal

Lichens of India." *Drugs from Plants* (P. C. Trivedi, ed.) p. 5 Avishkar Publishers, Distributors: Jaipur, India.

Nelsen, M. P., R. Lücking, C. K. Boyce, H. T. Lumbsch, and R. H. Ree. 2020. "No Support for the Emergence of Lichens Prior to the Evolution of Vascular Plants." *Gebiology* 18 (1): 3–13.

Nevitt, S. J., J. Thornton, C. S. Murray, and T. Dwyer. 2020. "Inhaled Mannitol for Cystic Fibrosis." *Cochrane Database of Systematic Reviews* 5 (5): CD008649.

Newcombe, C. F. 1897. *Unpublished Notes on Haida Plants.* C. F. Newcombe Accession 1897–1947, New York: Department of Anthropology (Belinda Kaye, Registrar for Loans and Archives), American Museum of Natural History.

Nguyen, H. T., H. Polimati, S. S. P. Annam, E. Okello, Q. M. Thai, T. Y. Vu, and V. B. Tatipamula. 2022. "Lobaric Acid Prevents the Adverse Effects of Tetramethrin on the Estrous Cycle of Female Albino Wistar Rats." *PloS ONE* 17 (7): e0269983.

Nguyen, T. B. L., O. Delalande, I. Rouaud, S. Ferron, Laura Chaillot, R. Pedeux, and S. Tomasi. 2018. "*Tert*-Butylphenolic Derivatives from *Paenibacillus odorifer*—A Case of Bioconversion." *Molecules* 23 (8): 1951.

Nguyen, T. T., S. Yoon, Y. Yang, H. B. Lee, S. Oh, M. H. Jeong, et al. 2014. "Lichen Secondary Metabolites in *Flavocetraria cucullata* Exhibit Anti-cancer Effects on Human Cancer Cells through the Induction of Apoptosis and Suppression of Tumorigenic Potentials." *PLoS ONE* 9 (8): e111676.

Nguyen, T. T., S. Nallapaty, G. S. N. K. Rao, S. T. Koneru, et al. 2021. "Evaluating the In Vitro Activity of Depsidones from *Usnea subfloridana* Stirton as Key Enzymes Involved in Inflammation and Gout." *Pharmaceutical Sciences* 27 (2): 291–96.

Nguyen, T. T., T. N. Q. Chau, H. M. Van, T. P. Quoc, et al. 2021. "A New Hopane Derivative from the Lichen *Dirinaria applanata*." 35 (7): 1167–71.

Nguyen, V. K., H. V. Nguyen-Si, A. P. Devi, et al. 2022. "Eumitrins F–H: Three New Xanthone Dimers from the Lichen *Usnea baileyi* and Their Biological Activities." *Natural Product Research* 37 (9): 1480–90.

Nguyen, V. K., P. S. N. Dong, H. V. Nguyen-Si, E. Sangvichien, et al. 2023. "Eumitrins I–K: Three New Xanthone Dimers from the Lichen *Usnea baileyi*." *Journal of Natural Medicine* 77 (2): 403–11.

Nishanth, K. S., R. S. Sreerag, I. Deepa, C. Mohandas, and B. Nambisan. 2015. "Protocetraric Acid: An Excellent Broad-Spectrum Compound from the Lichen *Usnea albopunctata* against Medically Important Microbes." *Natural Product Research* 29 (6): 574–77.

Nishikawa, Y., K. Ohki, G. Takahashi, F. Fukuoka, and M. Emori. 1974. "Studies on the Water Soluble Constituents of Lichens II. Antitumor Polysaccharides of *Lasallia, Usnea* and *Cladonia* Species." *Chemical and Pharmaceutical Bulletin* 22: 2692–702.

Nithyanand, P., R. M. B. Shafreen, S. Muthamil, and S. K. Pandian. 2015. "Usnic Acid, a Lichen Secondary Metabolite Inhibits Group A *Streptococcus* Biofilms." *Antonie Van Leuwenhoek* 107 (1): 263–72.

Nugraha, A. S., L. F. Untari, A. Laub, et al. 2020. "Anthelmintic and Antimicrobial Activities of Three New Depsides and Ten Known Depsides and Phenols from Indonesian Lichen: *Parmelia cetrata*. Ach." *Natural Product Research* 35: 5001–10.

Nylander, W. 1866. "Les Lichens du Jardin du Luxembourg." *Bulletin de la Societé botanique de France* 13: 364–72.

Odabasoglu, F., et al. 2005. "Antioxidant Activity, Reducing Power and Total Phenolic Content of Some Lichen Species." *Fitoterapia* 6 (2): 216–19.

Oettl, S. K., J. Gerstmeier, S. Y. Khan, K. Wiechmann, et al. 2013. "Imbricaric Acid and Perlatolic Acid: Multi-targeting Anti-inflammatory Depsides from *Cetrelia monachorum*." *PloS ONE* 8 (10): e76929.

Ogmundsdóttir, H. M., G. M. Zoëga, S. R. Gissurarson, and K. Ingólfsdóttir. 1998. "Anti-proliferative Effects of Lichen-Derived Inhibitors of 5-lipoxygenase on Malignant Cell-Lines and Mitogen-Stimulated Lymphocytes." *Journal of Pharmacy and Pharmacology* 50 (1): 107–15.

Oh, J. M., Y. J. Kim, H. S. Gang, J. Han, H. H. Ha, and H. Kim. 2018. "Antimicrobial Activity of Divaricatic Acid Isolated from the Lichen *Evernia mesomorpha* against Methicillin-Resistant *Staphylococcus aureus*." *Molecules* 23 (12): 3068.

Olafsdottir, E. S., S. Omarsdottir, B. S. Paulsen, K. Jurcic, and H. Wagner. 1999. "Rhamnopranosylgalactofuranan, a New Immunologically Active Polysaccharide from *Thamnolia subuliformis*." *Phytomedicine* 6 (4): 273–79.

Omar, S. I., and J. Tuszynski. 2015. "Ranking the Binding Energies of p53 Mutant Activators and Their ADMET Properties." *Chemical Biology and Drug Design* 86 (2): 163–72.

Omarsdottir, S., J. Freysdottir, H. Barsett, B. Smestad, and E. S. Olafsdottir. 2005. "Effects of Lichen Heteroglycans on Proliferation and IL-10 Secretion by Rat Spleen Cells and IL-10 and TNF-Î⁺ Secretion by Rat Peritoneal Macrophages In Vitro." *Phytomedicine* 12 (6–7): 461–67.

Osawa, T., H. Kumon, C. A. Reece, and T. Shibamoto. 1991. "Inhibitory Effect of Lichen Constituents on Mutagenicity Induced by Heterocyclic Amines." *Environmental and Molecular Mutagenesis* 18 (1): 35–40.

Oswalt, W. H. 1957. "A Western Eskimo Ethnobotany." *Anthropology Papers of the Anchorage: University of Alaska* 6: 16–36.

Ouahiba, B., Y. Karima, B. Narimen, L. Razika, and A. Karim. 2018. "Preventive Effect of *Xanthoria parietina* Polyphenols on the Complications of Diabetes in White Rat." *Pakistan Journal of Pharmaceutical Science* 31 (1[Supp.1]): 317–24.

Özenver, N., M. Dawood, E. Fleischer, A. Klinger, and T. Efferth. 2020. "Chemometric and Transcriptomic Profiling, Microtubule Disruption and Cell Death Induction by Secalonic Acid in Tumor Cells." *Molecules* 25 (14): 3224.

Ozgencli, I., H. Budak, M. Ciftci, and M. Anar. 2018. "Lichen Acids May Be Used as a Potential Drug for Cancer Therapy; by Inhibiting Mitochondrial Thioredoxin Reductase Purified from Rat Lung." *Anticancer Agents in Medicinal Chemistry* 18 (11): 1599–605.

Ozturk, S., M. Erkisa, S. Oran, E. Ulukaya, S. Celikler, and F. Ari. 2021. "Lichens Exert an

Anti-proliferative Effect on Human Breast and Lung Cancer Cells through Induction of Apoptosis." *Drug and Chemical Toxicology* 44(3): 259–67.

Pagano, C., M. R. Ceccarini, P. Calarco, et al. 2019. "Bioadhesive Polymeric Films Based on Usnic Acid for Burn Wound Treatment: Antibacterial and Cytotoxicity Studies." *Colloids and Surfaces B Biointerfaces* 178: 488–99.

Paguirigan, J. A., R. D. Liu, S. M. Im, J. S. Hur, and W. Y. Kim. 2022. "Evaluation of Antimicrobial Properties of Lichen Substances against Plant Pathogens." *Plant Pathology Journal* 38 (1): 25–32.

Palacios-Moreno, J., C. Rubio, W. Quilhot, M. F. Cavieres, E. de la Peño, N. V. Quiñones, et al. 2019. "Epanorin, a Lichen Secondary Metabolite, Inhibits Proliferation of MCF-7 Breast Cancer Cells." *Biological Research* 52 (1): 55.

Palmer, A. L. 2023. *The Lichen Museum*. Minneapolis: University of Minnesota Press.

Paluszczak, J., R. Kleszcz, E. Studzinska-Sroka, et al. 2018. "Lichen-Derived Caperatic Acid and Physodic Acid Inhibit Wnt Signaling in Colorectal Cancer Cells." *Molecular and Cellular Biochemistry* 441: 109–24.

Pan, X. P., C. Wang, Y. Li, and L. H. Huang. 2018. "Physcion Induces Apoptosis through Triggering Endoplasmic Reticulum Stress in Hepatocellular Carcinoma." *Biomedicine and Pharmacotherapy* 99: 894–903.

Pang, M. J., Z. Yang, X. L. Zhang, Z. F. Liu, J. Fan, and H. Y. Zhang. 2016. "Physcion, a Naturally Occurring Anthraquinone Derivative, Induces Apoptosis and Autophagy in Human Nasopharyngeal Carcinoma." *Acta Pharmacologica Sinica* 37 (12): 1623–40.

Pant, R., A. Joshi, T. Joshi, P. Maiti, M. Nand, T. Joshi, V. Pande, and S. Chandra. 2021. "Identification of Potent Antigen 85C Inhibitors of *Mycobacterium tuberculosis* via In-House Lichen Library and Binding Free Energy Studies Part-II." *Journal of Molecular Graphics and Modelling* 103: 107822.

Papadopoulou, P., O. Tzakou, C. Vagias, P. Kefalas, and V. Roussis. 2007. "Beta-orcinol Metabolites from the Lichen *Hypotrachyna revolta*." *Molecules* 12 (5): 997–1005.

Papazi, A., E. Kastanaki, S. Pirintsos, and K. Kotzabasis. 2015. "Lichen Symbiosis: Nature's High Yielding Machines for Induced Hydrogen Production." *PLoS ONE* 10 (3): e0121325.

Papierska, K., V. Krajka-Kuzniak, J. Paluszczak, R. Kleszcz, et al. 2021. "Lichen-Derived Depsides and Depsidones Modulate the Nrf2, NF-kB and STAT3 Signaling Pathways in Colorectal Cancer Cells." *Molecules* 26 (16): 4787.

Paranagama, P. A., E. M. K. Wijeratne, A. M. Burns, M. T. Marron, et al. 2007. "Heptaketides from *Corynespora* sp. Inhabiting the Cavern Beard Lichen, *Usnea cavernosa*: First Report of Metabolites of an Endolichenic Fungus." *Journal of Natural Products* 70 (11): 1700–05.

Park, J. S., I. U. Rehman, K. Choe, R. Ahmad, H. J. Lee, and M. O. Kim. 2023. "A Triterpenoid Lupeol as an Antioxidant and Anti-Neuroinflammatory Agent: Impacts on Oxidative Stress in Alzheimer's Disease." *Nutrients* 15 (13): 3059.

Parrot, D., N. Legrave, D. Delmail, M. Grube, M. Suzuki, and S. Tomasi. 2016.

"Review—Lichen-Associated Bacteria as a Hot Spot of Chemodiversity: Focus on Uncialamycin, a Promising Compound for Future Medicinal Applications." *Planta Medica* 82 (13): 1143–52.

Paudel, B., H. D. Bhattarai, J. S. Lee, S. G. Hong, H. W. Shin, and J. H. Yim. 2008. "Antibacterial Potential of Antarctic Lichens against Human Pathogenic Gram-Positive Bacteria." *Phytotherapy Research* 22 (9): 1269–71.

Pejin, B. G. Tommonaro, C. Iodice, V. Tesevic, and V. Vajs. 2012. "Acetylcholinesterase Inhibition Activity of Acetylated Depsidones from *Lobaria pulmonaria.*" *Natural Products Research* 26 (17): 1634–37.

Pejin, B., C. Iodice, G. Bogdanovic, V. Kojic, and V. Tesevic. 2017. "Stictic Acid Inhibits Growth of Human Colon Adenocarcinoma HT-29 Cells." *Arabian Journal of Chemistry* 10 (Suppl 1): S1240–S1242.

Pennington, C. W. 1963. *The Tarahumar of Mexico: Their Environment and Material Culture.* Salt Lake City: University of Utah Press.

Pereira, M. I., A. C. Ruthes, E. R. Carbonero, R. Marcon, C. H. Baggio, et al. 2010. "Chemical Structure and Selected Biological Properties of a Glucomannan from the Lichenized Fungus *Heterodermia obscurata.*" *Phytochemistry* 71 (17–18): 2132–39.

Perez, Llano, G. A. 1944. "Lichens, Their Biological and Economic Significance." *Botanical Review* 10:1.

Perry, N. B., M. H. Benn, N. J. Brennana, E. J. Burgess, et al. 1999. "Antimicrobial, Antiviral and Cytotoxicity of New Zealand Lichens." *Lichenologist* 31 (6): 627–36.

Pham, N. K. T., H. T. Nguyen, T. B. N. Dao, K. L. Vu-Huynh, et al. 2022. "Two New Phenolic Compounds from the Lichen *Parmotrema cristiferum* Growing in Vietnam." *Natural Product Research* 36 (15): 3854–71.

Phan, H. V. T., A. P. Devi, H. D. Le, T. T. Nguyen, et al. 2021. "Dilatatone, a New Chlorinated Compound from *Parmotrema dilatatum.*" *Natural Products Research* 35 (21): 3608–12.

Phi, K. H., M. J. Shin, S. Lee, J. E. So, J. H. Kim, S. S. Suh, et al. 2022. "Bioactive Terphenyls Isolated from the Antarctic Lichen *Stereocaulon alpinum.*" *Molecules* 27 (7): 2363.

Piska, K., A. Galanty, P. Koczurkiewicz, P. Zmudzki, et al. 2018. "Usnic Acid Reactive Metabolites Formation in Human, Rat, and Mice Microsomes. Implication for Pepatoxicity." *Food and Chemical Toxicology* 120: 112–18.

Pompilio, A., S. Pomponio, V. di Vincenzo, V. Crocetta, M. Nicoletti, et al. 2013. "Antimicrobial and Antibiofilm Activity of Secondary Metabolite against Methicillin-Resistant *Staphylococcus aureus* Strains from Cystic Fibrosis Patients." *Future Microbiology* 8 (2): 281–92.

Popovoci, V., E. Matei, G. C. Cozaru, et al. 2022. "Evaluation of *Usnea barbata* (L.) Weber ex F. H. Wigg Extract in Canola Oil Loaded in Bioadhesive Oral Films for Potential Applications in Oral Cavity Infections and Malignancy." *Antioxidants* (Basel) 11 (8): 1601.

Popovoci, V., E. Matei, G.C. Cozaru, L. Bucur, C.E. Gird, et al. 2022a. "In Vitro Anticancer

Activity of Mucoadhesive Oral Films Loaded with *Usnea barbata* (L.) F. H. Wigg Dry Acetone Extract, with Potential Applications in Oral Squamous Cell Carcinoma Complementary Therapy." *Antioxidants* (Basel) 11 (10): 1934.

Posner, B., and G. B. Feige. 1992. "Studies on the Chemistry of the Lichen Genus *Umbilicaria* Hoffm." *Zeitschrift fur Naturforschung, C Journal of Bioscience* 47: 1–9.

Powers, S. 1877. *Aboriginal Botany. Indian Tribes of California,* 419–31. Washington, DC: Government Printing House.

Prateeksha, M. A. Yusuf, B. N. Singh, S. Sudheer, et al. 2019. "Chrysophanol: A Natural Anthraquinone with Multifacted Biotherapeutic Potential." *Biomolecules* 9 (2): 68.

Prateeksha, R. Bajpai, M. A. Yusuf, D. K. Upreti, V. K. Gupta, and B. N. Singh. 2020. "Endolichenic Fungus, *Aspergillus quandricinctus* of *Usnea longissima* Inhibits Quorum Sensing and Biofilm Formation of *Pseudomonas aeruginosa* PAO1." *Microbial Pathogenesis* 140: 103933.

Pringle, A., D. Chen, and J. W. Taylor. 2003. "Sexual Fecundity Is Correlated to Size in the Lichenized Fungus *Xanthoparmelia cumberlandia*." *Bryologist* 106 (2): 221–25.

Printzen C., and H. T. Lumbsch. 2000. "Molecular Evidence for the Diversification of Extant Lichens in the Late Cretaceous and Tertiary." *Molecular Phylogenetics and Evolution* 17 (3): 379–87.

Pulat, S., L. Subedi, P. Pandey, S. R. Bhoste, J. S. Hur, J. H. Shim, et al. 2023. "Topical Delivery of Atraric Acid Derived from *Stereocaulon japonicum* with Enhanced Skin Permeation and Hair Regrowth Activity for Androgenic Alopecia." *Pharmaceutics* 15 (2): 340.

Qi, F. F., W. Zhang, Y. Y. Xue, C. Geng, Z. G. Jin, J. B. Li, Q. Guo, et al. 2022. "Microbial Production of the Plant-Derived Fungicide Physicon." *Metabolic Engineering* 74: 130–38.

Quave, C. L. 2021. *The Plant Hunter: A Scientist's Quest for Nature's Next Medicines.* New York: Viking of Penguin Random House.

Racine, P. H., V. Harmann, and Y. Tollard D'Dudiffret. 1980. "Antioxidant Properties of Wax from Yugoslavian Oakmoss (*Evernia prunastri*)." *International Journal of Cosmetic Science* 2 (6): 305–13.

Rafika, B., and A. A. Monia. 2018. "Antibacterial Activity of the Chloroform, Acetone, Methanol and Aqueous Extracts of Algerian Lichens." *Jordan Journal of Pharmaceutical Sciences* 11 (2): 55–67.

Raggio, J., A. Pintado, C. Ascaso, R. de la Torre, et al. 2011. "Whole Lichen Thalli Survive Exposure to Space Conditions: Results of *Lithopanspermia* Experiment with *Aspicilia fruticulosa*." *Astrobiology* 11 (4): 281–92.

Raggio, J., D. S. Pescador, B. Gozalo, V. Ochoa, et al. 2023. "Continuous Monitoring of Chlorophyll as Fluorescence and Microclimatic Conditions Reveal Warming-Induced Physiological Damage in Biocrust-Forming Lichens." *Plant and Soil* 482 (1–2): 261–76.

Raj, P. S., A. Prathapan, J. Sebastian, A. K. Antony, M. P. Riya, et al. 2014. "*Parmotrema tinctorum* Exhibits Antioxidant, Antiglycation and Inhibitory Activities against Aldose Reductase and Carbohydrate Digestive Enzymes: An In Vitro Study." *Natural Products Research* 28 (18): 1480–84.

Rankovic, B, M. Misic, and S. Sukdolak. 2007. "Evaluation of Antimicrobial Activity of the Lichens *Lasallia pustulata, Parmelia sulcata, Umbilicaria crustulosa* and *Umbilicaria cylindrica.*" *Mikrobiologlya* 76 (6): 817–21.

Rankovic, B., M. Misic, and S. Sukdolak. 2008. "The Antimicrobial Activity of Substances Derived from the Lichens *Physcia aipolia, Umbilaria polyphylla, Parmelia caperata* and *Hypogymnia physodes.*" *World Journal of Microbiology and Biotechnology* 24: 1239–42.

Rankovic, B. R., M. M. Kosanic, and T. P. Stanojkovic. 2011. "Antioxidant, Antimicrobial and Anticancer Activity of the Lichens *Cladonia furcata, Lecanora atra* and *Lecanora muralis.*" *BMC Complementary and Alternative Medicine* 11: 97.

Rankovic, B., M. Kosanic, T. Stanojkovic, P. Vasiljevic, and N. Manojlovic. 2012. "Biological Activities of *Toninia candida* and *Usnea barbata* Together with their Norstictic Acid and Usnic Acid Constituents." *International Journal of Molecular Science* 13 (11): 14707–22.

Rankovic, B., ed. 2019. *Lichen Secondary Metabolites.* 2nd ed., 31–97. Cham. Switzerland: Springer International Publishing.

Rao, M. M. V., and T. Hariprasad. 2021. "In Silico Analysis of a Potential Antidiabetic Phytochemical Erythrin against Therapeutic Targets in Diabetes." *In Silico Pharmacology* 9 (1): 5.

Rashid, Z. M., M. Mormann, K. Steckhan, A. Peters, S. Esch, and A. Hensei. 2019. "Polysaccharides from Lichen *Xanthoria parietina*: 1,4/1,6-a-d-glucans and a Highly Branched Galactomannan with Macrophage Stimulating Activity via Dectin-2 Activation." *International Journal of Biological Macromolecules* 134: 921–35.

Raymond, M. 1945. "Notes ethnobotaniques sur les Tete-de Boule de manouan." *Etudes Ethnobotaniques Quebecoises* 55: 113–54.

Rebesca, M. A., D. Romie, M. Johnson, and J. Ryan. 1994. *Traditional Dene medicine part I: Report.* Lac La Martre, NWT, Canada: Dene Cultural Institute.

Reddy, R. G., L. Veeraval, S. Maitra, M. Chollet-Krugler, et al. 2016. "Lichen-Derived Compounds Show Potential for Central Nervous System Therapeutics." *Phytomedicine* 23 (12): 1527–34.

Reddy, S. D., B. Siva, K. Kumar, V. S. P. Babu, V. Sravanthi, et al. 2019. "Comprehensive Analysis of Secondary Metabolites in *Usnea longissima* (Lichenized Ascomycetes, Parmeliaceae) Using UPLC-ESI-QTOF-MS/MS and Pro-Apoptotic Activity of Barbatic Acid." *Molecules* 24 (12): 2270.

Reis, R. A., M. Iacomini, P. A. J. Gorin, L. M. de Souza, et al. 2005. "Fatty Acid Composition of the Tropical Lichen *Teloschistes flavicans* and Its Cultivated Symbionts." *FEMS Microbiology Letters* 247 (1): 1–6.

Rezanka, T., J. Jachymova, and V. Dembitsky. 2003. "Prenylated Xanthone Glucosides from Ural's Lichen *Umbilicaria proboscidea.*" *Phytochemistry* 62 (4): 607–12.

Rezanka, T., and V. M. Dembitsky. 2006. "The Colleflaccinosides, Two Chiral Bianthraquinone Glycosides with Antitumor Activity from the Lichen *Collema flaccidum* Collected in Israel and Russia." *Natural Products Research* 20 (10): 969–80.

Rezanka, T., and K. Sigler. 2007. "Hirtusneanoside, an Unsymmetrical Dimeric

Tetrahydroxanthone from the Lichen *Usnea hirta*." *Journal of Natural Products* 70 (9): 1487–91.

Ristic, S., B. Rankovic, M. Kosanic, T. Stanojkovic, S. Stamenkovic, P. Vasiljevic, I. Manojlovic, and N. Manojlovic. 2016. "Phytochemical Study and Antioxidant, Antimicrobial and Anticancer Activities of *Melanella subaurifera* and *Melanelia fuliginosa* Lichens." *Journal of Food Science Technology* 53 (6): 2804–16.

Ristic, S., B. Rankovic, and S. Stamenkovic. 2016a. "Biopharmaceutical Potential of Two *Ramalina* Lichens and Their Metabolites." *Current Pharmaceutical Biotechnology* 17 (7): 6561–658.

Róbertsdóttir, A. R. 2016. *Icelandic Herbs and Their Medicinal Uses*. Berkeley, CA: North Atlantic Books.

Rogers, R. D. 2011. *The Fungal Pharmacy: The Complete Guide to Medicinal Mushrooms and Lichens of North America*. Berkeley, CA: North Atlantic Books.

Rogers, R. D. 2016. *Mushroom Essences: Vibrational Healing from the Kingdom Fungi*. Berkeley, CA: North Atlantic Books.

Rogers, R. D. 2019. *Rejuvenate Your Brain Naturally*. Edmonton, AB: Prairie Deva Press.

Rogers, R. D. 2020. *Medicinal Mushrooms: The Human Clinical Trials*. Edmonton, AB: Prairie Deva Press.

Roser, L. A., P. Erkoc, R. Ingelfinger, et al. 2022. "Lecanoric Acid Mediates Anti-proliferative Effect by an M Phase Arrest in Colon Cancer Cells." *Biomedicine and Pharmacotherapy* 148: 112734.

Ross, A. C. G. 1970. "Two Neglected Remedies." *Homeopathy* 20 (6).

Roullier, C., M. Chollet-Krugler, E. M. Pferschy-Wenzig, A. Maillard, et al. 2011. "Characterization and Identification of Mycosporines-Like Compounds in Cyanolichens. Isolation of Mycosporine Hydroxyglutamicol from *Nephroma laevigatum* Ach." *Phytochemistry* 72 (11–12): 1348–57.

Russo, A., M. Piovano, L. Lombardo, L. Vanella, V. Cardile, and J. Garbarino. 2006. "Pannarin Inhibits Cell Growth and Induces Cell Death in Human Prostate Carcinoma DU-145 Cells." *Anticancer Drugs* 17 (10): 1163–69.

Russo, A., M. Piovano, L. Lombardo, J. Garbarino, and V. Cardile. 2008. "Lichen Metabolites Prevent UV Light and Nitric Oxide-Mediated Plasmid DNA Damage and Induce Apoptosis in Human Melanoma Cells." *Life Sciences* 83 (13–14): 468–74.

Russo, A., S. Caggia, M. Piovano, J. Garbarino, and V. Cardile. 2012. "Effect of Vicanicin and Protolichesterinic Acid on Human Prostate Cancer Cells: Role of Hsp70 Protein." *Chemico-Biologica Interactions* 195 (1): 1–10.

Ryan, F. 2002. *Darwin's Blind Spot: Evolution Beyond Natural Selection*. New York: Houghton Mifflin Harcourt.

Saenz, M. T., M. D. Garcia, and J. G. Rowe. 2006. "Antimicrobial Activity and Phytochemical Studies from Some Lichens from South of Spain." *Fitoterapia* 77 (3): 156–59.

Safak, B., I. H. Ciftci, M. Ozdemir, N. Kiyildi, et al. 2009. "In Vitro Anti-*Helicobacter pylori* Activity of Usnic Acid." *Phytotherapy Research* 23 (7): 955–57.

Safarkar, R., G. R. Rajaei, and S. Khjalili-Arjagi. 2020. "The Study of Antibacterial Properties of Iron Oxide Nanoparticles Synthesized Using the Extract of Lichen *Ramalina sinensis*." *Nanoscience and Nanotechnology–Asia* 3 (3): 157–66.

Sahin, E., S. D. Psav, I. Avan, M. Candan, Y. Sahinturk, and A. T. Koparal. 2019. "Vulpinic Acid, a Lichen Metabolite, Emerges as a Potential Drug Candidate in the Therapy of Oxidative Stress-Related Diseases, Such as Atherosclerosis." *Human and Experimental Toxicology* 38 (6): 675–84.

Saklani, A., D. K. Upreti. 1992. "Folk Uses of Some Lichens of Sikkim." *Journal of Ethnopharmacology* 37: 229–33.

Salem, S., E. Leghouchi, R. Soulimani, and J. Bouayed. 2021. "Reduction of Paw Edema and Liver Oxidative Stress in Carrageenan-Induced Acute Inflammation by *Lobaria pulmonaria* and *Parmelia caperata*, Lichen Species, in Mice." *International Journal of Vitamin and Nutrition Research* 91 (1–2): 143–51.

Salgado, F., L. Albornoz, C. Cortez, E. Stashenko, et al. 2017. "Secondary Metabolite Profiling of Species of the Genus *Usnea* by UHPLC-ESI-OT-MS-MS." *Molecules* 23 (1): 54.

Salgado, F., J. Caballero, R. Vargas, A. Cornejo, and C. Areche. 2020. "Continental and Antarctic Lichens: Isolation, Identification and Molecular Modeling of the Depside Tenuiorin from the Antarctic Lichen *Umbilicaria antarctica* as Tau Protein Inhibitor." *Natural Product Research* 34 (5): 646–50.

Salviano, T. L., D. C. Dos Santos Macedo, et al. 2021. "Fucoidan-Coated Liposomes: A Target System to Deliver the Antimicrobial Drug Usnic Acid to Macrophages Infected with *Mycobacterium tuberculosis*." *Journal of Biomedical Nanotechnology* 17 (8): 1699–710.

Sanchez, M., I. Urena-Vacas, E. Gonzalez-Burgos, P. K. Divakar, and M. P. Gomez-Serranillos. 2022. "The Genus *Cetraria* s. str.—A Review of Its Botany, Phytochemistry, Traditional Uses and Pharmacology." *Molecules* 27 (15): 4990.

Sand, G. 1870. *Conseulo*. Trans. Fayette Robinson. Philadelphia: T. B. Peterson and Brothers.

Sanjaya, A., A. Avidlyandi, M. Adfa, M. Ninomiya, and M. Koketsu. 2020. "A New Depsidone from *Teloschistes flavicans* and the Antileukemic Activity." *Journal of Oleo Science* 69 (12): 1591–95.

Santiago, K. A. A., R. Edrada-Ebel, T. E. E de la Cruz, Y. L. Cheow, and A. S. Y. Ting. 2021. "Biodiscovery of Potential Antibacterial Diagnostic Metabolites from the Endolichenic Fungus *Xylaria venustula* Using LC-MS-Based Metabolomics." *Biology* (Basel) 10 (3): 191.

Santos, L. C., N. K. Honda, I. Z. Carlos, and W. Vilegas. 2004. "Intermediate Reactive Oxygen and Nitrogen from Macrophages Induced by Brazilian Lichens." *Fitoterapia* 75 (5): 473–79.

Sanyaolu, A., C. Okorie, A. Marinkovic, A. F. Abbasi, et al. 2022. "*Candida auris*: An Overview of the Emerging Drug-Resistant Fungal Infection." *Infection and Chemotherapy* 54 (2): 236–46.

Sargsyan, R., A. Gasparyan, G. Tadevosyan, and H. Panosyan. 2021. "Antimicrobial and Antioxidant Potentials of Non-cytotoxic Extracts of Corticolous Lichens Sampled in Armenia." *AMB Express* 11 (1): 1–11.

Savale, S. A., C. S. Pol, R. Khare, N. Verma, S. Galkwad, B. Mandal, and S. C. Behera. 2016. "Radical Scavenging, Prolyl Endopeptidase Inhibitory, and Antimicrobial Potential of a Cultured Himalayan Lichen *Cetrelia olivetorum*." *Pharmaceutical Biology* 54 (4): 692–700.

Saver, A., J. P. Lulich, S. Van Buren, and E. Furrow. 2021. "Calcium Oxalate Urolithiasis in Juvenile Dogs." *Veterinary Record* 189 (3): e141.

Schinkovitz, A., A. Kaur, E. Urban, M. Zehl, et al. 2014. "Cytotoxic Constituents from *Lobaria scrobiculata* and a Comparison of Two Bioassays for Their Evaluation." *Journal of Natural Products* 77 (4): 1069–73.

Schneider, A. 1904. *A Guide to the Study of Lichens*. Boston: Knight and Miller.

Segatore, B., P. Bellio, D. Setacci, F. Brisdelli, et al. 2012. "In Vitro Interaction of Usnic Acid in Combination with Antimicrobial Agents against Methicillin-Resistant *Staphylococcus aureus* Clinical Isolates Determined by FICI and Pyramid/Triangle *E* Model Methods." *Phytomedicine* 19: 341–47.

Seklic, D. S., A. D. Obradovic, M. S. Stankovic, M. N. Zivanovic, T. L. Mitrovic, S. M. Stamenkovic, and S. D. Markovic. 2018. "Proapoptotic and Antimigratory Effects of *Pseudevernia furfuracea* and *Platismatia glauca* on Colon Cancer Cell Lines." *Food Technology and Biotechnology* 56 (3): 421–30.

Seklic, D. S., and M. M. Jovanovic. 2022. "*Platismatia glauca*—Lichen Species with Suppressive Properties on Migration and Invasiveness of Two Different Colorectal Carcinoma Cell Lines." *Journal of Food Biochemistry* 46 (7): e14096.

Semple, S. J., S. M. Pyke, G. D. Reynolds, and R. L. Flower. 2001. "In Vitro Antiviral Activity of the Anthraquinone Chrysophanic Acid against Poliovirus." *Antiviral Research* 49 (3): 169178.

Seo, C., J. H. Sohn, S. M. Park, J. H. Yim, H. K. Lee, and H. Oh. 2008. "Usimines A-C, Bioactive Usnic Acid Derivatives from the Antarctic Lichen *Stereocaulon alpinum*." *Journal of Natural Products* 71 (4): 710–12.

Seo, C., J. H. Sohn, J. S. Ahn, J. H. Kim, H. K. Lee, and H. Oh. 2009. "Protein Tyrosine Phosphate 1B Inhibitory Effects Depsidone and Pseudodepsidone Metabolites from the Antarctic Lichen *Stereocaulon alpinum*." *Bioorganic and Medicinal Chemistry Letters* 19 (10): 2801–3.

Seo, C., Y. H. Choi, J. S. Ahn, J. H. Yim, H. K. Lee, and H. Oh. 2009a. "PTP1B Inhibitory Effects of Tridepside and Related Metabolites Isolated from the Antarctic Lichen *Umbilicaria antarctica*." *Journal of Enzyme Inhibition and Medicinal Chemistry* 24 (5): 1133–37.

Sepahvand, A., E. Studzinska-Sroka, P. Ramak, and V. Karimian. 2021. "*Usnea* sp.: Antimicrobial Potential, Bioactive Compound, Ethnopharmacological Uses and Other Pharmacological Properties; a Review Article." *Journal of Ethnopharmacology* 268:113656.

Sepulveda, B., M. C. Chamy, M. Piovano, and C. Areche. 2013. "Lichens: Might Be Considered as a Source of Gastroprotective Molecules?" *Journal of the Chilean Chemical Society* 58 (2).

Sepulveda, B., D. Benites, L. Albornoz, M. Simirgiotis, O. Castro, O. Garcia-Beltran, and C. Areche. 2023. "Green Ultrasound-Assisted Extraction of Lichen Substances from

Hypotrachyna cirrhata. Ethyl Lactate, a Better Extracting Agent Than Methanol Toxic Organic Solvent?" *Natural Product Research* 37 (1): 159–63.

Shahi, S. K., M. Patra, A. Dikshit, and D. K. Upreti. 2003. "Botanical Antifungal Drug Fight Fungal Infection." *Proceedings of the First National Interactive Meeting on Medicinal and Aromatic Plants*, eds. A. Mathur, et al. London: CIMAP, 302–7.

Sharnoff, S. D. 1997. *Lichens and People*. Lichen (website).

Shcherbakova, A., A. A. Strömstedt, and U. Göransson, et al. 2021. "Antimicrobial and Antioxidant Activity of *Evernia prunastri* Extracts and Their Isolates." *World Journal of Microbiology and Biotechnology* 37: 129.

Sheldrake, M. 2020. *Entangled Life: How Fungi Make Our Worlds, Change Our Minds and Shape our Futures*. New York: Random House.

Shim, J. H. 2020. "Anti-aging Effects of Gyrophoric Acid on UVA-Irradiated Normal Human Dermal Fibroblasts." *Natural Products Communication* 15 (4): 1–8.

Shiromi, P., R. P. Hewawasam, R. G. U. Jayalal, H. Rathnayake, et al. 2021. "Chemical Composition and Antimicrobial Activity of Two Sri Lankan Lichens, *Parmotrema rampoddense*, and *Parmotrema tinctorum* against Methicillin-Sensitive and Methicillin-Resistant *Staphylococcus aureus*." *Evidence Based Complementary and Alternative Medicine* 2021: 9985325.

Shivanna, R., P. Hengameh, and H. G. Rajkumar. 2015. "Screening of Lichen Extracts for In-Vitro Anti-diabetic Activity Using Alpha Amylase Inhibitory Assay." *International Journal of Biological and Pharmaceutical Research* 6 (5): 364–67.

Shrestha, G., J. Raphael, S. D. Leavit, and L. L. St. Clair. 2014. "In Vitro Evaluation of Extracts from 34 Species of North American Lichens." *Pharmaceutical Biology* 52 (10): 1262–66.

Shrestha, G., A. M. El-Naggar, L. L. St. Clair, and K. L. O'Neill. 2015. "Anticancer Activities of Selected Species of North American Lichen Extracts." *Phytotherapy Research* 29 (1): 100–107.

Shrestha, G., L. L. St. Clair, and K. L. O'Neill. 2015a. "The Immune-Stimulating Role of Lichen Polysaccharides: A Review." *Phytotherapy Research* 29 (3): 317–22.

Shukla, I., L. Azmi, C. V. Rao, T. Jawaid, M. Kamal, A. S. Awaad, S. I. Alqasoumi, O. A. Alkhamees, and S. M. Alsanad. 2020. "Hepatoprotective Activity of Depsidone Enriched *Cladonia rangiferina* Extract against Alcohol-Induced Hepatotoxicity Targeting Cytochrome P450 2E1 Induced Oxidative Damage." *Saudi Pharmaceutical Journal* 28 (4): 519–27.

Si, K., L. L. Wei, X. Z. Yu, F. Wu, X. Q. Li, C. Li, and Y. B. Cheng. 2016. "Effects of (+)-Usnic and (+)-Usnic Acid-Liposome on *Toxoplasma gondii*." *Experimental Parasitology* 166: 68–74.

Sieteiglesias, V., E. González-Burgos, P. Bermejo-Bescós, P. K. Divakar, and M. P. Gómez-Serranillos. 2019. "Lichens of Parmeloid Clade as Promising Multitarget Neuroprotective Agents." *Chemical Research in Toxicology* 32 (6): 1165–77.

Silva, H. A. M. F., A. L. Aires, C. L. R. Soares, W. N. Siqueria, M. V. Lima, M. C. B. Martins, et al. 2021. "Schistosomicidal Effect of Divaricatic Acid from *Canoparmelia texana* (Lichen):

In Vitro Evaluation and Ultrastructural Analysis against Adult Worms of *Shistosoma mansoni*." *Acta Tropica* 222: 106044.

Simko, P., A. Leskanicova, M. Suvakova, A. Blicharova, et al. 2022. "Biochemical Properties of Atranorin-Induced Behavioral and Systematic Changes in Laboratory Rats." *Life* (Basel) 12 (7): 1090.

Singh, G., A. Calchera, D. Merges, H. Valim, J. Otte, I. Schmitt, and F. D. Grande. 2022. "A Candidate Gene Cluster for the Bioactive Natural Produce Gyrophoric Acid in Lichen-Forming Fungi." *Microbiology Spectrum* 10 (4): e0010922.

Singh, J, Y. Hussain, S. Luqman, and A. Meena. 2021. "Purpurin: A Natural Anthraquinone with Multifaceted Pharmacological Activities." *Phytotherapy Research* 35 (5): 2318–428.

Singh, N., D. Nambiar, R. K. Kale, and R. P. Singh. 2013. "Usnic Acid Inhibits Growth and Induces Cell Cycle Arrest and Apoptosis in Human Lung Carcinoma A549 Cells." *Nutrition and Cancer* 65 (suppl 1: 36–43).

Sisodia, R., M. Geol, S. Verma, A. Rani, and P. Dureja. 2013. "Antibacterial and Antioxidant Activity of Lichen Species *Ramalina roesleri*." *Natural Product Research* 27 (23): 2235–39.

Smith, G. C. S., and J. P. Pell. 2003. "Parachute Use to Prevent Death and Major Trauma Related to Gravitational Challenge: Systematic Review of Randomised Controlled Trials." *British Medical Journal* 327 (7429): 1459–61.

Smith, G. W. 1973. "Arctic Pharmacognosia." *Arctic* 26: 324–33.

Smith, H. H. 1923. "Ethnobotany of the Menomini Indian." *Bulletin of the Public Museum of Milwaukee* 4: 1–174.

Smith, H. H. 1929. "Materia Medica of the Bella Coola and Neighbouring Tribes of British Columbia." *Bulletin of the National Museum of Canada* 56: 47–68.

Smith, H. H. 1932. "Ethnobotany of the Ojibwe Indians." *Bulletin of the Public Museum of the City of Milwaukee* 4: 327–525.

Smith, H. H. 1933. "Ethnobotany of the Forest Potawatomi Indians." *Bulletin of the Public Museum of the City of Milwaukee* 7: 1–230.

Smriga, M., and H. Saito. 2000. "Effect of Selected Thallophytic Glucans on Learning Behavior and Short-Term Potentiation." *Phytotherapy Research* 14 (3): 153–55.

Snell, A. H. *A Taste of Heritage: Crow Indian Recipes and Herbal Medicines*. Lincoln: University of Nebraska Press.

Sohag, A. A. M., T. Hossain, A. Rahaman, P. Rahman, et al. 2022. "Molecular Pharmacology and Therapeutic Advances of the Pentacyclic Triterpene Lupeol." *Phytomedicine* 99: 154012.

Sökmen, B. B., K. Kinalioglu, and S. Aydin. 2012. "Antimicrobial and Antioxidant Activities of *Pseudevernia furfuracea* (L.) Zopf var. *furfuracea* and *Evernia prunastri* Lichens Collected from Black Sea Region." *Gazi University Journal of Science* 25 (3): 557–65.

Sokolov, D. N., V. V. Zarubaev, A. A. Shtro, M. P. Polovinka, et al. 2012. "Anti-viral Activity of (-) and (+)-Usnic Acids and Their Derivatives against Influenza Virus A(H1N1)2009." *Bioorganic and Medicinal Chemistry Letters* 22 (23): 7060–64.

Solár, P., G. Hrcková, L. Koptašiková, S. Velebný, Z. Solárová, and M. Backor. 2016. "Murine Breast Carcinoma 4T1 Cells Are More Sensitive to Atranorin Than Normal Epithelial NmuMG Cells In Vitro: Anticancer and Hepatoprotective Effects of Atranorin In Vivo." *Chemico-Biological Interactions* 250: 27–37.

Solárová, Z., A. Liskova, M. Samec, P. Kubatka, et al. 2020. "Anticancer Potential of Lichens' Secondary Metabolites." *Biomolecules* 10 (1): 87.

Soldan, S. S., and P. M. Lieberman. 2023. "Epstein-Barr Virus and Multiple Sclerosis." *Nature Reviews Microbiology* 21 (1): 51–64.

Somphong, A., V. Poengsungnoen, K. Buaruang, et al. 2022. "*Actinomadura parmotrematis* sp. nov., Isolated from the Foliose Lichen, *Parmotrema praesorediosum* (Nyl.) Hale." *International Journal of Systematic and Evolutionary Microbiology* 72 (7).

Spribille, T., V. Tuovinen, P. Resi, D. Vanderpool, et al. 2016. "Basidiomycete Yeasts in the Cortex of Ascomycete Macrolichens." *Science* 353: 488–92.

Spribille, T. 2018. "Relative Symbiont Input and the Lichen Symbiotic Outcome." *Current Opinion in Plant Biology* 44: 57–63.

Srimani, S., C. X. Schmidt, M. P. Gomez-Serranillos, H. Oster, and P. K. Divakar. 2022. "Modulation of Cellular Circadian Rhythms by Secondary Metabolites of Lichens." *Frontiers in Cellular Neuroscience* 16: 907308.

Srinivasan, M., K. Shanmugam, B. Kedike, S. Narayanan, S. Shanmugam, and H. G. Neelakantan. 2020. "Trypethelone and Phenalenone Deriviates Isolated from the Mycobiont Culture of *Trypethelium eluteriae* Spreng. and Their Anti-mycobacterial Properties." *Natural Product Research* 34 (23): 3320–27.

Stahl, J. L., and J. L. Bagot. 2020. "Beryllium Metallicum." *La Revue D'Home'opathie* 11 (2): 15–17.

Stehlow, W., and G. Hertzka. 1987. *Hildegard of Bingen's Medicine*. Santa Fe, NM: Bear & Company.

Stevens, J., and J. Palliser. 1984. *Traditional Medicine Project: Project sur la medicine traditionelle*. Avataq Cultural Institute, Inukjuak, QC.

Stojanovic, G., I. Zlatanovic, I. Zrnzevic, M. Stankovic, V. S. Jovanovic, and B. Zlatkovic. 2018. "*Hypogymnia tubulosa* Extracts: Chemical Profile and Biological Activities." *Natural Products Research* 32 (22): 2735–39.

Stojanovic, G., I. Zrnzevic, I. Zlatanovic, M. Stankovic, et al. 2020. "Chemical Profile and Biological Activities of *Peltigera horizontalis* (Hudson) Baumg. Thallus and Apothecia Extracts." *Natural Products Research* 34 (4): 549–52.

Stojanovic, I. Z., S. Najman, O. Jovanovic, G. Petrovic, J. Najdanovic, P. Vasiljevic, and A. Smelcerovic. 2014. "Effects of Depsidones from *Hypogymnia physodes* on HeLa Cell Viability and Growth." *Folia Biol* (Praha) 60 (2): 89–94.

Stratev, D., and O. A. Odeyemi. 2016. "Antimicrobial Resistance of *Aeromonas hydrophila* Isolated from Different Food Sources: A Mini-Review." *Journal of Infection and Public Health* 9 (5): 535–44.

Stubbs, R. D. 1966. "An Investigation of the Edible and Medicinal Plants Used by the Flathead Indians." MA thesis, University of Montana.

Studzinska-Sroka, E. Hoderna-Kedzia, A. Galanty, W. Bylka, K. Kacprzak, and K. Cwiklinska. 2015. "In Vitro Antimicrobial Activity of Extracts and Compounds Isolated from *Cladonia uncialis*." *Natural Products Research* 29 (24): 2302–7.

Studzinska-Sroka, E., H. Piotrowska, M. Kucinska, M. Murias, and W. Bylka. 2016. "Cytotoxic Activity of Physodic Acid and Acetone Extract from *Hypogymnia physodes* against Breast Cancer Cell Lines." *Pharmaceutical Biology* 54 (11): 2480–85.

Studzinska-Sroko, E., A. Galanty, and W. Bylka. 2017. "Atranorin—An Interesting Lichen Secondary Metabolite." *Mini-Reviews in Medicinal Chemistry* 17 (17): 1633–45.

Studzinska-Sroka, E., H. Tomczak, N. Malinska, M. Wronska, R. Kleszcz, et al. 2019. "*Cladonia uncialis* as a Valuable Raw Material of Biosynthetic Compounds against Clinical Strains of Bacteria and Fungi." *Acta Biochimica Polonica* 66 (4): 597–603.

Studzinska-Sroka, E., A. Majchrzak-Celinska, P. Zalewski, et al. 2021. "Lichen-Derived Compounds and Extracts as Biologically Active Substances with Anticancer and Neuroprotective Properties." *Pharmaceuticals* 14: 1293.

Studzinska-Sroka, E., A. Majchrzak-Celinska, P. Zalewski, D. Szwajgier, E. Baranowska-Wojcik, M. Zarowski, T. Plech, and J. Clelecka-Piontek. 2021. "Permeability of *Hypogymnia physodes* Extract Component-Physodic Acid through the Blood-Brain Barrier as an Important Argument for Its Anticancer and Neuroprotective Activity within the Central Nervous System." *Cancers* (Basel) 13 (7): 1717.

Studzinska-Sroka, E., A. Majchrzak-Celinska, M. Bandurska, N. Rosiak, et al. 2022. "Is Caperatic Acid the Only Compound Responsible for Activity of Lichen *Platismatia glauca* within the Nervous System?" *Antioxidants* (Basel) 11 (10): 2069.

Stuelp-Campelo, P. A., M. B. M. de Oliveira, et al. 2002. "Effect of a Soluble Alpha-D-glucan from the Lichenized Fungus *Ramalina celastri* on Macrophage Activity." *International Immunopharmacology* 2 (5): 691–98.

Su, Z. Q., Y. H. Liu, H. Z. Guo, C. Y. Sun, et al. 2017. "Effect-Enhancing and Toxicity-Reducing Activity of Usnic Acid in Ascitic Tumor-Bearing Mice Treated with Bleomycin." *International Immunopharmacology* 46: 146–55.

Subrahmanian, S. S., and S. Ramakrishnan. 1964. "Amino Acids of *Peltigera canina*." *Current Science* 33: 522.

Süleyman, H., D. Yildirim, A. Aslan, F. Göcer, et al. 2002. "An Investigation of the Anti-inflammatory Effects of an Extract from *Cladonia rangiformis* HOFFM." *Biological and Pharmaceutical Bulletin* 25 (1): 10–13.

Sun, C. L., F. Liu, J. Sun, J. Li, and X. Wang. 2016. "Optimisation and Establishment of Separation Conditions of Organic Acids from *Usnea longissima* Ach. by pH-Zone-Refining Counter-Current Chromatography: Discussion of the Eluotropic Sequence." *Journal of Chromatography A* 1427: 96–101.

Sun, T. X., M. Y. Li, Z. H. Zhang, J. Y. Wang, Y. Xing, et al. 2021. "Usnic Acid Suppresses Cervical Cancer Cell Proliferation by Inhibiting PD-L1 Expression and Enhancing T-Lymphocyte Tumor-Killing Activity." *Phytotherapy Research* 35 (7): 3916–35.

Sun, W., B. Zhang, H. Zheng, et al. 2017. "Trivaric Acid, a New Inhibitor of PTP1b with Potent Beneficial Effect on Diabetes." *Life Sciences* 169: 52–64.

Sun, W., C. Zhuang, X. Li, B. Zhang, et al. 2017. "Varic Acid Analogues from Fungus as PTP1B Inhibitors: Biological Evaluation and Structure-Activity Relationships." *Bioorganic and Medicinal Chemistry Letters* 27: 3382–85.

Takahashi, K., T. Takeda, S. Shibita, M. Inomata, and F. Fukroka. 1974. "Polysaccharides of Lichens and Fungi VI. Antitumor Active Polysaccharides of Lichens in Stictaceae." *Chemical and Pharmaceutical Bulletin* 22 (2): 404–8.

Talapatra, S. K., O. Rath, E. Clayton, S. Tomasi, and F. Kozielski. 2016. "Depsidones from Lichens as Natural Product Inhibitors of M-Phase Phosphoprotein 1, a Human Kinesin Required for Cytokinesis." *Journal of Natural Products* 70 (6): 1576–85.

Tan, C. Y., F. R. Wang, G. D. Anaya-Eugenio, J. C. Galllucci, et al. 2019. "A-Pyrone and Sterol Constituents of *Penicillium aurantiacobrunneum*, a Fungal Associate of the Lichen *Niebla homalea*." *Journal of Natural Products* 82 (9): 2529–36.

Tan, M. A., S. G. Castro, P. M. P. Oliva, P. R. J. Yap, A. Nakayama, H. D. Magpantay, and T. E. E. D. Cruz. 2020. "Biodiscovery of Antibacterial Constituents from the Endolichenic Fungi Isolated from *Parmotrema rampoddense*." *3 Biotech* 10 (5): 212.

Tanas, S., F. Odabasoglu, Z. Halici, A. Cakir, H. Aygun, A. Asian, and H. Suleyman. 2010. "Evaluation of Anti-inflammatory and Antioxidant Activities of *Peltigera rufescens* Lichen Species in Acute and Chronic Inflammation Models." *Journal of Natural Medicine* 64 (1): 42–49.

Tang, R., A. Kimishima, A. Setiawan, and M. Arai. 2020. "Secalonic Acid D as a Selective Cytotoxic Substance on the Cancer Cells Adapted to Nutrient Starvation." *Journal of Natural Medicine* 74 (2): 495–500.

Tapalsky, D. V., D. R. Petrenev, O. M. Khramchenkova, and A. S. Doroshkevich. 2017. "Antimicrobial and Antifungal Activity of Lichens Prevalent in Belarus." *Zhurnal Mikrobiologii Epidemiologii Immunobiologii* 2: 60–65.

Tas, I., A. B. Yildirim, G. C. Ozyigitoglu, et al. 2017. "Determination of Biological Activities (Antibacterial, Antioxidant and Antiproliferative) and Metabolite Analysis of Some Lichen Species from Turkey." *European Journal of Biomedical and Pharmaceutical Sciences* 4 (4): 13–20.

Tas, I., J. Han, S. Y. Park, Y. Yang, R. Zhou, et al. 2019. "Physciosporin Suppresses the Proliferation, Motility and Tumourigenesis of Colorectal Cancer Cells." *Phytomedicine* 56: 10–20.

Tas, I., M. Varli, Y. Son, J. Han, D. Kwak, Y. Yang, et al. 2021. "Physciosporin Suppresses Mitochondrial Respiration, Aerobic Glycolysis, and Tumorigenesis in Breast Cancer." *Phytomedicine* 91:153674.

Tatipamula, V. B., S. S. P. Annam, H. T. Nguyen, H. Polimati, and R. P. Yejella. 2021. "Sekikaic Acid Modulates Pancreatic ß-Cells in Streptozotocin-Induced Type 2 Diabetic Rats by Inhibiting Digestive Enzymes." *Natural Product Research* 35 (23).

Tatipamula, V. B., H. T. Nguyen, and B. Kukavica. 2022. "Beneficial Effects of Liposomal Formulations of Lichen Substances: A Review." *Current Drug Delivery* 19 (3): 252–59.

Tay, T., A. O. Türk, M. Yilmaz, H. Türk, and M. Kivanc. 2004. "Evaluation of the Antimicrobial Activity of the Acetone Extract of the Lichen *Ramalina farinacea* and Its (+)-Usnic Acid, Norstictic Acid, and Protocetraric Acid Constituents." *Zeitschrift für Naturforschung C Journal of Biosciences* 59 (5–6): 384–88.

Taylor, J., and T. Fourie. 2019. "Antimicrobial Properties from Lichens: An Evaluation of the Antimicrobial Properties of English Churchyard Lichens." *Acccess Microbiology* 1 (10).

Taylor, T. N., H. Hass, W. Remy, and H. Kerp. 1995. "The Oldest Fossil Lichen." *Nature* 378: 244.

Teit, J. A., and F. Boas. 1900. "The Thompson Indians of British Columbia." *American Museum of Natural History Memoirs* 2: 163–392. New York: American Museum of Natural History.

Thadhani, V. M., and V. Karunaratne. 2017. "Potential of Lichen Compounds as Anti-diabetic Agents with Antioxidative Properties: A Review." *Oxidative Medicine and Cellular Longevity.*

Thompson, R. Q., D. Katz, and B. Sheehan. 2019. "Chemical Comparison of *Prunus africana* Bark and Pygeum Products Marketed for Prostate Health." *Journal of Pharmaceutical and Biomedical Analysis* 163: 162–69.

Thorsteinsdottir, U. A., M. Thorsteinsdottir, and L. H. Lambert. 2016. "Protolichesterinic Acid, Isolated from the Lichen *Cetraria islandica*, Reduce LRRC8A Expression and Volume-Sensitive Release of Organic Osmolytes in Human Lung Epithelial Cancer Cells." *Phytotherapy Research* 30 (1): 97–104.

Throop, P. 1998. *Hildegard von Bingen's Physica. The Complete English Translation of Her Classic Work on Health and Healing.* (Trans. from Latin). Rochester, VT: Healing Arts Press.

Thuan, N. H., H. Polimati, R. Alluri, and V. B. Tatipamula. 2022. "Bioassay-Guided Isolation of Anti-mycobacterial Substances from the Traditionally Used Lichen *Cladonia pyxidata* (L.) Hoffm." *3 Biotech* 12 (4): 95.

Todd, D. A., C. P. Parlet, H. A. Crosby, C. L. Malone, et al. 2017. "Signal Biosynthesis Inhibition with Ambuic Acid as a Strategy to Target Antibiotic-Resistant Infections." *Antimicrobial Agents and Chemotherapy* 61 (8): e00263–17.

Tokiwano, T., H. Satoh, T. Obara, H. Hirota, Y. Yoshizawa, and Y. Yamamoto. 2009. "A Lichen Substance as an Antiproliferative Compound against HL-60 Human Leukemia Cells: 16-O-acetyl-leucotylic Acid Isolated from *Myelochroa aurulenta*." *Bioscience Biotechnology and Biochemistry* 73 (11): 2525–27.

Torres, A., M. Hochberg, I. Pergament, R. Smoum, V. Niddam, V. M. Dembitsky, et al. 2004. "A New UV-B Absorbing Mycosporine with pPhoto Protective Activity from the Lichenized Ascomycete *Collema cristatum*." *European Journal of Biochemistry* 271 (4): 780–84.

Torres-Benitez, A., J. E. Ortega-Valencia, M. Sanchez, P. K. Divakar, M. J. Simirgiotis, M. P. Gomez-Serranillos. 2022. "Metabolomic Profiling, Antioxidant and Enzyme Inhibition Properties and Molecular Docking Analysis of Antarctic Lichens." *Molecules* 27 (22): 8086.

Torres-Benitez, A., J. E. Ortega-Valencia, M. Sanchez, M. Hillmann-Eggers, et al. 2022a. "UHPLC-MS Chemical Fingerprinting and Antioxidant, Enzyme Inhibition,

Anti-Inflammatory In Silico and Cytoprotective Activities of *Cladonia chlorophaea* and *C. gracilis* (Cladoniaceae) from Antarctica." *Antioxidants* (Basel) 12 (1): 10.

Tozatti, M. G., D. S. Ferreria, L. G. B. Flauzino, et al. 2016. "Activity of the Lichen *Usnea steineri* and Its Major Metabolites against Gram-Positive, Multidrug-Resistant Bacteria." *Natural Product Communications* 11 (4): 493–96.

Trybus, W., T. Król, E. Trybus, and A. Stachurska. 2021. "Physcion Induces Potential Anticancer Effects in Cervical Cancer Cells." *Cells* 10 (8): 2029.

Tuong, T. L., V. T. Nga, D. T. Huy, et al. 2014. "A New Depside from *Usnea aciculifera* Growing in Vietnam." *Natural Product Communications* 9 (8): 1179–80.

Tuong, T. L., T. Aree, L. T. M. Do, P. K. P. Nguyen, et al. 2019. "Dimeric Tetrahydroxanthones from the Lichen *Usnea aciculifera*." *Fitoterapia* 137: 104194.

Tuong, T. L., L. T. M. Do, T. Aree, P. Wonganan, and W. Chavasiri. 2020. "Tetrahydroxanthone-Chromanone Heterodimers from Lichen *Usnea aciculifera* and Their Cytotoxic Activity against Human Cancer Cell Lines." *Fitoterapia* 147: 104732.

Tuovinen, V., A. M. Millanes, S. Freire-Rallo, A. Rosling, and M. Wedin. 2021. "*Tremella macrobasidiata* and *Tremella variae* Have Abundant and Widespread Yeast Stages in *Lecanora* Lichens." *Environmental Microbiology* 23 (5): 2484–98.

Türk, H., et al. 2003. "The Antimicrobial Activity of Extracts of the Lichen *Cetraria aculeata* and Its Protolichesterinic Acid Constituents." *Zeitschrift fur Naturforschung* 59 (11–12): 850–54.

Turkez, H., E. Aydin, T. Sisman, and A. Aslan. 2012. "Role of *Peltigera rufescens* (Weis) Humb. (a Lichen) on Imazalil-Induced Genotoxicity: Analysis of Micronucleus and Chromosome Aberrations In Vitro." *Toxicology and Industrial Health* 28 (6): 492–98.

Turkez, H., E. Aydin, and A. Aslan. 2012a. "Effects of Lichenic Extracts (*Hypogymnia physodes*, *Ramalina polymorpha* and *Usnea florida*) on Human Blood Cells: Cytogenetic and Biochemical Study." *Iranian Journal of Pharmaceutical Research* 11 (3): 889–96.

Turkez, H., E. Aydin, and A. Aslan. 2012b. "*Xanthoria elegans* (Link) (Lichen) Extract Counteracts DNA Damage and Oxidative Stress of Mitocycin C in Human Lymphocytes." *Cytotechnology* 64 (6): 679–86.

Turkez, H., E. Aydin, and A. Aslan. 2014. "Role of Aqueous *Bryoria capillaris* (Ach.) Extract as a Genoprotective Agent on Imazalil-Induced Genotoxicity In Vitro." *Toxicology and Industrial Health* 30 (1): 33–39.

Turner, N. J. 1973. *The Ethnobotany of the Bella Coola Indians of British Columbia*. Syesis, publication of Royal Museum of BC. 6: 193–220.

Turner, N. J., R. Bouchard, and D. I. D. Kennedy. 1980. *Ethnobotany of the Okanagan-Colville Indians of British Columbia and Washington*. Occasional Paper 21. Victoria: British Columbia Provincial Museum Publications.

Turner, N. J., and B. S. Efrat. 1982. *Ethnobotany of the Hesquiat Indians of Vancouver Island*. Cultural Recovery Paper 2, Victoria: British Columbia Provincial Museum Publications.

Turner, N. J., J. Thomas, B. F. Carlson, and R. T. Ogilvie. 1983. *Ethnobotany of the Nitinaht*

Indians of Vancouver Island. Occasional Paper 24. Victoria: British Columbia Provincial Museum Publications 24: 1–165.

Turner, N. J., L. C. Thompson, M. T. Thompson, and A. Z. York. 1990. *Thompson Ethnobotany: Knowledge and Usage of Plants by the Thompson Indians of British Columbia.* Memoir 3. Victoria: Royal British Columbia Museum.

Turner, N. J. 1998. *Plant Technology of First Peoples in British Columbia.* Victoria: University of British Columbia Press and Royal British Columbia Museum.

Turner, N. J. 2004. *Plants of Haida Gwaii.* Winlaw, BC: Sononis Press.

Turner, N. J. 2004a. *Expert Report: Tsilhqot'in and Xeni Gwet'in Plant Use and Occupancy.* Presented in the William vs. Her Majesty the Queen, Xeni Gwet'in/Tsilqot'in Land Rights Trial. British Columbia Supreme Court, Canada.

Turner, N. J., and J. C. Thompson. 2006. *"Nwana" a lax Yuup: Plants of the Gitga' People.* Victoria, Canada: Cortex Consulting, School of Environmental Studies, and Coasts Under Stress.

Turner, N. J., and R. J. Hebda. 2012. *Saanich Ethnobotany: Culturally Important Plants of the WSANEC People.* Victoria: Royal British Columbia Museum.

Turney-High, H. H. 1937. *The Flathead Indians of Montana. Memoirs of the American Anthropological Association* 48. Menasha, WI: American Anthropological Assn.

Uprety, Y., H. Asselin, A. Dhakal, and N. Julien. 2012. "Traditional Use of Medicinal Plants in the Boreal Forest of Canada: Review and Perspectives." *Journal of Ethnobiology and Ethnomedicine* 8: 7.

Urbanska, N., P. Simko, A. Leskanicova, M. Karasova, Z. Jendzelovska, R. Jendzelovsky, et al. 2022. "Atranorin, a Secondary Metabolite of Lichens, Exhibited Anxiolytic/Antidepressant Activity in Wistar Rats." *Life* (Basel) 12 (11): 1850.

Ureña-Vacas, I., E. González-Burgos, S. De Vita, P. K. Divaker, G. Bifulco, and M. P. Gómez-Serranillos. 2022. "Phytochemical Characterization and Pharmacological Properties of Lichen Extracts from Cetrarioid Clade by Multivariate Analysis and Molecular Docking." *Evidence Based Complementary and Alternative Medicine* 2022: 5218248.

Ureña-Vacas, I., E. González-Burgos, P. K. Divakar, and M. P. Gómez-Serranillos. 2022a. "Lichen Extracts from Cetrarioid Clade Provide Neuroprotection against Hydrogen Peroxide-Induced Oxidative Stress." *Molecules* 27 (19): 6520.

Ureña-Vacas, I., E. González-Burgos, P. K. Divakar, and M. P. Gómez-Serranillos. 2023. "Lichen Depsides and Tridepside: Progress in Pharmacological Approaches." *Journal of Fungi* 9 (1): 116.

Váczi, P., Y. Gausiaa, and K. A. Solhaug. 2018. "Efficient Fungal UV-Screening Provides a Remarkably High UV-B Tolerance of Photosystem II in Lichen Photobionts." *Plant Physiology and Biochemistry* 132: 89–94.

Vaez, M., S. J. Davarpanah. 2021. "New Insights into the Biological Activity of Lichens; Bioavailable Secondary Metabolites of *Umbilicaria decussata* as Potential Anticoagulants." *Chemistry and Biodiversity* 18 (5): e2100080.

Valadbeigi, T. 2016. "Chemical Composition and Enzymes Inhibitory, Brine Shrimp Larvae Toxicity, Antimicrobial and Antioxidant Activities of *Caloplaca biatorina.*" *Zahedan Journal of Research in Medical Sciences* 18 (11): e4267.

Valadbeigi, T., and M. Shaddel. 2016. "Amylase Inhibitory Activity of Some Macro Lichens in Mazandaran Province, Iran." *Physiology and Pharmacology* 20: 215–219.

Valencia-Islas, N. A., J. J. Arguello, J. L. Rojas, et al. 2021. "Antioxidant and Photoprotective Metabolites of *Bunodophoron melanocarpum*, a Lichen from the Andean Paramo." *Pharmaceutical Sciences* 27 (2): 281–90.

Varli, M., H. T. Pham, S. M. Kim, I. Tas, C. D. B. Gamage, R. Zhou, S. Pulat, et al. 2022. "An Acetonic Extract and Secondary Metabolites from the Endolichenic Fungus *Nemania* sp. EL006872 Exhibit Immune Checkpoint Inhibitory Activity in Lung Cancer Cell." *Frontiers in Pharmacology* 13: 986946.

Varli, M., E. Y. Lee, Y. Yang, R. Zhou, et al. 2023. "1'O-methyl-averantin Isolated from the Endolichenic Fungus *Jackrogersella* sp. EL001572 Suppresses Colorectal Cancer Stemness via Sonic Hedgehog and Notch Signaling." *Scientific Reports* 13 (1): 2811.

Varol, A., M. Candan, T. Tay, and A. Türk. 2015. "Anti-cancer and Anti-angiogenic Activities of a Lichen Derived Substance: Alpha Collatolic Acid." Conference paper. Fifth International Congress of Molecular Medicine, May.

Varol, M., A. Türk, M. Candan, T. Tay, and A. T. Koparal. 2016. "Photoprotective Activity of Vulpinic and Gyrophoric Acids toward Ultraviolet B-Induced Damage in Human Keratinocytes." *Phytotherapy Research* 30 (1): 9–15.

Varol, M. 2018. "Anti-breast Cancer and Anti-angiogenic Potential of a Lichen-Derived Small-Molecule: Barbatolic Acid." *Cytotechnology* 70 (6): 1565–73.

Vartia, K. O. 1973. "Antibiotics in Lichens." In *The Lichens,* eds. V. Ahmadjian and M. E. Hale, 547–61. New York: Academic Press.

Vassari, M., L. Ponti, D. Degl'Innocenti, and M. C. Bergonzi. 2022. "Usnic Acid-Loaded Polymeric Micelles: An Optimal Migrastatic-Acting Formulation in Human SH-SY5Y Neuroblastoma Cells." *Pharmaceuticals* 15:1207.

Vassari, M., L. Ponti, D. Degl'Innocenti, and M. C. Bergonzi. 2024. "Liposomal Formulation Improves the Bioactivity of Usnic Acid in RAW 264.7 Macrophage Cells Reducing Its Toxicity." *Current Drug Delivery* 21 (1): 91–103.

Verma, N., B. C. Behera, A. Sonone, and U. Makhija. 2008. "Lipid Peroxidation and Tyrosinase Inhibition by Lichen Symbionts Grown In Vitro." *African Journal of Biochemistry Research* 2 (12): 225–31.

Verma, N., B. C. Behera, and B. Sharma. 2012. "Glucosidase Inhibitory and Radical Scavenging Properties of Lichen Metabolites Salazinic, Sekikaic and Usnic Acid." *Hacettepe Journal of Biology and Chemistry* 40 (1): 7–21.

Vinayaka, K. S., S. Karthik, K. C. Nandini, and T. R. P. Kedura. 2013. "Amylase Inhibitory Activity of Some Macrolichens of Western Ghats, Karnataka, India." *Indian Journal of Novel Drug Delivery* 5 (4): 225–28.

Vogel, V. J. 1970. *American Indian Medicine.* Norman: University of Oklahoma Press.

Vu, T. H., A. C. Le Lamer, C. Lalli, et al. 2015. "Depsides: Lichen Metabolites Active against Hepatitis C Virus." *PLoS ONE* 10e: 0120405.

Wang, F., S. Li, T. Y. Wang, G. A. Lopez, I. Antoshechkin, and T. F. Chou. 2022. "P97/VCP

ATPase Inhibitors Can Rescue p97 Mutation-Linked Motor Neuron Degeneration." *Brain Communications* 4 (4).

Wang, G., Y. Li, B. Wang, J. Gao, Z. Yan, and X. Li. 1991. "Anti-tumor Effect of *Cetraria laevigata* Rassad. Polysaccharides." *Zhongguo Zhong Yao Za Zhi* 16 (4): 242–44.

Wang, H. X., T. Yang, X. M. Cheng, S. F. Kwong, C. H. Liu, R. An, et al. 2018. "Simultaneous Determination of Usnic, Dffractaic, Evernicand Barbatic Acids in Rat Plasma by Ultra-High-Performance Liquid Chromatography-Quadrupole Exactive Orbitrap Mass Spectrometry and Its Application to Pharmacokinetic Studies." *Biomedical Chromatography* 32 (3).

Wang, J., H. Zhao, Q. X. Guo, and H. Y. Ding. 2022a. "Identification and Antibacterial Activity of *Thamnolia vermicularis* and *Thamnolia subuliformis*." *Journal of Microbiological Methods* 203: 106528.

Wang, J., X. H. Nong, X. Y. Zhang, X. Y. Xu, M. Amin, and S. H. Qi. 2017. "Screening of Anti-biofilm Compounds from Marine-Derived Fungi and the Effects of Secalonic Acid D on *Staphylococcus aureus* Biofilm." *Journal of Microbiology and Biotechnology* 27 (6): 1078–89.

Wang, L. S., T. Narui, H. Harada, C. F. Culberson, and W. L. Culberson. 2001. "Ethnic Uses of Lichens in Yunnan, China." *Bryologist* 104 (3): 345–49.

Wang, Q. X., L. Bao, X. L. Yang, et al. 2012. "Polyketides with Antimicrobial Activity from the Solid Culture of an Endolichenic Fungus *Ulocladium* sp." *Fitoterapia* 83 (1): 209–14.

Wang, S., X. M. Li. F. Teuscher, D. L. Li, A. Diesel, R. Ebel, et al. 2006. "Chaetopyranin, a Benzaldehyde Derivative, and Other Related Metabolites from *Chaetomium globosum*, an Endophytic Fungus Derived from the Marine Red Alga *Polysiphonia urceolata*." *Journal of Natural Products* 68 (11): 1622–25.

Wang, T., C. Shen, F. Guo, Y. Q. Zhao, J. Wang, et al. 2021a. "Characterization of a Polysaccharide from the Medicinal Lichen, *Usnea longissima*, and Its Immunostimulating Effect In Vivo." *International Journal of Biological Macromolecules* 181: 672–82.

Wang, W. J., S. Niu, L. X. Qiao, F. L. Wei, J. M. Yin, S. S. Wang, Y. Ouyang, and D. Chen. 2021. "Usnea Acid as Multidrug Resistance (MDR) Reversing Agent against Human Chronic Myelogenous Leukemia K562/ADDR Cells via an ROS Dependent Apoptosis." *BioMed Research International* 2021: 9808613.

Wang, X. C., S. Biswas, N. Paudval, H. Pan, et al. 2019. "Antibiotic Resistance in *Salmonella typhimurium* Isolates Recovered from the Food Chain through National Antimicrobial Resistance Monitoring System between 1996 and 2016." *Frontiers in Microbiology* 10: 985.

Wang, Y. C., Z. H. Zheng, S. C. Liu, H. Zhang, E. Li, et al. 2010. "Oxepinochromenones, Furochromenone, and Their Putative Precursors from the Endolichenic Fungus *Coniochaeta* sp." *Journal of Natural Products* 73 (5): 920–24.

Warren, E., K. Morgan, T. J. Toward, M. Schwenkglenks, and J. Leadbetter. 2019. "Cost Effectiveness of Inhaled Mannitol (Bronchitol®) in Patients with Cystic Fibrosis." *Pharmacoeconomics* 37 (3): 435–46.

Wassman, C. D., R. Baronio, O. Demir, B. D. Wallentine, C. K. Chen, L. V. Hall, et al. 2013. "Computational Identification of a Transiently Open L1/S3 Pocket for Reactivation of Mutant p53." *Nature Communications* 4: 1407.

Watt, J. M., and M. R. Breyer-Brandwijk. 1962. *The Medicinal and Poisonous Plants of Southeastern and Eastern Africa*. Edinburgh: E. and S. Livingstone.

Weaver, W. W. trans., ed. 2001. *Sauer's Herbal Cures: America's First Book of Botanic Healing 1762–1778*. New York: Routledge.

Wedin, M., S. Maier, S. Fernandez-Brime, B. Cronholm, M. Westberg, and M. Grube. 2016. "Microbiome Change by Symbiotic Invasion in Lichens." *Environmental Microbiology* 18 (5): 1428–39.

Weissbuch, B. K. 2014. "Medicinal Lichens: The Final Frontier." *Journal of the American Herbalists Guild* 12 (2): 22–28.

Weiss-Penzias, P. S., M. S. Bank, D. L. Clifford, A. Torregrosa, B. Zheng, W. Lin, and C. C. Wilmers. 2019. "Marine Fog Inputs Appear to Increase Methylmercury Bioaccumulation in a Coastal Terrestrial Food Web." *Scientific Reports* 9 (1): 17611.

Wennekens, A. J. 1985. "Traditional Plant Usage by Chugach Natives around Prince William Sound and the Lower Kenai Peninsula, Alaska." MA thesis, University of Alaska.

Whang, W. K., H. S. Park, I. H. Ham, M. Y. Oh, H. Namkoong, et al. 2005. "Methyl Gallate and Chemicals Structurally Related to Methyl Gallate Protect Human Umbilical Vein Endothelial Cells from Oxidative Stress." *Experimental and Molecular Medicine* 37 (4): 343–52.

Whiting, A. F., 1939. *Ethnobotany of the Hopi*. Museum of Northern Arizona Bulletin 15.

Widhelm, T. J., F. R. Bertoletti, M. J. Asztalos, J. A. Mercado-Diaz, et al. 2018. "Oligocene Origin and Drivers of Diversification in the Genus Sticta (Lobariaceae, Ascomycota)." *Molecular Phylogenetics and Evolution* 126: 58–73.

Wigger, G. W., T. C. Bouton, K. R. Jacobson, et al. 2022. "The Impact of Alcohol Use Disorder on Tuberculosis: A Review of the Epidemiology and Potential Immunologic Mechanisms." *Frontiers in Immunology* 13: 864817.

Wijeratne, E. M. K., B. P. Bashyal, M. X. Liu, D. D. Rocha, et al. 2012. "Geopyxins A-E, Ent-kaurane Diterpenoids from Endolichenic Fungal Strains *Geopyxis* aff. majalis and *Geopyxis* sp. AZ0066: Structure-Activity Relationships of Geopyxins and Their Analogues." *Journal of Natural Products* 75 (3): 361–69.

Wijeratne, E. M. K., G. M. Kamal, B. Gunaherath, V. M. Chapla, J. Tillotson, et al. 2016. "Oxaspirol B with p97 Inhibitory Activity and Other Oxaspirols from *Lecythophora* sp. FL1275 and FL1031, Endolichenic Fungi Inhabiting *Parmotrema tinctorum* and *Cladonia evansii*." *Journal of Natural Products* 79 (2): 340–52.

Williams, D. E., J. Davies, B. Patrick, et al. 2008. "Cladoniamides A-G Tryptophan-Derived Alkaloids Produced in Culture by *Streptomyces uncialis*." *Organic Letters* 10: 3501–4.

Wilson, M. R. 1978. "Notes on Ethnobotany in Inuktitut." *Western Canadian Journal of Anthropology* 8: 180–96.

Wise, J. R. 1863. *The New Forest: Its History and its Scenery*. London: Smith Elder.

Wu, G. Q., J. X. Xu, Q. Y. Wang, Z. Y. Fang, et al. 2023. "Methionine-Restricted Diet: A Feasible Strategy against Chronic or Aging-Related Diseases." *Journal of Agricultural and Food Chemistry* 71 (1): 5–19.

Wyman, L. C., and S. K. Harris. 1941. "Navajo Indian Medical Ethnobotany." *University of New Mexico Bulletin Anthropology Series* 3: 1–76.

Wyzewski, Z., M. B. Mielcarska, K. P. Gregorczyk-Zboroch, and A. Myszka. 2022. "Virus-Mediated Inhibition of Apoptosis in the Context of EBV-Associated Diseases: Molecular Mechanisms and Therapeutic Perspectives." *International Journal of Molecular Sciences* 23 (13): 7265.

Xiang, W. J., Q. Q. Wang, L. Ma, and L. H. Hu. 2013. "B-Orcinol-type Depsides from the Lichen *Thamnolia vermicularis*." *Natural Products Research* 27 (9): 804–8.

Xie, F., X. Y. Luan, Y. Gao, K. Xu, and H. X. Lou. 2020. "Cytotoxic Heptaketides from the Endolichenic Fungus *Ulospora bilgramii*." *Journal of Natural Products* 83 (5): 1623–33.

Xie, L. L., M. J. Li, D. S. Liu, X. Wang, P. Y. Wang, et al. 2019. "Secalonic Acid-F, a Novel Mycotoxin, Represses the Progression of Hepatocellular Carcinoma via MARCH1 Regulation of the PI3K/AKT/ß-catenin Signaling Pathway." *Molecules* 24 (3): 393.

Xiong, Y. X., L. Ren, Z. Q. Wang, Z. C. Hu, and Y. J. Zhou. 2015. "Anti-proliferative Effect of Physcion on Human Gastric Cell Line via Inducing ROS-Dependent Apoptosis." *Cell Biochemistry and Biophysics* 73 (2): 537–43.

Xue, L., H. L. Tang, J. W. Song, J. Y. Long, L. L. Zhang, and X. F. Li. 2019. "Chrysophanol: A Review of Its Pharmacology, Toxicity and Pharmacokinetics." *Journal of Pharmacy and Pharmacology* 71 (10): 1475–87.

Yamamoto, Y., et al. 1993. "Using Lichen Tissue Cultures in Modern Biology." *Bryologist* 96 (3): 384–93.

Yamamoto, Y., Y. Miura, Y. Kinoshita, et al. 1995. "Screening of Tissue Cultures and Thalli of Lichens and Some of Their Active Constituents for Inhibition of Tumor-Promoter-Induced Epstein-Barr Virus Activation." *Chemical and Pharmaceutical Bulletin* 43 (8): 1388–90.

Yamamoto, Y., Y. Kinoshita, H. Matsubara, et al. 1998. "Screening of Biological Activities and Isolation of Biological-Active Compounds from Lichens." *Recent Research Developments in Phytochemistry* 2:23–33.

Yamamoto, Y., Y. Kinoshita, G. R. Thor, M. Hasumi, K. Kinoshita, K. Koyama, K. Takahashi, and I. Yoshimura. 2002. "Isofuranoaphthoquinone Derivatives from Cultures of the Lichen *Arthronia cinnabarina* (DC.) Wallr." *Phytochemistry* 60 (7): 741–45.

Yamano, Y., and H. L. Rakotondraibe. 2022. "Understanding the Biosynthesis of Paxisterol in Lichen-Derived *Penicillium aurantiacobrunneum* for the Production of Fluorinated Derivatives." *Molecules* 27 (5): 1641.

Yañez, O., M. I. Osorio, E. Osorio, W. Tiznado, Lina Ruíz et al. 2023. "Antioxidant Activity and Enzymatic of Lichen Substances: A Study Based on Cyclic Voltammetry and Theoretical." *Chemico-Biological Interactions* 372: 110357.

Yang, Y., S. Y. Park, T. T. Nguyen, Y. H. Yu, et al. 2015. "Lichen Secondary Metabolite, Physciosporin, Inhibits Lung Cancer Cell Motility." *PLoS ONE* 10 (9): e0137889.

Yang, Y., T. T. Nguyen, M. H. Jeong, F. Crisan, Y. H. Yu, H. H. Ha, K. H. Choi, et al. 2016. "Inhibitory Activity of (+)-Usnic Acid against Non-small Cell Lung Cancer Cell Motility." *PloS ONE* 11 (1): e0146575.

Yang, Y., Y. H. Yu, H. H. Ha, et al. 2017. "Inhibitory Activity of Lichen Secondary Metabolite Physciosporin, against Lung Cancer Cell Motility." *Cancer Research* 77 (13) Abstract 4209.

Yang, Y., W. K. Bae, S. J. Nam, M. H. Jeong, R. Zhou, et al. 2018. "Acetonic Extracts of the Endolichenic Fungus EL002332 Isolated from *Endocarpon pusillum* Exhibits Anticancer Activity in Human Gastric Cancer Cells." *Phytomedicine* 40: 106–15.

Yang, Y., S. R. Bhosle, Y. H. Yu, S. Y. Park, R. Zhou, et al. 2018. "Tumidulin, a Lichen Secondary Metabolite, Decreases the Stemness Potential of Colorectal Cancer Cells." *Molecules* 23 (11): 2968.

Yang, Y., T. T. Nguyen, I. Pereira, J. S. Hur, and H. G. Kim. 2019. "Lichen Secondary Metabolite Physciosporin Decreases the Stemness Potential of Colorectal Cancer Cells." *Biomolecules* 9 (12): 797.

Yangin, S., D. Cansaran-Duman, G. G. Eskiler, S. Aras. 2022. "The Molecular Mechanisms of Vulpinic Acid Induced Programmed Cell Death in Melanoma." *Molecular Biology Reports* 49 (9): 8273–80.

Yaoi, X. Y., B. Y. Lu, C. T. Lü, Q. Bai, D. Z. Yan, and H. Xu. 2017. "Taraxerol Induces Cell Apoptosis through a Mitochondria-Mediated Pathway in HeLa Cells." *Cell Journal* 19 (3): 512–19.

Yayla, S. K., Z. Kocakaya, G. S. Karatoprak, S. Ilgün, and A. Ceylan. 2023. "Analyzing the Impact of *Ramalina digitellata*, *R. fastigiate*, *R. fraxinea*, and *R. polymorpha's* Usnic Acid Concentration on Antioxidant, DNA-Protective, Antimicrobial, and Cytotoxic Properties." *Chemistry and Biodiversity* 20 (1): e202200816.

Yeash, E. A., L. Letwin, L. Malek, Z. Suntres, K. Knudsen, and L. P. Christopher. 2017. "Biological Activities of Undescribed North American Lichen Species." *Journal of the Science of Food and Agriculture* 97 (14): 4721–26.

Yilmaz, M., T. Tay, M. Kivanc, H. Türk, and A. O. Türk. 2005. "The Antimicrobial Activity of Extracts of the Lichen *Hypogymnia tubulosa* and Its 3-hydroxyphysodic Acid Constituent." *Zeitschrift fur Naturforschung Section C Journal of Biosciences.* 60 (1–2): 35–38.

Yilmaz, M., N. Y. Sanözlü, M. Candan, and N. Tay. 2017. "Screening of Antibacterial, Antituberculosis and Antifungal Effects of Lichen *Usnea florida* and Its Thamnolic Constituent." *Biomedical Research* 28: 3108–13.

Yoshikawa, K., N. Kokudo, M. Tanaka, T. Nakano, et al. 2008. "Novel Abietane Diterpenoids and Aromatic Compounds from *Cladonia rangiferina* and Their Antimicrobial Activity against Antibiotics Resistant Bacteria." *Chemical and Pharmaceutical Bulletin* 56 (1): 89–92.

Youn, D. H., J. B. Park, H. L. Kim, Y. N. Jung. J. W. Kang, et al. 2017. "Chrysophanic Acid Reduces Testosterone-Induced Benign Prostatic Hyperplasia in Rats by Suppressing 5*a*-reductase and Etracellular Signal-Regulated Kinase." *Oncotarget* 8 (6): 9500–12.

Young, D., G. Ingram, and Lise Swartz. 1989. *Cry of the Eagle: Encounters with a Cree Healer.* Toronto: University of Toronto Press.

Young, D., R. Rogers, and R. Willier. 2015. *A Cree Healer and His Medicine Bundle: Revelations of Indigenous Wisdom.* Berkeley CA: North Atlantic Books.

Yu, X. L., X. Y. Yang, X. L. Gao, R. F. Bai, X. Yin, et al. 2016. "Phenolic Constituents from Lichen *Usnea longissima*." *Zhongguo Zhong Yao Za Zhi* 41 (10): 1864–69.

Yu, X. L., Q. Guo, G. Z. Su, A. Yang, et al. 2016a. "Usnic Acid Derivatives with Cytotoxic and Antifungal Activities from the Lichen *Usnea longissima*." *Journal of Natural Products* 79 (5): 1373–80.

Yu, X. B., Y. S. Cai, X. Zhao, C. Y. Wu, J. Q. Liu, T. T. Niu, X. Shan, Y. J. Lu, Y. Ruan, and J. W. He. 2022. "Investigation of the Chemical Structure of Anti-amyloidogenic Constituents Extracted from *Thamnolia vermicularis*." *Journal of Ethnopharmacology* 289: 115059.

Yuan, W. H., M. T. Teng, Y. F. Yun, N. Jiang, et al. 2020. "Talarolactone A, an Isocoumarin Derivative Fused with Dihydrothiophene with Selective Antimigratory Activity from the Endolichenic Fungus *Talaromyes* sp." *Journal of Natural Products* 83 (5): 1716–20.

Yuan, X. L., and S. H. Xiao. 2005. "Lichen-Like Symbiosis 600 Million Years Ago." *Science* 308 (5724): 1017–20.

Yurdacan, B., U. Egeli, G. G. Eskiler, I. E. Eryilmaz, G. Cecener, and B. Tunca. 2019. "The Role of Usnic Acid-Induced Apoptosis and Autophagy in Hepatocellular Carcinoma." *Human and Experimental Toxicology* 38 (2): 201–15.

Zaghi, D., and J. R. Griffin. 2016. "Defining 'Lichen' from Greek Mycology to Modern Dermatology." *JAMA Dermatology* 152 (10): 1136.

Zambare, V. P., and L. P. Christopher. 2012. "Biopharmaceutical Potential of Lichens." *Pharmaceutical Biology* 50 (6): 778–98.

Zeytinoglu, H., Z. Incesu, B. A. Tuylu, A. O. Turk, and B. Barutca. 2008. "Determination of Genotoxic, Antigenotoxic and Cytotoxic Potential of the Extract from Lichen *Cetraria aculeata* (Schreb.) Fr. In Vitro." *Phytotherapy Research* 22 (1): 118–23.

Zhai, M. M., C. X. Jiang, Y. P. Shi, et al. 2016. "The Bioactive Secondary Metabolites from *Talaromyces* Species." *Natural Products and Bioprospecting* 6 (1): 1–24.

Zhang, H., L. Y. Huang, L. Y. Tao, J. Y. Zhang, F. Wang, X. Zhang, and L. W. Fu. 2019. "Secalonic Acid D Induces Cell Apoptosis in Both Sensitive and ABCG2-Overexpressing Multidrug Resistant Cancer Cells through Upregulating c-Jun Expression." *Acta Pharmaceutica Sinica* B. 9 (3): 516–25.

Zhang, J. Y., L. Y. Tao, Y. J. Liang, Y. Y. Yan, et al. 2009. "Secalonic Acid D Induced Leukemia Cell Apoptosis and Cell Cycle Arrest of G(1) with Involvement of GSK-3beta/beta-catenin/c-Myc Pathway." *Cell Cycle* 8 (15): 2444–50.

Zhang, L. P., R. T. Dong, Y. Wang, L. X. Wang, et al. 2021. "The Anti-breast Cancer Property of Physcion via Oxidative Stress-Mediated Mitochondrial Apoptosis and Immune Response." *Pharmaceutical Biology* 59 (1): 303–10.

Zhang, Q., R. L. Luan, H. X. Li, Y. Liu, et al. 2018. "Anti-inflammatory Actions of Ambuic Acid, a Natural Product Isolated from Solid Culture of *Pestalotiopsis neglecta*, through Blocking ERK/JNK Mitogen-Activated Protein Kinase Signaling Pathway." *Experimental and Therapeutic Medicine* 16 (2): 1538–46.

Zhang, X., Z. W. Gao, K. Chen, et al. 2022a. "Lupeol Inhibits the Proliferation and Migration of MDA-MB-231 Breast Cancer Cells via a Novel Crosstalk Mechanism between Autophagy and EMT." *Food and Function* 13 (9): 4967–76.

Zhang, Y., J. Shi, Y. Zhao, H. Cui, and S. Liu. 2012. "An Investigation of the Anti-diabetic Effects of an Extract from *Cladonia humilis*." *Pakistan Journal of Pharmaceutical Sciences* 25 (3): 509–12.

Zhang, Y., C. Y. Tan, R. W. Spjut, J. R. Fuchs, A. D. Kinghorn, and L. H. Rakatondraibe. 2020. "Specialized Metabolites of the United States Lichen *Niebla homalea* and Their Antiproliferative Activities." *Phytochemistry* 180: 112521.

Zhang, Y. Y., J. Clancy, J. Jensen, R. T. McMullin, L. S. Wang, and S. D. Leavitt. 2022. "Providing Scale to a Known Taxonomic Unknown—At Least a 70-Fold Increase in Species Diversity in a Cosmopolitan Nominal Taxon of Lichen-Forming Fungi." *Journal of Fungi* (Basel) 8 (5): 490.

Zhao, L., J. C. Kim, M. J. Paik, W. J. Lee, and J. S. Hur. 2016. "A Multifunctional and Possible Skin UV Protectant, (3*R*)-5-Hydroxymellein, Produced by an Endolichenic Fungus Isolated from *Parmotrema austrosinense*." *Molecules* 22 (1): 26.

Zhao, L., J. C. Kim, and J. S. Hur. 2022. "7-Hydroxy-2-octenoic acid-ethyl Ester Mixture as an UV Protectant Secondary Metabolite of an Endolichenic Fungus Isolated from *Menegazzia terbrata*." *Archives of Microbiology* 204 (7): 395.

Zheng, Z., S. Zhang, X. Lu, Y. Ma, Y. Fan, et al., 2012. "Trivaric Acid, a Potent Depside Human Leukocyte Elastase Inhibitor." *Biological and Pharmaceutical Bulletin* 35: 2247–51.

Zhou, B. X, X. L. Liang, Q. T. Feng, J. Li, X. P. Pan, et al. 2019. "Ergosterol Peroxide Suppresses Influenza A Virus-Induced Pro-inflammatory Response and Apoptosis by Blocking RIG-1 Signaling." *European Journal of Pharmacology* 860: 172543.

Zhou, Q., H. Liu, B. Qi, X. Y. Shi, W. H. Guo, et al. 2021. "Emodin Alleviates Intestinal Barrier Dysfunction by Inhibiting Apoptosis and Regulating the Immune Response in Severe Acute Pancreatitis." *Pancreas* 50 (8): 1202–11.

Zhou, Y. F., H. X. Shi, K. Hu, J. W. Tang, et al. 2017. "Gypmacrophin A, a Rare Pentacyclic Sesterterpenoid, Together with Three Depsides, Functioned as New Chemical Evidence for *Gypsoplaca macrophylla* (Zahlbr.) Timdal Identification." *Molecules* 22 (10): 167.

Zhu, J. L., X. M. Zhang, X. Chen, Y. Sun, Y. Dai, et al. 2017. "Studies on the Regulation of Lipid Metabolism and the Mechanism of the Aqueous and Ethanol Extracts of *Usnea*." *Biomedicine and Pharmacotherapy* 94: 930–936.

Directory of Common Names

This book is arranged in alphabetical order by genus. The list below is provided for readers who may know a species by its common name but who do not know its genus. The page number given is where the genus description begins.

Abraded camouflage lichen, see *Melanelia*, 143
Alpine bloodspot lichen, see *Ophioparma*, 154
Alpine camouflage lichen, see *Melanelia*, 143
Alpine coral lichen, see *Stereocaulon*, 221
Alpine foam lichen, see *Stereocaulon*, 221
Arctic finger lichen, see *Dactylina*, 76
Arctic kidney lichen, see *Nephroma*, 149
Arctic rag lichen, see *Asahinea*, 25
Arctic rock tripe lichen, see *Umbilicaria*, 233
Arctic tumbleweed, see *Masonhalea*, 142
Armored fog lichen, see *Niebla*, 151
Ascerbic rock tripe lichen, see *Umbilicaria*, 233

Ballpoint rock tripe lichen, see *Umbilicaria*, 233
Bark rash lichen, see *Pyrenula*, 197
Beaded tube lichen, see *Hypogymnia*, 106
Bearded jellyskin lichen, see *Leptogium*, 126
Bearded rim lichen, see *Lecanora*, 118
Beard lichen, see *Usnea*, 239
Bitter wart lichen, see *Pertusaria*, 180
Black-edged leaf lichen, see *Parmotrema*, 161
Black-eye lichen, see *Tephromela*, 227
Black-eyed rim lichen, see *Lecanora*, 118
Black-foot Cladonia lichen, see *Cladonia*, 61
Black stone flower, see *Parmotrema*, 161
Black tree hair lichen, see *Bryoria*, 29
Blistered jellyskin lichen, see *Leptogium*, 126

Blistered rock tripe lichen, see *Umbilicaria*, 233
Blister lichen, see *Toninia*, 231
Bloodspot lichen, see *Haematomma*, 100
Bloody comma lichen, see *Arthonia*, 24
Blue felt lichen, see *Pectenia*, 171
Blue-gray rosette lichen, see *Physcia*, 182
Blue jellyskin lichen, see *Leptogium*, 126
Blue oilskin lichen, see *Leptogium*, 126
Blushing rock tripe lichen, see *Umbilicaria*, 233
Blushing scale lichen, see *Psora*, 193
Boreal beard lichen, see *Usnea*, 239
Boreal oakmoss lichen, see *Evernia*, 87
Boreal pixie cup lichen, see *Cladonia*, 61
Born-again pelt lichen, see *Peltigera*, 171
Borrer's speckled-back lichen, see *Punctelia*, 194
Bright cobblestone lichen, see *Acarospora*, 16
Bristly beard lichen, see *Usnea*, 239
Bristly loop lichen, see *Hypotrachyna*, 112
British soldiers lichen, see *Cladonia*, 61
Broom moss lichen, see *Pseudoparmelia*, 192
Brown beret lichen, see *Baeomyces*, 27
Brown cobblestone lichen, see *Acarospora*, 16
Brown-eyed rim lichen, see *Lecanora*, 118
Brown-eyed sunshine lichen, see *Vulpicida*, 254
Brown-eyed wolf lichen, see *Letharia*, 128
Brown-head stubble lichen, see *Chaenotheca*, 52
Brownish monk's hood lichen, see *Hypogymnia*, 106

Index of Lichens and Medicinal Applications

Lichens listed under medical conditions represent the most relevant genus entries for that condition. Other passing references to these conditions can be found in the text.